Aging, Autonomy, and Architecture
Advances in Assisted Living

Edited by

BENYAMIN SCHWARZ

and RUTH BRENT

Aging,
Autonomy,
and Architecture

Advances in Assisted Living

The Johns Hopkins University Press
Baltimore and London

© 1999 The Johns Hopkins University Press
All rights reserved. Published 1999
Printed in the United States of America on acid-free paper
9 8 7 6 5 4 3 2 1

The Johns Hopkins University Press
2715 North Charles Street
Baltimore, Maryland 21218-4363
www.press.jhu.edu

ISBN 0-8018-6033-4 pbk.

Terrestrial shelters, tortuous roads, tenable places
Concatenated in time and age and habitat.

A DEDICATION TO THOSE WITH WHOM WE LOVE TO DWELL

Contents

Foreword   **ix**
M. POWELL LAWTON

Acknowledgments   **xi**

Contributors   **xiii**

Introduction   **xv**

PART I   **IDEALISM AND REALISM**

Chapter 1   The Definition and Evolution of Assisted Living within a
Changing System of Long-Term Care   **3**
VICTOR REGNIER

Chapter 2   Assisted Living: The Current State of Affairs   **21**
RONALD K. TINSLEY AND KENNETH E. WARREN

Chapter 3   The Promise of Assisted Living as a Shelter and Care Alternative
for Frail American Elders: A Cautionary Essay   **32**
STEPHEN M. GOLANT

PART II   **ATTRIBUTES OF PLACE AND BEHAVIORS OF PEOPLE**

Chapter 4   Gerontopia: A Place to Grow Old and Die   **63**
RUTH BRENT

Chapter 5   Personal Rituals: Identity, Attachment to Place,
and Community Solidarity   **81**
LEON A. PASTALAN AND JANICE E. BARNES

Chapter 6   Integrating Cultural Heritage into Assisted-Living Environments   **90**
URIEL COHEN AND KEITH DIAZ MOORE

Chapter 7   Life-Quality Alzheimer Care in Assisted Living   **110**
JOHN ZEISEL

Chapter 8   Models for Environmental Assessment   **130**
MARGARET P. CALKINS AND GERALD D. WEISMAN

PART III   **THE PROVISION AND CONSUMPTION OF CARE**

Chapter 9   Dementia Care in Assisted Living: A Case Study of Copper Ridge   **143**
CAROL L. KERSHNER, CARMEL ROQUES, AND CYNTHIA D. STEELE

Chapter 10   Primary Care in Assisted Living: A Geriatrician's Perspective   **156**
PAMELA Z. CACCHIONE AND JOHN E. MORLEY

Chapter 11   "I Live Here, but It's Not My Home":
Residents' Experiences in Assisted Living   **166**
JACQUELYN FRANK

PART IV   **DESIGN: WHO CARES?**

Chapter 12   Assisted Living: An Evolving Place Type   **185**
BENYAMIN SCHWARZ

Chapter 13   Communicating Homeyness from the Outside:
Elderly People's Perceptions of Assisted Living   **207**
JOHN P. MARSDEN AND RACHEL KAPLAN

Chapter 14   Designing to Meet the Needs of People with Alzheimer's Disease   **229**
J. DAVID HOGLUND AND STEFANI D. LEDEWITZ

Chapter 15   Place Makes a Difference: A Case Study in Assisted Living   **262**
DANIEL J. CINELLI

Chapter 16   Hospice: A Case Study Making a Difference   **278**
GREGORY J. SCOTT AND MARTIN S. VALINS

Epilogue   Emerging Themes, Further Reflections   **291**
BENYAMIN SCHWARZ AND RUTH BRENT

Index   **307**

Foreword

Dr. Schwarz and Dr. Brent have moved the state of the art of ecological gerontology ahead considerably by providing this multiauthored book on assisted living. The scholarly underpinnings of the entire book make it the first on assisted living that has called equally upon theory and application to characterize assisted living and to set goals for this housing form's future development.

My purpose is less to praise the book, however, than to view its message within the framework of the forty years of development of housing forms tailored to the needs of older people. At that time, we knew only the home for the aged and were just beginning to see "independent housing" emerge as a new form. That was when the dichotomy of the medical model and the social model became defined. That issue is revisited in the editors' introduction, in which the necessity for such a choice is questioned. "Congregate housing" was the next arrival, simultaneously with "life care," in which the ideal of filling in parts of the independence-dependence continuum with residential environments to which the in-betweeners might move was articulated. As the editors note, this points-on-the-continuum model of long-term residential care demanded the continued movement of people as their health declined.

Aging, Autonomy, and Architecture argues forcefully that such segmentation and necessity for relocation are not necessary to achieve a sense of security, individuality, and positive environmental features such as homelike quality. The idea of tailoring a package of services to the individual's needs is the functional equivalent of transfer to a more supportive environment while at the same time avoiding the dysfunctionality of aging in place in which the context remains inflexible. Heterogeneity among a resident population is better preserved by the unbundled services aspects of assisted living than by the rigid buy-the-whole-package approach of earlier congregate housing.

There are costs to unbundling. Schwarz and Brent and chapter authors are forthright in their acknowledgment of cost as a persistent issue. No matter how much better the efficiency of the individually tailored service package, the unpleasant fact remains that there is virtually no overlap between the financial capability of the people who populate Section 202/Section 8 congregate housing (low-income) and of those who live in nonsubsidized assisted living. The ability to serve the poor is a criterion for the success of the assisted-living housing model that we cannot afford to ignore. And we should praise the states that are leading the way in daring to apply tax funds to reduce the socioeconomic inequities that burden assisted living as a type.

The ideal of individualization remains to be tested to its fullest. Such a test can come only after we have had a couple of decades of experience to see how early assisted-living environments develop, as their original residents age, as the physical plant changes, and as the outside community's perception of those residences changes. Will residents be encouraged to remain as they become more frail physically and mentally? Will older buildings and aging surrounding neighborhoods contribute negative perceptions to potential residents?

It will be difficult for assisted-living sponsors and management to avoid a trend toward the kind of segmentation of the market and procrustean service provision that have characterized earlier housing forms. Even now, assisted-living clients are notably more frail than the modal resident in nominally independent housing. At the present time, however, there is more overlap between assisted-living residents and nursing home residents, as is clearly desirable. There are predictions that the nursing home may be a dying breed or at least that it dwindle in size of population served and evolve into a residential location in which only the medically needy will live. Such a change would put pressure on assisted-living environments to serve increasing numbers of activities-of-daily-living-impaired and cognitively impaired people. Will assisted living eventually become a new name for the nursing home? Will such residences be able to handle ever-larger resident populations with the individualistic, autonomy-respecting, and homelike quality of the forerunners of assisted living of today? Will continuing pressure to assist frail people in these environments with government tax supports erode the individualized aspects of assisted living that give it such high quality?

These anxieties, and the questions raised about assisted living of the future, point to the need for vigilance about the services offered, and the way they are offered, in assisted living. If the characterization of this genre of environment and its distinctions from other types of residence, especially in well-meaning accreditation and licensing efforts, become too much the focus of our attention, we shall be insufficiently attuned to maintenance and fortification of the quality innovations brought thus far into the care scene by assisted living. Adaptation to changes in the individual, maintenance of heterogeneity of the resident population as a whole, individualization of care, studied risk taking, and provision of some low-cost care are the ingredients of quality. They are also at risk of compromise as the vanguard type of the present becomes the entrenched model of the future. By far the greatest proportion of this book is devoted to these essences of quality. I hope that this message of the book will live, along with those essences themselves.

M. Powell Lawton
PHILADELPHIA GERIATRIC CENTER

Acknowledgments

Designers are committed to the belief that place makes a difference in human life. This élan vital, or life force, drives their professional lives. With this same zeal, monuments are molded, sacred places are created, and homes are actualized. Thus, when the places for the most vulnerable people in our society, old and frail persons, are so removed from where they want to reside, the challenge presents itself to designers. As a result, the propitious theme "Place Makes a Difference: Advances in Assisted Living" piques the attention of researchers and practitioners in social gerontology and environmental design. This was the title of two symposia and one workshop at two conferences, and it was the guiding force for and precursor to this book. This volume can be seen as a result of the interest at these gatherings among researchers and practitioners in social gerontology and in environmental design.

We wish to thank the presenters for the Gerontological Society of America symposia: Rosalie Kane, Robert Mollica, Victor Regnier, Connie Baldwin, David Hoglund, Uriel Cohen, and Leon Pastalan; and for the 1996 Environmental Design Research Association: Margaret Calkins, Gerald Weisman, Victor Regnier, Connie Baldwin, Stefani Ledewitz, Uriel Cohen. M. Powell Lawton served as an impromptu discussant.

We are grateful to many others who helped bring this book to fruition. First, we owe particular thanks to our editor at the Johns Hopkins University Press, Wendy Harris, whom we met at the GSA convention in Los Angeles. From the very beginning and throughout the process, she supported our work. We also wish to acknowledge Peg Thompson, Jon Pynoos, Keren Brown Wilson, and Joan Hyde for their own pioneering work and interest in our mission, and Carol Zimmerman, Diane Hammond, and the rest of the staff of the Johns Hopkins University Press.

To David Smith, whose motto is "The answer is yes. What's the question?" we are especially thankful. David opened his St. Louis facility, The Gatesworth, to us and our students and confirmed our belief that an ideal assisted-living setting is possible.

We also owe much to our colleagues at the University of Missouri. David Barry, Barbara O'Gorman, and Carla Harris helped in the reading and production process. Bea Smith, Steve Zweig, David Oliver, and Toni Sullivan gave their amity and assistance.

Our families provided patience, encouragement, and beneficence. Thank you Rachel, Guy, Mor, and Tom. Thank you Ed, Jessica, and Jonathan.

Finally, acknowledgment is given to the elders in our personal lives. The wills of our aging mothers and the memories of our paragon fathers continue to guide.

Contributors

Janice E. Barnes, doctoral candidate, College of Architecture and Urban Planning, University of Michigan, Ann Arbor

Ruth Brent, Ph.D., professor and chair, Department of Environmental Design, University of Missouri, Columbia

Pamela Z. Cacchione, R.N., Ph.D., geriatric nurse practitioner, St. Louis University School of Medicine

Margaret P. Calkins, Ph.D., president, IDEAS (Innovative Designs in Environments for an Aging Society, Inc)., Cleveland Heights, Ohio

Daniel J. Cinelli, A.I.A., director of geriatric environments, OWP&P Architects, Inc., Chicago

Uriel Cohen, D.Arch., professor and associate dean, School of Architecture and Urban Planning, University of Wisconsin, Milwaukee

Jacquelyn Frank, Ph.D., assistant professor, Department of Sociology and Anthropology, Illinois State University, Normal

Stephen M. Golant, Ph.D., professor, Department of Geography, and adjunct professor of Urban and Regional Planning, University of Florida, Gainesville

J. David Hoglund, A.I.A., principal-in-charge, Pittsburgh office of the New York-based architectural firm Perkins Eastman Architects PC

Rachel Kaplan, professor, School of Natural Resources and Department of Psychology, University of Michigan, Ann Arbor

Carol L. Kershner, vice president and executive director, Copper Ridge, Sykesville, Maryland

Stefani D. Ledewitz, A.I.A., adjunct professor of architecture, Carnegie Mellon University, and senior associate, Perkins Eastman Architects PC, Pittsburgh

John P. Marsden, Ph.D., project associate, IDEAS (Innovative Designs in Environments for an Aging Society, Inc.), Cleveland Heights, Ohio

Keith Diaz Moore, fellow, Institute on Aging and Environment, School of Architecture and Urban Planning, University of Wisconsin, Milwaukee

John E. Morley, M.B.B.Ch., professor of gerontology and director, Division of Geriatric Medicine, St. Louis University Medical School

Leon A. Pastalan, Ph.D., professor, College of Architecture and Urban Planning, University of Michigan, Ann Arbor

Victor Regnier, F.A.I.A., professor, School of Architecture, Leonard Davis School of Gerontology, University of Southern California, Los Angeles

Carmel Roques, director of resident services, Copper Ridge, Sykesville, Maryland

Benyamin Schwarz, Ph.D., associate professor, Department of Environmental Design, University of Missouri, Columbia

Gregory J. Scott, A.I.A., partner, Reese, Lower, Patrick & Scott, Ltd. Architects, Lancaster, Pennsylvania

Cynthia D. Steele, R.N., M.P.H., assistant professor, Department of Psychiatry and Behavioral Sciences, Johns Hopkins School of Medicine, Baltimore; co-director, Copper Ridge Education and Research Institute, Sykesville, Maryland

Ronald K. Tinsley, national director, Senior Living and Post–Acute Care Services, PricewaterhouseCoopers, St. Louis

Martin S. Valins, senior associate, OWP&P Architects, Inc., Chicago; former director of research, Reese, Lower, Patrick & Scott, Ltd. Architects, Lancaster, Pennsylvania

Kenneth E. Warren, M.B.A., president, Avatar Group, a senior living consulting firm, Sarasota, Florida

Gerald D. Weisman, Ph.D., professor, School of Architecture and Urban Planning, University of Wisconsin, Milwaukee

John Zeisel, Ph.D., president, Hearthstone Alzheimer Care Ltd., Lexington, Massachusetts. He has taught social science and design at Harvard, Yale, and McGill Universities and at the University of Minnesota

Introduction

BENYAMIN SCHWARZ
RUTH BRENT

As we near the end of the millennium, American society is faced with a formidable challenge. The proportion of elderly people aged 80 years or older is projected to increase by nearly 300 percent between now and the year 2040 (U.S. Congress, 1991). Given the association between advanced old age and functional disabilities, these numbers will affect corresponding individual and societal problems. Although institutionalization befalls only 5 percent of elderly persons, among those who reach the age of eighty, this percentage rises to more than 30 percent. The debate on long-term care often focuses on the nursing home. And even though the nursing home is only one social response to the needs of the elderly, and a considerable amount of care is delivered in the home by family, friends, or home-care services, "of those in the 65+ age bracket in 1990, 43 percent will eventually reside for some period of time in a nursing home and two-thirds of them will be female" (Agich, 1993:5). This percentage is high enough to make us think about the places we might prefer to reside and about the way we want to be treated when long-term care touches our lives.

Alluding to the premise of assisted living, the title of this book links the themes of *aging*, *autonomy*, and *architecture*, combining notions of the lifelong process of aging with the inevitable dependency resulting from old age. *Security* and *autonomy* in long-term care are addressed in this book not as alternatives but rather as basic human needs both of which need to be satisfied if we are to optimize outcome (Parmelee and Lawton, 1990). The continuum of autonomy-security characterizes the search for an ideal architectural setting that keeps support and stimulation in equal focus.

Old age is a complex and elusive concept. As Cornman and Kingson (1996:19) note: "The concept is complex because it simultaneously raises questions for the individual (how am I going to age?), for families (who is going to take care of whom?), for professions (who will pay me how much to deliver services to "old" people?), and for social and economic policies (how many public dollars should we spend on which older people?)." The term *old age* can convey positive as well as negative notions—wisdom and respect or frailty and dependence. In the context of assisted living, aging is associated with persons whose activities are often restricted because of significant functional disabilities. This term refers to the degree to which illness or impairment interferes with meaningful daily living. "The loss or impairment of the ability to perform such basic daily functions as shopping or bathing strikes at what the elderly value most—independent living" (Pegels, 1981:5). Dependency, one of the most compelling problems of old age, is often seen as a product of decline and deterioration, as loss in both physical and mental functioning. However, behavioral dependency is not necessarily conjoined with old age. "Rather, the environment plays a dominant role in the development and maintenance of dependency in the elderly" (Baltes, 1996:152).

As elders become aware of restrictions in their own capacity, and the surrounding environmental influences become progressively more pervasive in limiting activity, they invariably resort to *selection* and *compensation*. Selection includes both environmental changes, such as relocation, and changes in active behavior, which can lead to passive adjustments or may be interpreted as a decrease in the number of commitments. When a sudden change, such as a stroke, severely impairs the elderly, decisions must be made. Staying at home may not be possible, but these elderly can select an appropriate alternative setting, or the kind of self-care needed, or the type of rehabilitation, or the kind of activities they want to perform. Whether they have other mechanisms to accomplish the same objectives in a specific domain, despite their lost or reduced capacities, represents the second component—compensation. Similar to the idea of prosthetics, compensation deals with technical as well as human means that make up for impairments in order to support autonomy. Relative independence can be achieved through devices such as canes or handrails or through human assistance. These aids may range from help with activities of daily living, such as housework, food preparation, and hygiene, to highly skilled nursing and medical care. Compensation might require the acquisition of new skills, new means, and new technology to enable the elderly to pursue their lives as fully as possible. Obviously, though, optimization in situations of increasing loss is limited by what is possible, particularly with regard to frail elders in need of long-term care. "The reality of long-term care apparently forces even the staunchest proponents of autonomy as independence to deal with reality of an impaired decision-making capacity or incompetence that is an ineliminable feature of long-term care" (Agich, 1993:10).

Agich raises two important questions with regard to autonomy and long-term care. First, he asks whether the choices afforded to individuals in long-term care are meaningful or worth making: "Ideally, choice that enhances autonomy is choice that is meaningful for individuals and allows them to express and develop their own individuality. If such is not the case, then the true sense of autonomy of persons is not enhanced" (107). The kinds of choice typically afforded to nursing home residents, for example, are rather limited and do not include choices that preserve and enhance their individuality and identity. Being able to identify with one's choice is a prerequisite for true autonomy.

The second question is whether the lifestyle available to elders in long-term care settings is something with which elders can identify. Life in a group setting introduces people to a heterogeneous, complex sociocultural system in a proximity that is very different from the places in which most residents lived before their institutionalization. This situation creates fertile ground for potential conflicts and confrontations. Kane (1990) summarizes this predicament in the nursing home: "The nursing home typically affords little privacy, personal space, or opportunity to use public space. The policy of enforced roommates minimizes the chance for personal autonomy. Even though special units for senile dementia are becoming more common, in most nursing homes the interspersing of the confused and the lucid can create a world of the absurd for cognitively intact residents. And too often nursing home residents are literally tied or otherwise physically restrained, a crude and extreme form of behavioral control" (16).

One of the challenges for institutional long-term care is to maintain residents' lifestyle in ways coherent with these elders' own views of self and their current abilities. In addition to physical ailments and disabilities, frailty and old age bring many fears, sorrows, losses, and frustrations. The task of a long-term care facility is to become a truly therapeutic environment, in which treatments that ameliorate discomfort and help maintain integrated functioning are provided. Furthermore, it should attend to the everyday routine and quality of experience of its residents. In this context, the physical environment plays a pivotal role.

Architecture can have a considerable impact on the lifestyles and well-being of frail elders. Long-term care arrangements must respond to the changing characteristics of their resident populations and the variations within individuals over time. The physical environment should be able to provide for more than a single, narrowly defined stage of frailty at any given time. In general, facilities for this population should balance efforts at selection, compensation, and optimization of individual elders (Baltes, 1996), and designers of this milieu should strive to do more than produce settings that merely satisfy functional efficiency, marketing needs, construction costs, and building codes.

The controversy over the choice between the medical model and the social model for long-term care has shifted to a debate over the physical qualities of the setting and the services provided. However, the intention of this book is not to make a distinction between the medical model and the social model as if they are two diametrically opposed ways of structuring assisted living or any other type of residential environment. Furthermore, most of the principles highlighted in this book are applicable to the nursing home as well as to independent housing. Nursing homes and assisted-living environments do not necessarily represent, respectively, the medical model and the social model. The choice is not between two models. Rather, the attributes of environments created for long-term care are determined by initial decisions regarding the characteristics of the people the environment attempts to serve; these environments are then adjusted as residents age in place.

In discussing these issues, the contributors to this book agree that long-term care settings should first have a residential rather than an institutional character. The common notion is that the residential qualities of "home" and the normalized life patterns that they imply should be used in all kinds of environment for frail elders. In addition, the therapeutic environment should promote wellness and support residents in coping with the stresses that accompany their conditions. The task is to establish limits to support and challenge, consistent with the characteristics of the residents. Accordingly, many policy makers, researchers, and providers now see social care for impaired older people as being as important as medical treatment. This assertion applies to all levels of care short of those in which life is threatened by physical illness. Thus, the premise of assisted living is one representation of a relatively recent trend that strives to make the setting of long-term care a place that "makes the world right again" (Kastenbaum, 1983:12).

In its essence, assisted living is a model of long-term care for people who conform to the same profile as nursing home residents. As one of the fastest growing options for providing long-term care today, assisted living is a response to the way we medicalize, institutionalize, and professionalize long-term care facilities in ways never originally envisioned. This blend of services and housing serves people with a range of impairments and functional capacities. Many of the residents have significant physical and mental health problems. Residents may be afflicted with dementia, may have impaired mobility or incontinence, may need care during the night, or may lack the cognitive ability to live without continuous supervision. Programs of assisted living offer frail elders a broad set of choices by separating the "nursing" component from the room-and-board component. By unbundling services from housing, older persons do not necessarily need to move along the continuum of care to more dependent care facilities. This philosophy separates assisted living from models that combine housing with varying levels of oversight and care. Frequently, the facilities offer self-contained apartments and supportive services, which may be purchased separately or included in the monthly fee. However, for the residents, the crucial difference is the chance to avoid institutionalization and maintain their remaining functional independence in a residential environment that provides affordable, secure, and supportive dwellings.

The primary goal of assisted living is to provide services tailored to individual needs in a residential and normalized setting. Individuality is the fundamental premise underlying this model of care. Residents are treated as individuals with differing personal needs. Routines and service plans are flexible and can be modified in response to changing individual needs. Services are provided on the basis of the competence of each individual served. The care and aid options may include three meals a day, assistance with housekeeping, laundry, and bathing, as well as personal and functional support services related to activities of daily living. Skilled nursing tasks such as the giving of injections, changing of dressings, monitoring of medications, and diagnosis and assessment of clinical symptoms can also be arranged as needed. While many facilities are not prepared to give long-term medical care, most of them have 24-hour emergency response programs on-site.

These essential constituents are frequently provided in self-contained private apartments, each with a kitchen, bathroom, and sleeping and living areas. In most cases, the facilities consist of a cluster of apartments in a single building with common areas, including a common dining room. These generate a sense of family, community, and belonging; the residents feel comfortable, secure in a setting that evokes memories and feelings of being at home. Design features, such as lockable doors, individual temperature controls, intercom systems, and personal furniture and decorations, are critical attributes of this environment.

In response to both consumer demand and dwindling federal and state resources, several states now allow the development of new models of long-term care. At the moment, however, such options are more likely to be available to middle- and upper-income people who can afford to pay privately for the services or to people who maintain insurance policies that allow for the payment of nonmedical needs. Unfortunately, lowered income and frailty tend to lead elders to subsidized housing, in which professional nursing or therapy is not provided, or to medically oriented, long-term care institutions.

This collection of writings is a reflection of the hopes and tensions between the theory and practice in the field of assisted living. While the contributors come from a variety of disciplines, their common perspective is grounded in the domain of environments for the aging. The significance of the discourse is evident in the breadth of the cross-disciplinary exchange on the environmental context of aging in assisted living from the physical, social, commercial, cultural, clinical, and psychological perspectives.

The chapters in this book are grouped into four parts, arranged in a thematic progression, and are followed by an epilogue.

Part I. Idealism and Realism

The authors in Part I express both idealism and realism with regard to assisted living in the United States. The attitudes toward this new, burgeoning, type of residential long-term care runs the gamut from acceptance of the current model, to the promise of this housing and service combination model, to skepticism about the future of this model. In a balanced and informed perspective, the evolution of assisted living is charted.

Victor Regnier, a long-time leader in assisted living, carries the flag of idealism for assisted living. He systematically discusses the definition and evolution of this long-term care alternative and presents ten factors that have influenced the growth of assisted living. Regnier lists the growth in the numbers of the older old population, the continuing increase in the cost of long-term care, the changing preferences of consumers and advocates, the questions regarding the concepts of institutionalization, and the interests of corporate America in the new industry. He highlights normative attributes of a "best practices" assisted-living model and future trends that will influence assisted living.

Ron Tinsley and Ken Warren portray the reality of the industry from the viewpoint of the market, based on responses to two surveys distributed to assisted-living and senior housing providers throughout the United States. Citing data on the aging of the population, the affordability of assisted living, and the characteristics of current residences, the authors report on the growth of the assisted-living industry. Using charts and tables, Tinsley and Warren discuss issues such as the percentage of residents needing assistance with activities of daily living (ADLs), the distances of assisted-living facilities from original homes, and the referral sources for assisted-living residences. Extrapolating from these data, the authors attempt to predict the future of the industry, reflecting the views of the Assisted-Living Federation of America (ALFA).

Stephen Golant directly confronts the feasibility of assisted living as a shelter and care alternative for frail Americans. Acknowledging a justifiable optimism for this alternative, he considers individual and societal forces that may cause it to fall short of its promise. He does not accept the superficial criticisms of this form of care but digs deeper to find economic, social, political, and health care delivery concerns. He concludes with penetrating questions on the future of assisted living. Golant feels that the social model of care may be threatened by its own ideals. It is not whether the ideal of assisted living will exist but rather whether it will be available only to a small group of high-income elderly consumers or also to the majority of low- and middle-income frail elders seeking an alternative to the nursing home.

Part II. Attributes of Place and Behaviors of People

Part II emphasizes the environmental and behavioral perspectives of studies on settings for long-term care. The authors cover the territory from where people grow old and die to personal rituals, cultural heritage, life quality, and comprehensive models for the assessment of group housing for elderly people. Focusing on the attributes of place and the behaviors of people, contributors in this section convey a spirit of altruistic advocacy that naturally leads to design intervention.

Ruth Brent reviews stories about frail elders and their journey through the last chapter of life, beginning with a place in which no one wants to die. The case studies illustrate attributes and dimensions that developers of assisted-living arrangements attempt to translate into the sociophysical environment of their facilities. The case is made, through poignant life stories and humanistic literature, that the attributes of the places where we grow old and where we die are essentially the same. Brent, an advocate of aging in place, explains that the ideal place where life and death meet is a residence that maximizes personal autonomy. Brent anticipates assisted-living arrangements to become this kind of place.

Leon Pastalan and Janice Barnes ask the fundamental question concerning residential environments, How much like home is it? They build the case for attention to personal rituals that help give meaning to people's daily lives. This is neither an exercise in trivia nor a common approach to understanding how we dwell in the place we call home. The chapter increases our appreciation for the manner in which each person routinely goes about performing activities in a set time and place. While most people wish to age in place, changes in household composition typically occur at one or more points in the aging process, forcing elders to find alternative housing solutions. That is when the importance of personal rituals is perceived. It is only after these individual behavior patterns have been altered or eliminated due to a change in personal lives that they become noticeable. The discussion can provide new perspectives on the connections among personal rituals, self-identity, place attachment, and community solidarity. It is expected that the arguments can foster a greater understanding by families, significant others, and caregivers of the need to maintain rituals that are important to individuals so that their personal identity and quality of life will be preserved or enhanced.

Uriel Cohen and Keith Diaz Moore present a conceptual framework that facilitates discussion about the transaction between the unique needs of elderly persons and a culturally responsive environmental design, given that all individuals are part of a particular culture, with unique positions within their social world and possessing their own unique histories. Self-identity, self-worth, dignity, and respect are defining characteristics of an elder's self-image. Phenomena experienced through culture provide resources for creating more therapeutic programs and more meaningful environments for an aging society. The chapter addresses the need for a more thoughtful consideration of schemata behind the physical expression: the spatial organization of the environment and its responsiveness to lifestyles, social structures, daily activities, and rituals, among other factors, all of which hold meaning and significance to those particular users. The authors identify the key issues that integrate cultural heritage in diverse habitats: an Oneida longhouse, a special care unit, a Jewish home, a traditional Japanese *takanoma*, and a Pennsylvania Dutch home.

John Zeisel, wearing the two hats of scholar and care provider, pursues life quality in facilities for persons with Alzheimer's disease by asking the question, Do we care for these people as if they were dying or as if they were living? The author discusses the life quality (L-Q) model, which organizes a comprehensive design and management approach for providing high-quality care to people with Alzheimer's disease and related disorders. It includes two distinct parts that relate intimately in practice. The first part is a model for the physical design of special care units and assisted-living residences for people with dementia. The second part refers to a model for managing organizations that provide care in assisted-living and other settings for people with dementia. The individual organization (I-O) model focuses on the needs and dignity of the individual with dementia. This is essential to successful caregiving, especially in community and group settings. Based on a case study at Hearthstone Alzheimer's care treatment residences, Zeisel argues that, without careful management of the organization that provides the context for caregivers, they will be unable to provide the individualized care that is needed.

Margaret Calkins and Gerald Weisman trace the development of conceptual models and propose a new model of assessment in assisted-living settings. Eventually, such a model could be used by regulators and clients. Although licensed differently from skilled nursing care facilities, assisted living can be broadly defined to include services that range from light personal care to 24-hour nursing care. This makes it difficult to differentiate between these two forms of supportive residential setting. This chapter asserts that what differentiates assisted living from traditional skilled nursing care is different therapeutic goals. Increased emphasis on personal control and autonomy, continuity with past routines and patterns of behavior, and supporting independence are but a few of the basic tenets of assisted living. With the proliferation of assisted living, there is increased interest, from both regulators and clients, in being able to assess the quality of these settings. The authors argue that to be meaningful, an assessment must be based on the underlying therapeutic goals. Analysis of several environmental assessment protocols for residential settings for the elderly suggests that different environments have different therapeutic goals as their frameworks. The differences in the goals stem, in part, from the ways in which they were derived. The chapter is based on recent research conducted to establish a comprehensive set of therapeutic goals for residential care settings for people with dementia. This set of therapeutic goals form the foundation of a comprehensive environmental assessment protocol that provides both descriptive and evaluative information about assisted-living settings in this context.

Part III. The Provision and Consumption of Care

The authors in Part III describe assisted living from the perspectives of both providers and consumers. They render the rewards and frustrations in the daily operation of assisted-living facilities as well as the benefits and the difficulties of residing in such settings. Although the contributors focus on diverse aspects of the social dimensions of assisted living, the chapters reinforce the notion that the social context determines the symbiotic relationships between elders, staff, and the environment. Providers and consumers have wisdom to share aspects of care programs and the generally elusive meanings of the sociophysical environment for caregivers and residents.

Carol Kershner, Carmel Roques, and Cynthia Steele discuss their experiences as care providers in a purpose-built assisted-living facility for frail elders with memory-impairing illnesses. Assisted living for the memory impaired, they claim, is an entity unlike any other care setting. It is neither a typical assisted-living environment nor a nursing home. The setting must account for parameters associated with both settings while replicating neither. Care in such a setting can significantly improve quality of life for both residents and their families. The authors argue that, while protection against consequences of altered judgment or the burden inherent in providing daily care are usually the incentives for seeking placement, once the adjustment to the new living arrangements has occurred, the benefits of assisted-living environments emerge. The chapter reviews the basic elements of dementia care in an assisted-living setting. It addresses the building and design features, staff training requirements, assessment and treatment protocols, systems of support for families, and programming for meaningful involvement for residents, including activities that promote daily living skills and socialization.

Pamela Cacchione and John Morley voice the rarely heard view of the geriatrician who practices primary care in an assisted-living setting. Eliminating the need for residents and their families to travel long distances to their primary care provider is an advantage and a positive marketing tool for the facility. Revealing the problems and successes of this model, the authors describe their practice in assisted living, located in a housing arrangement geared to independent living. Residents of this facility are frail elders who suffer from combinations of chronic conditions. The diagnosis and treatment of chronic diseases often include a poor prognosis, with its concomitant fears. Chronic illness can be accompanied by a pervasive feeling of powerlessness and dependence. Because many of these illnesses offer little or no chance of cure, ill people and their families may become desperate. The importance of this chapter stems from the medical perception of the contributors and their unique view of a different set of problems pertaining to residents in assisted-living arrangements.

Jacquelyn Frank takes the consumers' perspective to heart, as her title plainly states, "I live here, but it's not my home." From her fieldwork, she concludes that, while design should not be downplayed, providers must realize that creating a place that is "homelike" does not necessarily make it "home" to assisted-living residents. Residents perceive architecture and interior design to be the only differences between assisted living and nursing homes. Frank claims that, regardless of the alterations that are made to the physical design, the majority of residents seem unable to make it their home. In addressing this dilemma, she notes that philosophy of care is enmeshed with the physical structure and hopes this fact challenges researchers and developers to find ways of translating assisted-living ideals into livable realities.

Part IV. Design: Who Cares?

Grounded in the well-known metaphorical need for bridging the gap between environmental behavior research and architectural practice, the authors in Part IV believe that place makes a difference. Contributors to this section come from two related disciplines: practicing architects and theoreticians interested in environments for the aging. The section opens with two theory-oriented chapters, which are followed by three chapters that discuss several recently built assisted-living facilities. Through the images and the postoccupancy evaluations of the settings, one realizes the breadth and diversity of assisted-living architecture. However, there is a common thread between the architects who discuss their work in this section: they wish to address the needs and wants of residents, staff, and operators. An architectural firm can do good work in various ways. It can be strong in ideas, service, or delivery (Cuff, 1991). This group of architects are professionals who make a conscious effort through their work to advance the design of assisted living to the next level. In this sense, they produce design that cares.

Benyamin Schwarz explores assisted living as a place type for the provision of long-term care. He delves into this special blend of shelter and personal care with special attention to the association between the concept of home and the homelike model of care. Schwarz attempts to show that the concept of assisted living is ambiguous and, therefore, cannot be taken for granted. He argues that the single most important factor that designers can influence in creating housing arrangements for frail elders is the degree of autonomy and individual choice allowed to the residents. The architectural framework can provide or inhibit opportunities for privacy, independence, control, and choice. Thus, it is important to study attributes of assisted living that attempt to translate combinations of resident characteristics, staff attributes, program philosophy, and physical features into a place type that supports the personal autonomy of residents.

John Marsden and Rachel Kaplan systematically examine whether the exterior appearance of assisted-living settings is perceived by elder people as homelike. The authors discuss the elusiveness of the concept of home and the framework for studying the communication of "homeyness" in assisted living. Using the results of two studies, the authors compare and contrast the homeyness framework of "supportive protection," "human scale," and "naturalness." Through preference ratings and homelike ratings, Marsden and Kaplan attempt to determine the commonalties underlying these perceptions. They focus on three categories: entryways, massing or building height, and sense of "institutional" or "homelike."

David Hoglund and Stefani Ledewitz approach design for persons with Alzheimer's disease with seven basic premises. As with any premier design research team, proof is in praxis. The much acclaimed, purpose-built, Woodside Place is that proof. Hoglund and Ledewitz review the history of Woodside Place in Oakmont, Pennsylvania, and discuss results from their three-year study of the place their architectural firm designed. The authors comment on the influence of the environment on the behavior of residents. Among other issues, they refer to behaviors, such as sundowning and wandering. The authors approach the process of design with the assumption that knowledge derived from social and behavioral science research can improve predictions of the congruence between design and use. Accordingly, they begin their work with the existing knowledge and research, followed by the programming stage, which specifies the social knowledge to be incorporated into the building, and then proceed to the final design stage and building construction. Their last step is conducted after users inhabit the building. A postoccupancy evaluation completes the circle, providing new knowledge to inform the design process for the next round of projects.

Daniel Cinelli tells the story of a design process for an assisted-living addition to Heritage Village, an intermediate and sheltered care community in northeastern Illinois. He walks the reader through the strategic vision statement, market feasibility study, master plan, programming and design criteria, design solutions for assisted living, marketing issues, and preliminary postoccupancy evaluation. Criticizing his own successful project, the author-architect discusses problems in the design process. Toward the end of the chapter, he refers to the fact that Heritage House was developed in a nonlicensed environment, using common sense and consumer input as its driving force. The author voices his concern about restrictive regulations for assisted living, which he believes will force designers to produce deficient settings that will not meet resident expectations. He offers solutions to the problem, emphasizing the need for a dialogue among residents, providers, designers, and regulators to ensure that future settings meet the needs of elder care consumers.

Gregory Scott and Martin Valins claim that assisted living is increasingly becoming the focus for long-term care providers, as the role of the nursing home begins to fall out of the continuum in long-term care. An important care model that has traditionally been placed in the medical camp is the inpatient hospice. As with environments for people with dementia, inpatient hospice programs have more to do with care and support than with medicine. Thus, the assisted-living concept begins to embrace the hospice environment. The result is a radical, volte-face from traditional nursing home design. As a result of intensive programming and research into the essence of hospice, a recently completed stand-alone hospice building in Lancaster County, Pennsylvania, is offered as a case study in innovation, design, and programming that moves forward the debate regarding the roles of the residential model vis-à-vis the therapeutic care model. The authors combine both theory and practice in discussing an inpatient hospice building, detailing both the architectural and, more important, the behavioral objectives of the Essa Flory Hospice. Profile information, project background, and design concepts are disclosed. In their conclusions, the authors develop more intangible therapeutic goals, including the use of daylight and connections with nature. Photographs of this hospice, which looks and feels like a home, help the reader to imagine how it may contribute to stress-free last days of tenants' lives.

Epilogue: Emerging Themes, Further Reflections

In the epilogue, we provide a short summary of the themes that have emerged and point toward directions worthy of concentration in future research. Our interpretations are, naturally, colored by our environment-behavior research background. The rationale for this discipline stems from "the gap between designers' prediction or claim of how their designs will work and how they *do* work" (Lang, 1987:vii). In other words, researchers are uncomfortable with designers' inability to predict the performance of their buildings in relation to human activity. For the same reason, we believe in the need to study the phenomenon of assisted living within this scholarly context. We have faith in assisted living as an innovative blend of housing and services for older, frail Americans. It represents for us a manifestation of a broad, and inevitable, transformation in the provision of long-term care. The Chinese, who have always had a thoroughly dynamic worldview, seem to be well aware of this profound linkage between crisis and change. One of humanity's oldest books of wisdom, the *I Ching*, or Book of Changes, depicts this kind of systemic transition: "The movement is natural, arising spontaneously. For this reason the transformation of the old becomes easy. The old is discarded and the new is introduced. Both measures accord with the time; therefore no harm results" (Wilhelm, 1968:97). Assisted living symbolizes this shift, and for that reason it deserves further serious research with the domain of environment-behavior studies.

References

Agich, G. 1993. *Autonomy and Long-Term Care*. New York: Oxford University Press.

Baltes, M. 1996. *The Many Faces of Dependency in Old Age*. New York: Cambridge University Press.

Cornman, J., and E. Kingson. 1996. Trends, issues, perspectives, and values for the aging of the baby boom cohorts. *Gerontologist* 36:15–26.

Cuff, D. 1991. *Architecture: The Story of Practice*. Cambridge: MIT Press.

Kane, R. 1990. Everyday life in nursing homes: "The way things are." In R. Kane and A. Caplan, eds., *Everyday Ethics: Resolving Dilemmas in Nursing Home Life*. New York: Springer.

Kastenbaum, R. 1983. Can the clinical milieu be therapeutic? In G. Rowles and R. Ohta, eds., *Aging and Milieu: Environmental Perspectives on Growing Old*. New York: Academic.

Lang, J. 1987. *Creating Architectural Theory: The Role of the Behavioral Sciences in Environmental Design*. New York: Van Nostrand Reinhold.

Parmelee, P., and M. Lawton. 1990. The design of special environments for the aged. In J. Birren and K. Schaie, eds., *Handbook of the Psychology of Aging*, 3d ed. New York: Academic.

Pegels, C. 1981. *Health Care and the Elderly*. Rockville, Md.: Aspen.

U.S. Congress, Senate, Special Committee on Aging. 1991. *Aging America: Trends and Projections*. Washington, D.C.: Government Printing Office.

Wilhelm, R. 1968. *I Ching*. London: Routledge & Kegan Paul.

Aging, Autonomy, and Architecture
Advances in Assisted Living

PART I   IDEALISM AND REALISM

The Definition and Evolution of Assisted Living within a Changing System of Long-Term Care

VICTOR REGNIER

The future of assisted living might be compared to speculation about the career potential of a bright and promising young teenager: the possibility of great achievement is clear; how well it can live up to that potential depends a great deal on what occurs in the next decade. The maturation of assisted living could be thwarted by regulatory impediments or assisted by strong competition among sponsors intent on serving consumer demand.

This chapter provides a foundation for understanding more about where assisted living is going in the near term. It starts with a general definition. Next, ten factors associated with its growth are identified. Following that, nine normative characteristics associated with the best examples of assisted living are described, and eight future trends and issues are detailed.

The current strong demand for assisted-living arrangements and the long-term success of assisted-living dwellings in northern Europe bodes well for its development. The major cloud on the horizon is the enormous increase in the number of older frail people and the potential economic burden they pose, which will clearly challenge our ability to respond effectively to future demand.

The Definition of Assisted Living

The definition of *assisted living* has never been and perhaps never will be precise. Assisted living means to some people a care philosophy, to others a building type, and to still others a regulatory category. The following definition is a hybrid, assembling elements from the work of Kane and Brown (1993) and Regnier (1994). *Assisted living is a long-term care alternative that involves the delivery of professionally managed personal and health care services in a group setting that is residential in character and appearance; it has the capacity to meet unscheduled needs for assistance, while optimizing residents' physical and psychological independence.*

This definition assumes that assisted living is a *long-term care alternative;* in other words, a potential replacement for some aspects of skilled nursing care. Being *professionally managed,* assisted living is different from traditional board-and-care homes. Providers of assisted living are generally better trained and have a more sophisticated understanding of how to deal with a range of behavioral and medical problems. Both personal care and health care services are included. Even though an assisted living setting may not provide in-depth, 24-hour health care monitoring, as in a nursing home, health monitoring and health services are provided. This assistance is over and above what is normally considered the standard in a personal care or congregate setting. Rosewood Estate, in Highland Park, Minnesota, is an example of such an assisted-living arrangement (see figure 1.1).

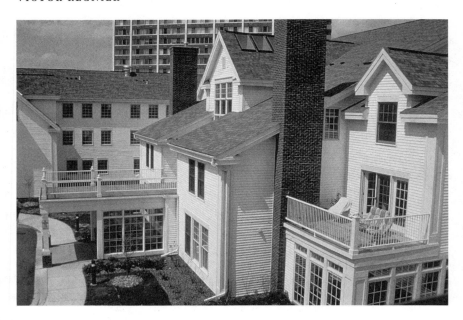

FIGURE 1.1. Rosewood Estate, Highland Park, Minnesota

Group setting assumes that services are being delivered to several individuals at a single location, not to older people living in separate dwelling units in the community. *Residential in character and appearance* describes the overall sense of the environment, which should resemble a housing environment, not a health care institution. *Meeting unscheduled needs* means that systems (electronic or personnel) are in place to connect the older person with a staff that is made available on a 24-hour basis. Finally, *optimizing residents' physical and psychological independence* is an important outcome measure. Assisted living should support individuals at their margin of need while at the same time challenging their competence. This is the essence of independence, which involves choice and control over one's own environment.

Although this definition seems relatively specific, there is a great deal more to assisted living than is easily communicated through a definition. As assisted living evolves in its capability to manage frailer individuals, these defining characteristics will also change.

Ten Factors affecting the Growth of Assisted Living

A number of factors are responsible for the meteoric rise of assisted living as the current long-term care alternative of choice. Many of these are very basic and represent underlying considerations that have been present in long-term care decision making for years. However, in the last decade these forces have individually and collectively reached a tipping point that has forced a rethinking of what defines long-term care in the United States. The following ten factors are among the most powerful influences affecting the growth of assisted living.

Growth in the Numbers of the Older Old

Perhaps the greatest influence on the growth of assisted living is the enormous increase in the number of people over the age of 85 and the projections showing that these numbers will continue to grow well into the next century. Conservative demographic projections show that the number of people over the age of 85 will double between 1990 and 2010 and then double again between 2010 and 2040 (Spencer, 1989). Other, more plausible projections, which use assumptions such as a continuing 2 percent yearly decrease in mortality (Guralnik, Yanagishita, and Schneider, 1988), predict that the growth in numbers by 2040 may be close to seven times the 1990 population. These trends not only relate to the United States but also are characteristic of what is happening throughout the world in both industrialized societies and Third World countries. Many of the these older old are not acutely ill but are simply very old and frail. To maintain independence, these individuals require a range of supportive personal and health care services like those made available in assisted living.

The Continuing Upward Spiral of Long-Term Care Costs

One of the major challenges to long-term care is making it affordable. The continuing increase in long-term care costs has concerned both policy makers and consumers. Policy makers and politicians see the cost of long-term care burgeoning out of control. Consumers are increasingly questioning the value of the services provided by nursing homes, especially in the light of other growing alternatives. Rivlin and Weiner (1988) estimate that long-term care costs will triple in the 1990s and will increase exponentially beyond that unless we discover new ways to care for an increasingly dependent older-old population. Assisted living has been shown to be 20–30 percent less expensive than conventional nursing home care. Through the use of more efficient technologies, it may have the capacity to be made even more affordable in the future.

The Changing Preferences of Consumers and Their Advocates

Older consumers, many of whom themselves have put a parent into an institution, are increasingly reluctant to accept such placement for themselves. Many have grown accustomed to the choice, control, autonomy, and privacy that living at home provides. The increased cost and the institutional lifestyle associated with conventional nursing homes facilities is unappealing to the vast majority. Furthermore, the children of the elderly, who are increasingly making decisions about placement, are seeking value and responsiveness from service providers. They feel that delaying placement as long as possible is generally the best approach. Therefore, concepts like continuing-care retirement communities that encourage a move earlier in old age grow less appealing. These family members are seeking an environment that is residential in character and is friendly and appealing to visit. Nursing homes so resemble hospitals that many older people and their families avoid this alternative at all costs.

Questioning the Hospital-Based Care Model

Changes in minimal hospital stays brought about by tough-minded utilization committees and insurance reimbursement analyses have forced hospitals into rethinking the balance between outpatient and inpatient care. This same movement has also called into question the appropriateness of the nursing home as a model for long-term care. Just as the minimum hospital stay was challenged by diagnosis-related groups (DRGs), so has nursing home care been questioned for those who are not sick but are nonetheless placed in an expensive, very institutionalized health care environment. At the same time, nursing homes are experiencing an increase in the number of extremely ill older people. When these residents are intermixed with financially indigent lighter care residents and with people with dementia, questions about the appropriateness of nursing home environments arise. Increasingly, nursing homes see themselves as subacute settings oriented toward medically indigent residents in need of rehabilitation services or special medical care. Regulations that recognize this increasing level of dependency have encouraged nursing homes to continue their reliance on an institutional, hospital-based, platform of care. The result is a greater mismatch between populations, making it less sensible to place a mentally or physically frail older person in this type of health care environment.

The Growth of New Technologies and Care Systems

The last decade has seen an explosion in electronic communication technology, personal computers, fax machines, modems, remote sensing devices, noninvasive medical diagnostic equipment, and information systems like the Internet. These increases in technology have also had profound impacts on medical care. Incontinence, once considered a rationale for institutionalization, has been redefined by incontinence products and self-managed incontinence programs. Electronic communications systems such as Lifeline, Wanderguard, and TeleAlarm are redefining the way older people are monitored and receive care in a range of housing environments. Portable medical devices are allowing more older people to die at home. Given the monitoring and sensing technologies available in buildings today, they are increasingly safe. Living in a sprinkled building is much safer than driving a car or boarding an airplane. Decentralized technologies have made it increasingly feasible to safely care for older, sicker people in noninstitutional environments.

Questioning of the Concept of Institutionalization

The deinstitutionalization movement over the last twenty years has successfully placed many institutionalized people in more effective, community-based housing and service arrangements. As a result of the success of such movements, older residents and their families are increasingly questioning whether it is necessary to enter a nursing home. The availability of community-based care and the increasing number of other options have older people and their families pondering if nursing home placement is a concept of the past. Many older people see themselves "aging in place" until they can no longer care for themselves. At that point, an assisted-living environment might seem a better fit for their needs. A nursing home does not make sense unless they require sophisticated, 24-hour medical care monitoring, which is necessary for only a relatively small number of aging individuals.

A Lack of Informal, Family-Based Care Opportunities

Middle-aged women, who have traditionally been caregivers for their parents, are increasingly engaged in work outside of the home. As a result, they do not have the available time that previous generations had to care for ailing and dependent parents. Many of these children of the elderly are seeking housing and service alternatives that allow them to be involved with their parents' care but in ways that provide them greater flexibility. This has long been an issue in northern European countries, which have some of the highest female workforce participation rates in the world. Their system of elder care is highly dependent on assisted-living-type housing alternatives for the frail segment of their population.

Changing Attitudes regarding Regulation

The increasingly stringent nursing home regulations implemented over the last twenty years in response to abuses have failed to deliver better, more attractive facilities. Consumers in search of cost-effective and humane residential care environments generally avoid highly regulated nursing homes. Policy makers who question the effectiveness of current nursing home regulations to produce attractive alternatives have encouraged states and service providers to seek other approaches. Oregon and Washington started what has since become a widespread movement by introducing a special licensing category for assisted living. According to Mollica (1995), nearly 60 percent of the states are considering, are developing, or have new regulations that apply to assisted living. Another factor encouraging the development of new standards for assisted living is the growth in unlicensed facilities seeking to satisfy the demand for more flexible housing and service arrangements.

An Awareness of Cross-Cultural Solutions

In today's world, countries located thousands of miles from one another find themselves interconnected through finance, political cooperation, and world trade. Greater familiarity with other cultures through world travel has also allowed us to appreciate and understand how other countries deal with similar problems. Most countries are struggling with the problem of a burgeoning older-old population. In the last several decades, northern Europeans have devised systems to deal creatively with the needs and preferences of older people for noninstitutional supportive housing. These buildings and service systems are more influential today, as we seek to learn from one another through cross-cultural examinations. As the United States struggles to understand how best to deal with its aging population, so do other countries. Our ability to learn from one another increases the probability that new models will borrow ideas from other cultures.

The Response of Corporate America

Corporate America has responded aggressively to the creative opportunities that are developing as society continues to age. Of particular interest is the mismatch between what consumers want and what is available. In response to the perceived need for more assisted-living units, new public companies have formed, hospitality organizations are formulating national programs, and nursing home providers are shifting their inventory toward assisted-living facilities. *Provider* magazine in its October 1995 issue profiled ten major providers and their plans to build more than 250 facilities in the following ten years. Estimates show that assisted-living housing will become an $8–12 billion industry over the next ten to fifteen years.

Nine Attributes of an Ideal Assisted-Living Model

Defining what constitutes an assisted-living model is a challenge, especially at a time when consumer demand and the continuing refinement of physical models and operational systems have led to enormous variety. The following nine attributes have been identified from innovative projects in Europe and the United States. Even though few, if any, projects embrace all nine of these concepts, they serve as objectives against which we can measure the inventiveness and creativity of assisted-living facilities.

Residential Appearance

The overall residential look of the building is an important first step in presenting the philosophy that assisted living combines housing and services. The architectural precedent for design should be the single-family house or the multiple-family dwelling, not a hospital. Nursing homes are related by code and occupancy to hospitals, and their design follows some of the same principles. Furthermore, the assisted-living building should use scale elements that relate the building in appearance to a large manor house. Techniques like using a sloped roof, residentially scaled attached porches, traditional residential materials, and residential door and window details give the building a friendly, approachable look and feeling. Sunrise assisted living is an example of such a building (see figure 1.2).

Smaller-Scale Arrangements

Lessening the scale of a building by reducing height, mass, and bulk is another way to make the setting more familiar and less overwhelming. This is commonly done by breaking the building into small unit clusters and arraying these on the site. In general, buildings of between twenty and sixty units are the most successful at reducing to a residential scale. The aggregation of units should be large enough to meet minimum economies of scale for services like meal production and medical service delivery but small enough to accommodate residents in comfortable and familiar residential common spaces. For example, when the dining room grows beyond sixty chairs, the scale of the room becomes less residential and more institutional. Sunrise of Severna Park, Maryland, for example, has several small-scale living spaces oriented toward the garden and outdoor views (see figure 1.3).

The Person as a Unique Individual

The program should deal with every resident as a distinct person. The assessment and treatment plan, the activities offered, and the role of that person in the ecology of the setting should be recognized as unique. This means that the staff must know each resident well and that the plan for activities should not be routine or center on the convenience of the staff but should center on resident interests. This may mean that several smaller activities are implemented in place of one large event.

Family Involvement

Family members should be encouraged to participate in the lives of their parents and grandparents, not only socially but also through techniques such as family-based assessments that involve family members as active partners in the caregiving process. A few key common spaces in the build-

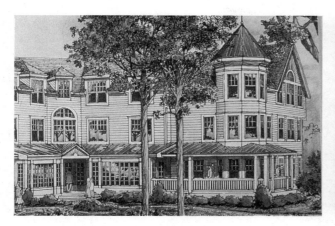

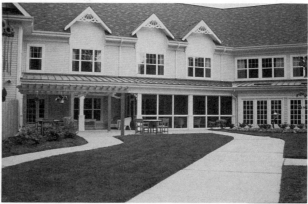

FIGURE 1.2. *Sunrise Assisted Living, Alexandria, Virginia*

FIGURE 1.3. *Sunrise, Severna Park, Maryland, Alzheimer's garden*

ing should be specifically designed to support family interaction. Also, outdoor patios and porches can be attractive areas to sit, talk, and watch the local scenery. Taking a meal together or helping with tasks, like washing personal laundry, builds interaction around a meaningful activity. At Heritage, in Newton, Massachusetts, such meeting places are popular (see figure 1.4).

Mental and Physical Stimulation

Activities that build competency by strengthening upper- and lower-body muscles or that stimulate mental acuity through a range of programs are desirable. Health restoration should involve older people in physical therapy and intellectually challenging activities. Activities that involve children in intergenerational programs have been particularly successful in some environments. The plaza in front of the Heritage, in Cleveland Circle, Massachusetts, is a meeting place in which residents can meet children or watch them at play (see figure 1.5).

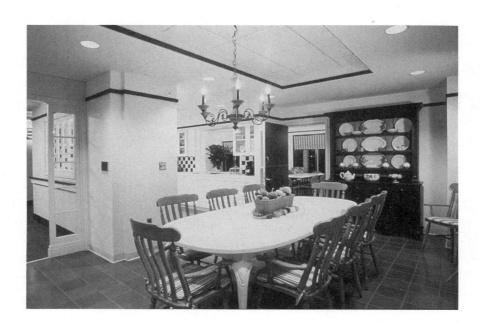

FIGURE 1.4. *The Heritage, Newton, Massachusetts*

9

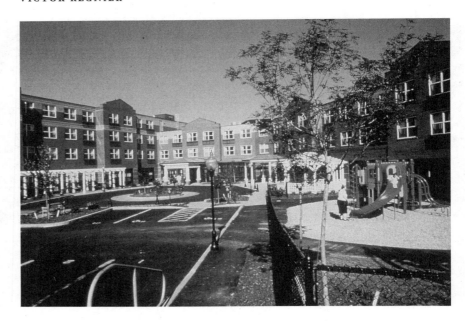

FIGURE 1.5. *The Heritage, Cleveland Circle, Massachusetts*

Residential Privacy and Completeness

The dwelling unit should be private, have at least a kitchenette for food storage and preparation, and be large enough to accommodate a family member for an overnight stay. An accessible full bathroom with a shower makes the unit complete and ensures privacy as well as safety and accessibility. A stove top or microwave oven can provide the resident with food preparation options; these applicances can be removed if the older person can not competently and safely manage them. It is important that the unit appear to be a complete housing unit and not a hospital room.

The Surrounding Community

The environment should strive to integrate residents into the surrounding community rather than isolate them from its resources and contacts. This can be implemented in two principal ways: by encouraging residents to make trips to services in the surrounding neighborhood, rather than bringing everything into the building; and by inviting community groups to visit. This has been done successfully with intergenerational programs. Programs like respite or adult day care encourage people in the community to think of the assisted-living facility as a community resource. In addition, spaces that encourage residents to meet with others outside of their residential community can be built (see figure 1.6).

Independence, Interdependence, and Individuality

The focus of care should be on self-maintenance with assistance. Residents should be encouraged to help one another and to be helped by others. Designing the setting to support friendships encourages helping behaviors, facilitates informal exchange, and builds a sense of community that makes residents feel good about their contribution to others.

The Frail Older Person

The facility should be targeted toward a frail and dependent population. The age range should be between 82 and 87. The population should meet

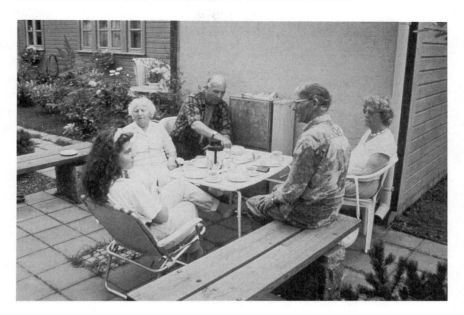

FIGURE 1.6. *Scandinavia Service House, Halmsted, Sweden*

the 40/40 rule (Regnier, Hamilton, and Yatabe, 1995): at least 40 percent of the population has difficulty with incontinence and 40 percent has some problems with memory loss or dementia.

Eight Future Trends and Issues

As assisted living evolves as a concept, a building type, and a lifestyle, we will continue to see shifts in its definition and purpose. The market niche that assisted living fills appears to be widening. Newer projects are capturing sicker and frailer individuals, who would normally have been placed in nursing homes. This continuing evolution effects not only how assisted living is defined but also how it is regulated, what new technologies are incubated, and how systems of care are refined.

Multiple Model Development

Assisted-living models are developing in a variety of ways. Some sponsors, like the American Association of Homes and Services for the Aging (AAHSA) prototype (see chapter 15) and the Minneapolis (Rosewood Estates) model (Regnier, 1994), are using larger unit sizes and services that are purchased on an as-needed basis. Other sponsors, like National Guest Homes, have chosen models that use primarily double-occupied units to reduce costs and to create a smaller, more compact physical footprint. Others, most notably Assisted Living Concepts and ADS Senior Housing, focus on building smaller-sized, single-occupied units. Sunrise Assisted Living and Marriott Corporation, on the other hand, have a more eclectic approach and mix unit sizes. Sunrise offers an enormous range, from double-occupied units to large, single-occupied, "turret" units.

Each of these sponsors seeks a specific target population, and each believes the strategy it employs is superior. The fact that there are still very few available units in most markets means that any true competitive test of philosophies has yet to take place. However, the enormous number of units currently being produced in suburban and ex-urban locations around major cities will allow consumers more choice. If a single model emerges as the most popular, we are likely to see other sponsors emulate that model.

However, we must remember that housing is one of the most unique building types in the world. The tremendous variety is spawned by differences in style, size, density, culture, region, socioeconomics, and lifestyle. A project constructed in downtown Chicago develops under different conditions from those that affect a project in Arlington Heights or in a sparsely populated area in the north. Such variety never had a chance to evolve in the overregulated nursing home industry, because the design of these buildings emulate hospitals. Institutional design is traditionally directed to support staff convenience and efficiency rather than to consider what it is like for residents to live there day after day.

It is also important to remember that housing design is not about style. Housing creates a context for living. The rooms, the sequences, the technology, the surrounding landscape, the amenities, and the features included in a typical housing environment conform to the way we choose to live. Housing more than any other building type reflects the nature of the society for which it has been constructed. As assisted living leans more heavily on the imagery and concept of housing for its future inspiration, so will it evolve to support different ideas about aging and about living in old age.

Affordability

Affordability has been at the forefront of assisted living as it developed from the beginning. Because most assisted living has been financed on a private payment platform, there has been concern about how moderate- to lower-income older people can afford it. Like the private versus public school debate over vouchers, assisted living has raised issues about the cost, quality, and appropriateness of entitlements for skilled nursing care environments. As new assisted-living models evolve that more effectively care for medically indigent individuals, the debate will become more heated. States like Washington and Oregon have been slowly encouraging the development of assisted living through entitlement vouchers that flow from waiver programs. These limited experiences have generally been successful and will most likely increase in size and type in the future.

There is currently a debate in the trade magazines of long-term care about "luxury creep" and the tendency for sponsors to add frills to a building to attract clients and protect it from adverse future competition (Moore, 1996). Questions are continually being raised about what consumers (especially families) are seeking in the design of these environments. Are we adding costly features with limited utility that consumers do not want? Or are these features ones that consumers appreciate and find well worth the extra cost?

Much of this debate centers upon exactly what the majority can afford or are willing to spend. Affordability is a relative concept, especially for a generation of older people who may have sizable equity in owner-occupied single-family houses. How much do they want to spend? How much are families willing to donate to make up the difference? What length of stay is appropriate for considering a strategy of spending down? How generous will insurance providers and government sources be in the future, as residents spend down and require subsidies? Answers to these questions are unavailable or uncertain.

Traditional approaches to housing finance involve interest subsidies. But these approaches, which are commonly used to create low-income apartment stock, have limited applicability to assisted living. This is because as much as three-fourths of the costs associated with assisted living involve the provision of health, food, personal care services, utilities, and maintenance. Thus, paying the amortized costs of land, building construction, and soft development costs is only one part of the overall cost burden.

A most interesting trend in assisted-living finance is the use of public finance mechanisms. As of December 1996, the eight largest producers of assisted-living facilities in the country were publicly owned. Among the twenty-five largest producers of assisted living, the majority are currently publicly owned and traded (Chain Reactions, 1996). This is in sharp contrast to the retirement housing industry, where only one of the twenty-five largest providers is a public company, and more like the nursing home industry, which shares a similar dependence on Wall Street for financial capital. Public ownership ties the industry to a powerful mechanism for expansion capital but also requires greater accountability to stockholders for returns and profitability.

There is fear that assisted living will evolve into a tiered system that uses different models for the haves and the have-nots. If this occurs, it will further distance itself from systems like traditional health care, in which equality governs the distribution of health care services among all income groups. The future of assisted-living subsidies will center on actions that governmental bodies like the Health Care Financing Agency (HCFA) take with regard to entitlement reimbursement. In the meantime, within the broader context of feasible arrangements, models are likely to develop that are targeted toward a range of income groups.

Loss of Acuity

One of the most interesting trends in the evolution of assisted living is the move toward servicing more acutely ill populations, although it is not universally embraced by providers. However, high profitability and greater consumer acceptance is often associated with assisted-living facilities that compete with nursing homes for residents. The newest wrinkle in this competition is the identification of Alzheimer's residents as a particularly appropriate resident population for assisted living.

Alzheimer's residents are a natural constituency for assisted living because they have primarily personal care needs. As they age and become more medically dependent, their need for more complex medical treatments increases, but this normally does not trigger nursing home placement until the last few months of life. Furthermore, there is some evidence that behavioral difficulties can result from the institutional setting. Swedish experiments (Kuller, 1991) carried out in the Varnhem psychogeriatric hospital demonstrate that creating smaller self-contained clusters of units designed and decorated to resemble small-group residential homes reduces the number of behavioral outbursts and the need for physical or chemical restraints.

After all, memory loss, like incontinence, is not an acute medical problem. A decade ago, residents were placed in nursing homes because they were incontinent. That logic today seems totally ridiculous, with drugstores that devote whole aisles to products for self-managed incontinence. But we continue to believe that memory loss requires institutionalization. This is just as shortsighted and antiquated as our thinking about incontinence a decade ago.

Some regulators interpret assisted living as a philosophy of care that centers on providing assistance in normalized residential environments. New Jersey, for example, has developed an assisted-living platform that conforms to nine levels of care, ranging from congregate assistance to subacute care (Mollica, 1995). In defining assisted living in this highly flexible way, New Jersey has allowed assisted-living providers to declare the level of care they want to provide, allowing the philosophy of assisted living to permeate to a much higher level of care while still using the traditional regulatory safeguards included in the building code and in various licensing codes.

What will keep assisted living from replacing nursing homes? Facilities are likely to self-declare the types of residents they will accept. No doubt, the efficiency and cost-effectiveness of operations are likely to play a major role in this decision. As technologies and care management systems progress, natural tipping points will emerge. As a resident becomes more severely impaired and requires more sophisticated life-sustaining interventions, another environment will fit his or her needs more effectively. Provider organizations will select the residents they manage based on whether the facility can safely, efficiently, and cost-effectively meet their needs.

Regulation

As the health care needs of residents in assisted living increase, so do the concerns about what constitutes appropriate regulatory oversight. Building design requirements are predicated on building categories that rely on specific resident profiles. These requirements are collected in the form of an occupancy category. In the Building Officials and Code Administrators code (BOCA) used to guide most construction in the eastern half of the United States, the occupancy category for most assisted living is called I-2. Building codes differ from state to state and can differ from municipality to municipality, and although most conform to the concepts and principles established in a general-use code like BOCA, they can vary depending on how they are interpreted by code officials. Local fire departments are also influential because they are responsible for saving residents and the building in case of fire. When a building is not designed to meet the exiting requirements for a mentally or physically frail person, then by law these individuals must move. Thus, designing a building so that it allows the older person to age in place requires forethought.

Multistory buildings constructed of steel and concrete frames are safer than buildings constructed solely of wood framing. Thus, these buildings do not require the same containment and firewall protections required for wood construction. Architecturally, these mitigations require fire doors and 1-hour corridor separations, which result in building designs that are primarily rooms connected to exit corridors. The flowing spaces created by

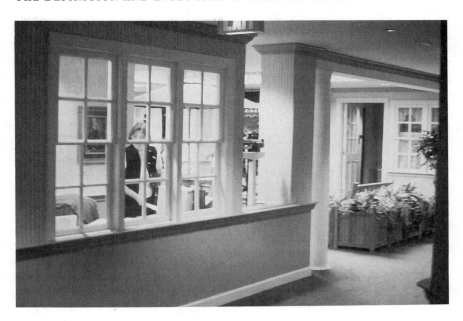

FIGURE I.7. Sunrise, Annapolis, Maryland

half-walls, pierced plane partitions, Dutch doors, interior windows, and open-plan configurations are difficult if not impossible to implement in wood construction. These limitations are avoided in steel construction; Sunrise in Annapolis, Maryland, features such half-walls and a Dutch door (see figure 1.7). The costs, it must be noted, of building with steel are often 10–15 percent higher than the costs of building with wood.

Most licensing regulations that govern health care, personal care, and food services are centered on the competency of the people who provide the service and how the service is rendered. However, building and licensing codes are intertwined, and often a change in the type of service provided triggers a more stringent building code requirement. Assisted living has traditionally been licensed by social care agencies, which in most states govern housing for developmentally disabled persons, day care for children, and adult board-and-care homes. The primary focus of board-and-care regulations has been on facilities serving fewer than twenty-five residents, but many of these are rapidly being replaced by larger, assisted-living facilities. Because board-and-care homes were established to provide personal care assistance, they have not been considered health care facilities. Most new assisted-living facilities, however, are constantly pushing the dependency envelope, and as a result they are considered in many states as health care facilities, which are regulated by state health care agencies. When these agencies are involved in the regulation of assisted-living housing, which are seen as just another type of nursing home, the regulations and requirements become much more stringent and narrow.

One of the reasons nursing homes are so unattractive and sterile is that they are regulated by rules similar to those that govern acute care hospitals, so the decision of where to place assisted living in the state regulatory system can have major consequences. Some health care agencies understand the differences between assisted living and nursing care and have established policies that seek to maintain the residential character of assisted-living facilities. The increase in dependency levels in assisted-living residents complicates these judgments. However, new technologies, safer fire and smoke systems, more effective electronic monitoring and communication systems, new training approaches, and smaller, self-contained, durable medical equipment make these environments safer and allow for more effective staff practices. In fact, buildings constructed under the proper building code and licensing categories are extremely safe. The National fire protection model code, NFPA 101, reports that no multiple death has ever been recorded in fire-sprinkled housing, except in the case of explosion. This is a far safer record than any automobile manufacturer or airline can offer.

Technology

New technologies are transforming the assisted-living environment in both operations and building construction. Communications technologies now make it easier to summon assistance, monitor building safety systems, contain and track residents with memory loss, and monitor specialty training for paraprofessionals. Computers, telephone systems, and multimedia will continue to have major impacts on the assisted-living industry, in part because many of the new companies attracted to assisted living are bringing with them systems of management and operations targeted on containing costs and increasing the amount and quality of information available. Electronic monitoring systems appear to be changing the most as interest in caring for Alzheimer's residents increases. Systems currently in use require residents to wear specially programmed bracelets that trigger alarms. Doors are locked or set with alarms, allowing residents to freely wander both inside and outside. Systems that track single individuals within a building, on the grounds, or in the neighborhood are under development. These new devices will be compatible with current alarm and building monitoring systems. The impact of this technology will give Alzheimer's residents even greater freedom, while further reducing the anxiety many experience when they are secured in one area of the building for a long time.

Communication systems, used to summon assistance when needed, help maintain the privacy and sanctity of the dwelling unit. Fee-for-service systems often use home care organizations to provide service in 15-minute increments. In the past, these providers have modified monitoring devices like Lifeline to provide a peripatetic service response system to residents. These systems have been combined with infrared portable telephone technologies and software for automatic billing. The inconveniences that made these ad hoc emergency call systems difficult to operate are being streamlined.

Staff training is also in the process of graduating from videos to multimedia applications. Computer-based learning programs that can randomly access knowledge in a custom-fitted program for specific task mastery have enormous potential for staff training and for family interaction. Learning about topics such as Alzheimer's disease through a custom-learning multimedia computer program will be the first step. This will be followed by the use of information for case analysis and the development of expert systems to guide patient care strategies. The high-touch, high-tech approach to monitoring residents will continue as monitoring becomes less labor-intensive, leaving time for interaction between residents and staff.

Family Involvement

The involvement of families may not seem like a new trend, but one of the most compelling reasons assisted living has become popular is due to the influence of family members. Family members select assisted-living environments over board-and-care facilities and nursing homes because these facilities are consistent with their own values and standards. They are seeking a management organization that is responsive to their requests and an environment that makes them feel welcome and at ease. Most successful assisted-living facilities have pursued a myriad of ways to involve family members, including volunteer activities, invitations to special events, and the provision of places in the building or on the grounds where family members can spend time with residents.

In the future, family-centered and family-friendly environments is likely to become even more popular as a higher percentage of residents come from Asian, Latino, and African American families, whose traditional, family-centered cultures have avoided nursing home placement in the past. In fact, small board-and-care homes have generally been the housing type of choice for these cultures and ethnic groups. Assisted-living facilities have sought ways to create a stronger legal and administrative bond with families. By avoiding the formal shifting of responsibility that occurs during the process of institutionalization, families of assisted-living residents have emerged with a deeper and more authoritative caregiving role. Innovations in acute health care, like the Planetree neighborhood cluster, are popular with minority families. Family members visit with residents (including children), bring special foods, and often spend long hours at the hospital.

In Europe, mixed-use housing arrangements that place family housing in the same building complex as housing for mentally and physically impaired persons have been very successful. Staff and family members alike find the convenience of living near the assisted-living residence an advantage. Housing that allows family members to share caregiving responsibilities through programs like adult day care, home health care, *aanluen woning* (Regnier, 1994: Dutch for housing electronically tethered to the emergency care system of an adjacent assisted living project), or respite placement will add flexibility and provide more options for families.

People with Dementia

As mentioned earlier, Alzheimer's residents are perhaps the most overlooked special-needs population in most assisted-living facilities (Regnier, 1997). The desire of care facilities to hold on to residents for as long as possible as they lose cognitive ability makes it necessary to design special accommodations. These generally involve placing individuals in a smaller-scale setting that is electronically monitored and that can be more effectively managed and controlled. Several trends in the design of Alzheimer's units are worth noting.

Focus on Residential Attributes: Features such as carpeted floors, memory-enhancing and thought-provoking accessories, familiar and comfortable furniture, generous daylight, incandescent (or color-corrected) artificial lighting, outdoor landscaping, and single-occupied dwelling units are being pursued in an effort to make these setting more homelike. These residential touches make residents feel comfortable and secure. When the set-

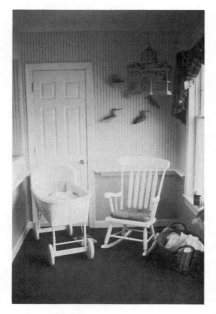

FIGURE 1.8. *Sunrise, Columbia, Maryland*

ting is familiar and comfortable, residents are also less likely to exhibit behavioral outbursts. Sunrise in Columbia, Maryland, has life skills stations (see figure 1.8), allowing dementia patients to recall positive events.

Neighborhood Clusters of Units: Splitting buildings into groups of eight to fifteen units creates intimate neighborhoods. Residents who take meals together and join one another in activities constitute "families," which become socially cohesive. Clustering units in self-contained "houses" reduces the scale of the setting, making it less overwhelming, easier to control, and more socially satisfying. The right size is large enough to stimulate sociability but small enough to contain the cascading effects of agitated behaviors.

Familiar Residential-Scaled Spaces and Activities: Creating spaces that are scaled and decorated like those in a typical single-family home allows providers to recreate elements of a residential lifestyle as part of the therapeutic program. For example, activities like setting the table or bussing dishes, in a residential-scale kitchen, reproduce habits and behaviors that are familiar and meaningful. Watching TV in a living room just like the one at home is reassuring and comforting.

Gardens and Outdoor Spaces: Places to walk and sit outside provide a way to exercise and also allow residents to be in contact with nature. This is a powerful and soothing experience that appears to have benefits for residents in both Sun Belt and Frost Belt locations. Agitation can sometimes be walked off, and the persistent desire to maintain movement benefits from the larger context outdoor spaces provide.

Family-Centered Environments: When family members feel welcome and participate in the daily life of residents, the setting gains a distinctive noninstitutional flavor. An environment that resembles the home a resident left is more enjoyable to visit and reduces the guilt a family member might experience in a setting that is less attractive or more institutional.

Encouraging Humor, Affection, and Emotional Attachment

One of the major complaints about skilled nursing environments is their sterility. Beyond the layout of rooms that resemble a hospital ward, visitors are almost always put off by the lack of normal residential furniture, finishes, wall coverings, floor coverings, and accessories. Nursing homes often experience criticism from regulators when attempts to humanize the environment like introducing plants, pets, or wall coverings are proposed. What is interpreted as legally appropriate is often what the regulator has seen in other facilities; deviations from the norm implies unacceptability.

However, nursing homes and assisted-living settings are questioning the exact meaning of ambiguously worded regulatory statements and are searching for more meaning and stimulation in the objects selected for display and decoration. The most effective humanizing interventions are those that stimulate positive affect. Among the most powerful are children, pets and plants, and the use of humor. In that regard, some of the most interesting work is that of Thomas (1996), who has vigorously pursued the use of pet birds, plants, and intergenerational programs in his Eden Alternative nursing home demonstration. Data from his research shows much lower incidents of psychotropic drug use, yearly infections per resident, and numbers of deaths when compared with a control facility.

The stimulation of positive feelings and emotion will continue to be a key element in the design of successful settings. Martha Child, known for her highly articulated interior designs, insists that each room should have a "huggability" index. Artwork subjects, the themes used to decorate unit clusters, color and pattern choices, and use of accessories to stimulate whimsy and emotional attachment should make a setting more emotionally stimulating. This result relies on the underlying perceptions and associations that residents and their families have with the objects and visual patterns that make up the decorated environment.

Conclusions

Assisted living is becoming a more widely recognized long-term care alternative, even though its form and organization appear to be evolving. As Paul Klaassen, CEO of Sunrise Assisted Living and industry leader, has frequently stated, we are in the beginning of the product development cycle of assisted living; "the best assisted-living environments have yet to be invented." One thing can be predicted: assisted living will continue to change as new opportunities for humanizing the provision of personal care services evolve. As a market-sensitive housing and service creation, assisted living will evolve in response to the needs of older residents and the desires and interests of family members.

References

Chain Reactions. 1996. *Contemporary Long Term Care* 19(12): 35–47.

Guralnik, J., M. Yanagishta, and E. Schneider. 1988. Projecting the older population of the United States: Lessons from the past and prospects for the future. *Milbank Quarterly* 66:283–308.

Kane, R., and K. Brown. 1993. *Assisted Living in the United States: A New Paradigm for Residential Care for Frail Older Persons?* Washington, D.C.: American Association of Retired Persons.

Kuller, R. 1991. Familiar design helps dementia patients cope. In W. Preiser, J. Vischer, and E. White, eds., *Design Intervention: Toward a More Humane Architecture.* New York: Van Nostrand Reinhold.

Mollica, R. 1995. *Guide to State Assisted-Living Policy.* Portland, Maine: National Academy for State Health Policy and the National Long-Term Care Resource Center.

Moore, J. 1996. *Assisted Living: Pure and Simple Development and Operating Strategies.* Fort Worth, Tex.: Moore Diversified Services.

Regnier, V. 1994. *Assisted Living Housing for the Elderly: Design Innovations from the United States and Europe.* New York: Van Nostrand Reinhold.

———. 1997. Design for assisted living. *Contemporary Long Term Care* 2(20): 50–56.

Regnier, V., J. Hamilton, and Y. Yatabe. 1995. *Assisted Living for the Aged and Frail: Innovations in Design, Management and Financing.* New York: Columbia University Press.

Rivlin, A., and J. Weiner. 1988. *Caring for the Disabled Elderly.* Washington, D.C.: Brookings.

Spencer, G. 1989. *Projections of the Population of the United States by Age, Sex, and Race, 1988 to 2080.* U.S. Bureau of the Census, Current Population Reports P-25. Washington, D.C.: Government Printing Office.

Thomas, W. 1996. *Life Worth Living: How Someone You Love Can Still Enjoy Life in a Nursing Home.* Acton, Mass.: VanderWyk and Burnham.

CHAPTER 2

Assisted Living
The Current State of Affairs

RONALD K. TINSLEY
KENNETH E. WARREN

**The Supply of and
Demand for Assisted Living**

The number of assisted-living residences in the United States has been the subject of considerable debate within the industry. Estimates of between 30,000 and 40,000 residences that serve up to 1 million residents have been used by the industry (PricewaterhouseCoopers, 1998). This estimate, however, has been contested, based on defining what residences or facilities should be included in such an inventory. Other industry sources indicate that there may be between 15,000 and 20,000 (*McKnight's Long-Term Care News*, 1997).

Larger estimates of the number of assisted-living residences may include small homes operated by a sole proprietor caring for two or more unrelated elderly individuals. These smaller residences may actually be converted family homes and typically provide limited care to their residents. Some industry sources further define assisted living to include only those residences offering a full range of support services, including but not necessarily limited to meals, transportation, activities programs, and assistance with personal care. The National Investment Conference (NIC) for the senior living and long-term care industries, a professional organization that provides quality research information related to this industry, has provided an analysis of assisted-living residence supply, which gives a further indication of the confusion over estimates of supply (see table 2.1).

Compounding the issue of the supply of assisted-living accommodations is the lack of common licensure, or even a common classification, for assisted living in the United States. Throughout the United States, assisted-living services are licensed by state regulatory bodies, which in 1996 referred to such housing and services by titles such as, but not limited to, residential care facilities, domiciliary care homes, personal care homes, adult congregate-living facilities, homes for the aged, foster care homes, adult foster care homes, catered living facilities, retirement homes, homes for adults, board-and-care homes, and community residences (see table 2.2). In 1997, twenty-two states had licensure regulations for assisted living, six states had regulations pending, and ten states were developing or otherwise studying assisted living (PricewaterhouseCoopers, 1998).

While there are differences regarding the number of assisted-living residences, there is a general consensus that this number will increase. The NIC estimates that the demand for assisted living, based on population data, will increase from a current estimate of 457,000 beds in 1996 to between a "conservative" estimate of 675,000 beds and an "optimistic" estimate of 1,164,000 beds by 2030 (Mueller and Laposa, 1997). During the twelve-month period ending June 30, 1996, many of the top assisted-living opera-

Table 2.1. Estimated Supply of Assisted-Living Facilities in the United States, 1996

Item	Number
Total facilities estimate (includes board and care, assisted living, and facilities for mentally retarded persons)	65,000
Less unlicensed board-and-care facilities	(33,569)
Equals subtotal of licensed facilities	31,431
Less board-and-care homes for mentally retarded persons	(13,169)
Equals licensed facilities for nonmentally retarded persons	18,262
Less residences with twenty-five or fewer units	(13,962)
Equals subtotal of licensed facilities for nonmentally retarded persons with greater than twenty-five units	4,300

Source: Data from Mueller and Laposa, 1997.

tors more than doubled their bed capacity. Much of the growth was fueled by Wall Street, as dozens of assisted-living companies tapped the public equities market. This, in turn, opened the industry to even more sources of funding, especially from real estate investment trusts (Industry may experience growing pains, 1997). The availability of financing for residences facilitates the growth of assisted-living residences; however, many underlying factors account for the current interest and growth in assisted living, including the aging population, an increasing need for assistance services, a continued increase in the number of persons who live alone, changes in the labor force, the affordability of assisted-living residences, and a desire for a residential-style health care living environment.

The Aging Population

Perhaps the most important factor in the growth of the assisted-living industry, as well as many other seniors-oriented industries, is the projected growth in the population aged 65 years and older. By the year 2050, as many as one in five Americans could be elderly. Most of this growth should occur between 2010 and 2030, when the baby boom generation achieves its elderly years (U.S. Bureau of the Census, 1995b). A major factor in the growth of the 65-years-and-older age group is the increase in life expectancy. Life expectancy in the United States rose from 47 years in 1900, to 68 years in 1950, to 76 years in 1991. There is also a difference in the life expectancy of men and women. In 1991, women had a life expectancy of 79 years, but men had a life expectancy of 72 years.

As with any type of projection, researchers differ in the magnitude of the growth that will occur in the older population in the United States. The U.S. Bureau of the Census has developed three estimates, or three series, of population projections based on three levels of mortality for persons aged 65 years and older. The estimates range from a low of approximately 18.2 million persons to a high of approximately 31.1 million persons by the year 2050 (U.S. Bureau of the Census, 1997a). The growth of age cohorts 65–74, 75–84, and 85 and older have also been analyzed using the Census Bureau's middle-series population projections (see figure 2.1). Although the growth in the 65-and-older age group is significant, it is the immediate

Table 2.2. State Classifications for Assisted Living, 1996

State	Classification
Alabama	Assisted-living facilities
Alaska	Assisted-living facilities
Arizona	Adult care homes
Arkansas	Residential care homes
California	Residential care facilities for the elderly
Colorado	Personal care boarding homes
Connecticut	Assisted-living services agencies
Delaware	Rest homes
Florida	Adult congregate living facilities, extended congregate care facilities
Georgia	Personal care homes
Hawaii	Assisted-living facilities
Idaho	Residential care facilities
Illinois	Sheltered care facilities
Indiana	Residential care facilities
Iowa	Residential care facilities
Kansas	Assisted-living facilities, residential health care facilities
Kentucky	Personal care homes
Louisiana	Adult residential care homes
Maine	Boarding homes
Maryland	Multifamily or group senior assisted-living housing
Massachusetts	Assisted living residences
Michigan	Homes for the aged
Minnesota	Elderly housing with services establishments
Mississippi	Personal care homes
Missouri	Residential care facilities
Montana	Personal care facilities
Nebraska	Residential care facilities
Nevada	Residential facilities for groups
New Hampshire	Residential care homes
New Jersey	Assisted-living residences
New Mexico	Adult residential sheltered care facilities
New York	Adult homes, enriched housing programs
North Carolina	Adult care homes, group homes for the developmentally disabled, multiple-unit assisted housing with services
North Dakota	Basic care facilities, assisted-living facilities
Ohio	Assisted-living facilities
Oklahoma	Residential care homes
Oregon	Assisted-living facilities
Pennsylvania	Personal care homes
Rhode Island	Residential care, assisted-living facilities
South Carolina	Community residential care facilities
South Dakota	Assisted-living centers
Tennessee	Assisted-care living facilities
Texas	Personal care facilities
Utah	Assisted-living facilities
Vermont	Residential care homes
Virginia	Adult care residences, assisted-living facilities
Washington	Boarding homes
West Virginia	Personal care homes
Wisconsin	Assisted-living facilities
Wyoming	Assisted-living facilities

Source: Information from the American Health Care Association.

Population in Thousands

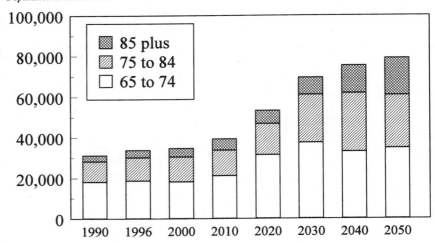

FIGURE 2.1. *Population aged 65 and older, by age group, 1990–2050*
SOURCE: *Data from U.S. Bureau of the Census, 1997a.*

growth trends in the oldest population (defined as those individuals 85 years of age and older) that has captured the interest of the assisted-living industry. This group is expected to experience a significant increase in population regardless of which census estimate series is considered (see figure 2.2).

The Increasing Need for Assistance

Assisted living fulfills the needs of individuals requiring supportive care. An industry survey completed in 1998 indicates that assisted-living residents, on average, needed assistance with three ADLs (PricewaterhouseCoopers, 1998). The population with the greatest need for assistance is the most prominent user of assisted-living services. Approximately 6.5 million older people (aged 65 and older) need assistance with activities of daily living (ADLs) or instrumental activities of daily living (IADLs). As the number of older Americans continues to increase (especially those 85 years of age and older), the number of people who need assistance with ADLs may double by the year 2020. In 1996, 50 percent of the population 85 years of age and older needed assistance with at least one ADL or IADL (see figure 2.3).

Population in Thousands

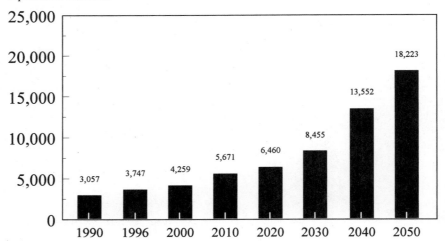

FIGURE 2.2. *Population aged 85 and older, 1990–2050*
SOURCE: *Data from U.S. Bureau of the Census, 1997b.*

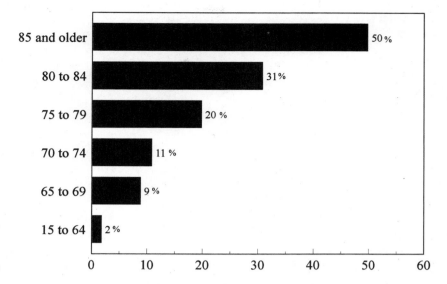

FIGURE 2.3. Percentage of persons needing assistance with everyday activities, by age, 1990–1991 (civilian noninstitutionalized population)
SOURCE: Data from U.S. Bureau of the Census, 1995b.

Persons Who Live Alone

The likelihood of living alone increases with age. Most of this increase is due to an aging population in which women outlive men. In 1993, 80 percent of noninstitutionalized elderly persons who lived alone were women. The likelihood of women living alone increases from 32 percent for the 65–74 age cohort to 57 percent for those 85 years of age and older. The trends for men are similar, with 13 percent of the 65–74 age cohort living alone, rising to 29 percent aged 85 and older (U.S. Bureau of the Census, 1995b). Societal changes, such as rising divorce rates and the growing numbers of persons choosing not to marry, have further increased the number of Americans living alone. This growth in the number of elderly persons living alone has resulted in increasing demand for services that historically were provided by a spouse, other family members, or live-in caregivers.

Changes in the Labor Force

The changing labor force in our society has influenced the availability of caregivers at home. In 1915, 20.5 percent of the total labor force were women. In 1996, the proportion of U.S. workers who were women had increased to more than 56 percent. The greater the percentage of the U.S. workforce that women occupy, the less time women have to fill what has been historically their role as caregivers. In 1995, among 55.7 percent of married couples both the husband and the wife worked (U.S. Bureau of the Census, 1995a). The increase in working women and in two-earner households places increasing pressure on the time available to care for elderly parents. While the time available to provide caregiving is being reduced, more and more individuals in their 50s and 60s are facing the concern and expense of caring for elderly relatives. The parent support ratio (the number of persons aged 85 and over per a hundred persons aged 50–64 years of age) increased from a ratio of 3:100 in 1950 to a ratio of 10:100 in 1993. This ratio may rise as high as 29:100 by 2050 (U.S. Bureau of the Census, 1995b).

The Affordability of Assisted Living

Table 2.3. Average Rates for Care (in dollars)

Type of Care	Average Rate
Assisted living	72[a] private room
Acute care	821
Subacute care	250
Skilled nursing	111 private bed/ private pay
Home health	83[b]

Source: Information from Marion Merrill Dow and Healthcare Financial Management Association
[a]Per diem.
[b]Per visit for nursing.

The Desire for a Residential-Style Care Environment

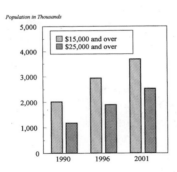

FIGURE 2.4. Household income of those aged 80 and older, 1990, 1997, 2002
SOURCE: *Information from Claritas, Inc.*

The Characteristics of Assisted-Living Residences

One of the attractions of assisted living is its relative affordability compared to skilled nursing care. In 1997, the average rate for a private room in an assisted-living residence was approximately $66 per day (Pricewaterhous Coopers, 1998). Compared to other levels of health care (see table 2.3), assisted living provides a cost-effective option for those frail elderly persons not in need of nursing or acute care. The number of persons 80 years of age and older with incomes sufficient to afford assisted living is increasing. More than 54 percent of individuals 80 years of age and older are estimated to have yearly incomes of $15,000 and above, and 35 percent are estimated to have incomes of $25,000 and above (see figure 2.4).

Managed care penetration and the continued development of integrated delivery systems will likely have an impact on the further development of the assisted-living industry. Managed care is expected to assess assisted living as a cost-effective alternative care setting. Control of the quality and escalating costs of health care is a significant objective of managed health care. In some areas of the country, managed care penetration in acute care as well as extended care settings has already begun to occur (PricewaterhouseCoopers, 1998).

A decision to move into an assisted-living residence is typically made during a time of crisis for the prospective resident. Families are often driven by the need to find a care setting for loved ones whose physical, emotional, or mental condition has forced them to seek more appropriate living environments. Many families are reluctant to place their loved one in an institutional setting, such as a nursing home, unless the individual requires 24-hour skilled medical care. Many older persons are placed in nursing homes because they or their families cannot find (or are not aware of) other, more appropriate residential care settings, in which 24-hour personal care is provided. Skilled care usually consists of medical care provided by technically trained medical staff in an institutional setting. Personal care, on the other hand, can be provided by well-trained, nonmedical aides in a residential setting such as an assisted-living residence. Research varies as to estimates of residents in nursing homes who could be appropriately cared for in an assisted-living setting. However, "numerous studies suggest that one-fifth to one-third of those in institutions are receiving an inappropriate level of care" (Johnson and Grant, 1985).

The number of units in an assisted-living residence varies: some residences are converted residential homes, some are freestanding assisted-living residences, and some are part of large retirement communities with multiple levels of care. Current industry practice is to build freestanding assisted-living residences averaging forty to a hundred units per facility. Facility size is influenced by several factors, including market forces, site constraints, and programs (Mueller and Laposa, 1997). One survey places the average number of units in an assisted-living facility at sixty-seven (Coopers & Lybrand, 1997b); another study indicates a median unit size of seventy-seven (Coopers & Lybrand, 1997a).

Table 2.4. Average Size of Unit (in square feet)

Type of Unit	Average Size
Semiprivate room	309
Private room (studio)	303
One bedroom	484
Two bedroom	769

Source: Data from PricewaterhouseCoopers L.L.P., 1998.

Table 2.5. Amenities in Resident Units

Amenity	Percentage of Units Providing Amenity
Stove in room	23.8
Microwave in room	39.1
Refrigerator in room	69.5
Sink in room (in addition to bathroom sink)	67.7
Private toilet	94.5
Private shower	79.6
Private bathtub	19.3

Source: See Table 2.4.

Assisted-living residences provide a variety of living arrangements, from semiprivate rooms to two-bedroom apartments. Private units (single-occupancy rooms or studio apartments) account for 52.9 percent of the total; one-bedroom units account for 26.2 percent; semiprivate units account for 11.4 percent; two-bedroom apartments account for 4.0 percent; and other units, including ward rooms (three beds or more), account for 5.5 percent. The average assisted-living residence, is 48,184 square feet in size.

Resident units range in size from an average of 303 square feet in a private unit to 769 square feet in a two-bedroom apartment (see table 2.4). The amenities provided in an assisted-living residence vary: nearly 95 percent provide private toilets in the resident's room; nearly 80 percent provide a private shower (see table 2.5). More than 30 percent of residences have dedicated Alzheimer's care units; the average Alzheimer's care unit had forty-two beds and an occupancy rate of 92.1 percent. Respite care, a short-term stay in an assisted-living residence, is provided by nearly 79 percent of assisted-living residences. These residences served an average of 1.7 respite care residents.

Who Lives in an Assisted-Living Residence?

Providers of assisted living describe their typical resident as an 84-year-old single or widowed woman requiring assistance with ADLs. This is not surprising, considering the longer life expectancy of women and the increase in elderly persons living alone. The average resident's age in an assisted-living residence is 80.9 years for men and 83.3 years for women. Approximately 78.4 percent of assisted-living residents are female. Married couples living together in an assisted-living residence account for 2.4 percent of residents. Residents require assistance with an average of three ADL deficiencies: 46.9 percent have some form of cognitive impairment, nearly 38 percent use a walker or wheelchair, and approximately 27 percent have daily incontinence.

Although some states provide Medicaid or state aid to residents, assisted living relies mainly on private-pay residents. Only 9.7 percent of assisted-living residents receive assistance from state Medicaid waiver programs, Supplemental Security Income, or other state assistance programs. As would be expected, assisted-living residents have a relatively high average

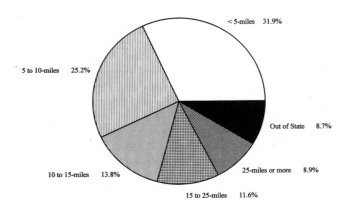

FIGURE 2.5. *Distance from which residents relocate (percentage)*

annual income of $30,800, which compares to an estimated 1996 median income of $17,000 for households of those aged 80 and older (estimates from Claritas, Inc.). In addition, average financial resources (assets) of assisted-living residents is $153,000.

Proximity is an important factor in choosing an assisted-living facility, both for the residents and for their families. More than 68 percent of assisted-living residents relocate from within fifteen miles of their assisted-living residence (see figure 2.5). As important as the resident's location is the family's proximity to the assisted-living residence: more than 78 percent of assisted-living residents had family living within twenty miles of the residence (see figure 2.6). The majority of assisted-living residents move from their own homes or from other family members' homes (see figure 2.7). Family members are a strong referral source for assisted-living residences. Hospitals and physicians, however, account for more than 26 percent of the referrals to assisted-living residences (see table 2.6).

The Future of the Assisted-Living Industry

Growth in the elderly population, changes in the labor force, and the increasing need for assistance are expected to drive the continued increase in the number of assisted-living residences. However, many factors may have

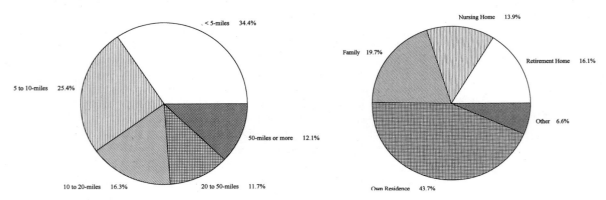

FIGURE 2.6. *Distance of the nearest family member to the residence (percentage)*

FIGURE 2.7. *Places from which residents relocate (percentage)*

Table 2.6. Sources of Referral for Assisted-Living Residences

Referral Source	Percentage
Family member	22.8
Hospital	12.7
Physician	7.9
Yellow pages or media advertisement	13.4
Other resident of the facility	5.7
Nursing home	6.7
Drive by the facility	8.2
Area agency on aging or other social service agency	4.8
Trustee/family legal adviser	2.2
Home health care agency	3.6
Church	1.6
Other	10.4

Source: See Table 2.4.

an impact on the operations of assisted-living residences in the future. The following list summarizes the probabilities:

— By the turn of the century, the number of assisted-living units in the United States will approach the number of nursing home units.

— The years 1996–2000 will provide a four-year window of opportunity for new construction, the conversion of existing retirement product, and the expansion of naturally occurring retirement communities.

— The years 2000–2005 will bring excellent opportunities to acquire many of the assisted-living residences built between 1996 and 2000 as the industry begins to consolidate.

— Hospitals will play a major role in the future development and success of the industry.

— Managed care systems will have a key role in the operations of assisted-living residences and use of the product and services.

— By the turn of the century, third-party reimbursement will be a major source of payment for assisted-living housing and services, as reimbursement dollars become more scarce, home health care inefficiencies come into focus, and all payers look for more cost-effective housing and care options.

— Assisted-living residences will replace nursing homes as the predominate site for residents with Alzheimer's disease and related dementias.

— The assisted-living industry will have a tremendous impact on the development of new regulations and will have effective certification and accreditation programs.

— The availability of hospice services in assisted living will become commonplace.

— The scope of skilled services permitted in assisted-living residences will increase dramatically, realizing the concept of aging in place.

— Building code standards for assisted-living residences will lessen only slightly due to health and safety concerns.

—Major legal battles will occur, dealing with such issues as negotiated risk, fair housing, individual freedom, right to privacy, zoning laws, and states' rights to protect individuals' health and safety.
—Those who choose assisted living as a profession are in "for a very exciting ride."
—The successful assisted-living companies of tomorrow will not be doing tomorrow what they are doing today.

Note

A significant portion of the data in this chapter was obtained from *An Overview of the Assisted Living Industry, 1998*, a research publication coproduced by the Assisted Living Federation of America (ALFA) and PricewaterhouseCoopers LLP. *An Overview* summarizes the results of an annual survey distributed to providers of assisted living throughout the United States. The survey has become a recognized resource for the assisted-living industry. During the summer of 1997, ALFA and PricewaterhouseCoopers mailed the survey to approximately 3,369 members of ALFA. Responses to the survey included 402 facilities from thirty-five states (with 23,525 units).

Certain financial statistical information in this chapter was obtained from *The State of Seniors Housing, 1996*, a research publication coproduced by the American Seniors Housing Association and Coopers & Lybrand LLP. This report summarizes the results of an annual survey distributed to providers of senior housing throughout the United States and includes information on continuing care retirement communities, congregate living facilities, and assisted-living facilities. Approximately 252 facilities, representing over 40,000 units, responded to this survey in 1996.

References

Coopers & Lybrand. 1997a. *The State of Seniors Housing, 1996*. Washington, D.C.: American Seniors Housing Association.

———. 1997b. *An Overview of the Assisted Living Industry, 1996*. Fairfax, Va.: Assisted-Living Federation of America.

Industry may experience growing pains in 1997. 1997. *Provider*, February 27.

Johnson, C., and L. Grant. 1985. *The Nursing Home in American Society*. Baltimore: Johns Hopkins University Press.

McKnight's Long-Term Care News. 1997. February 6.

Mollica, R., and K. Snow. 1996. *State Assisted-Living Policy, 1996*. Portland, Maine: National Academy for State Health Policy.

Mueller, G., and S. Laposa. 1997. *The Investment Case for Senior Living and Long-Term Care Properties in an Institutional Real Estate Portfolio, 1996*. Annapolis, Md.: National Investment Conference for the Senior Living and Long-Term Care Industries.

PricewaterhouseCoopers. 1998. *An Overview of the Assisted Living Industry, 1998*. Fairfax, Va.: Assisted-Living Federation of America.

U.S. Bureau of the Census. 1995a. *Household and Family Characteristics, March 1995*. Washington, D.C.: Government Printing Office.

———. 1995b. *Statistical Brief, Sixty-five Plus in the United States*. Washington, D.C.: Government Printing Office.

————. 1997a. *Population Projections of the United States by Age, Sex, Race, and Hispanic Origin, 1995 to 2050*. Current Population Reports P25-1130. Washington, D.C.: Government Printing Office.

————. 1997b. *Resident Population of the United States: Middle Series Projections, 1996–2000, by Age and Sex*. Current Population Reports P25–1130. Washington, D.C.: Government Printing Office.

CHAPTER 3

The Promise of Assisted Living as a Shelter and Care Alternative for Frail American Elders

A Cautionary Essay

STEPHEN M. GOLANT

Experts have proclaimed the assisted-living facility as a highly promising group shelter and care setting that can accommodate physically and mentally frail older Americans who require a protective environment, regular and unscheduled assistance with the activities of daily living, and some nursing care. Some proponents further argue that the assisted-living facility can accommodate many of the elder occupants now found in nursing homes but without subjecting them to a highly institutionalized, medical, and regimented living environment. Rather, the assisted-living facility, at least as it is ideally portrayed, offers residents a social, or residential, model of shelter and care. This implies an architectural setting that more resembles a residence, an inn, or a hotel than a hospital or nursing home and an organizational environment that as much as possible allows residents to retain their dignity, independence, control, individuality, and privacy.

Unlike more medically oriented long-term care settings or very small, traditional board-and-care facilities, assisted-living facilities provide residents with their own apartments, where they can lock their doors and have their own bathroom and kitchen facilities. Residents have much more say about how they conduct their everyday activities, such as when they eat or recreate, and have a more active role in deciding what services they receive and when they receive them. Quality of care is judged less on staff resources, physical plant, and organizational practices and standards than on resident care outcomes. Terms such as *residents, units,* and *services,* rather than *patients, beds,* and *care* are used to describe this long-term care option (Regnier, Hamilton, and Yatabe, 1995; Klaassen, 1994). The private sector is now the predominant provider of assisted care, which is the fastest growing group housing alternative for frail elders and is being lauded as a much less expensive alternative to the nursing home.

The optimism for this alternative form of long-term care is clearly justified. However, it is important to consider some of the individual and societal forces that may cause it to fall short of its lofty expectations. This chapter addresses two concerns: first, that the availability and attributes of these facilities will be inconsistent with the preferences and demands of most consumers; second, that a social model of care cannot be widely achieved in practice.

A Mismatch between Supply and Demand

The initial demand for assisted-living housing has been relatively strong as older persons, family members, and professionals averse to nursing homes look to more homelike and humane facilities to accommodate their higher care needs. States have imposed constraints on nursing home expansion, but state regulations and licensing standards for the assisted-living alternative are relatively limited and uncomplicated and have encouraged its development. Catering primarily to a growing, higher-income, elderly consumer market, assisted-living housing providers have not been hampered by government restrictions on the pricing of their shelter and care products (Hambrook, 1990). As one professional group puts it: "Unlike other long-term care options, appropriate access to supportive service and health care in seniors housing is not determined by government formulas, third-party reimbursement, or federally mandated regulatory requirements" (ASHA, 1994). An increased demand has also been spurred by some state governments, which have subsidized the service costs of this alternative to accommodate poor frail elders who might otherwise have occupied more expensive nursing home beds, paid for by Medicaid.

Although the growth in the availability of assisted-living facilities seems assured, the match between the supply and demand for this alternative may be far from perfect. Housing providers in some markets will overestimate the number of elders in their late 70s and older who will be consumers of their products. This prospect becomes more likely as the number of new players—nursing homes, hotel chains, and large developers—enter the market and substantially increase the supply of this shelter and care alternative (Howell, 1996). This may unfortunately result in some providers of this housing alternative experiencing the same financial downfalls as congregate housing developers did in the 1980s, who also incorrectly read the size and attributes of the elderly consumer market. The following sections elaborate on these concerns.

The Negative Side of Assisted Living

Whatever may be the virtues of the assisted-living facility as a shelter and care environment, most older Americans consider it an unattractive choice, for two reasons: they must relocate from their current housing, and they would be living in age-segregated housing, a social situation having some very strong negative connotations (Golant, 1985, 1995).

THE NEED TO MOVE

Even though older persons often occupy dwellings more compatible with their lifestyles as younger adults, most demonstrate little desire to move (AARP, 1990). Many factors account for this residential inertia, but central is the importance of living in a familiar setting. Older people's sense of competence and control and overall emotional well-being are greatly enhanced when they know their surroundings, can maintain their social relationships and long-established routines and activities, and can keep their valued possessions. Many are unwilling to make environmental changes that require emotionally demanding adaptation. They do not want the stress of learning about a new environment, nor do they not want to confront the potentially humbling experience of educating the occupants of a new setting about "who they are" to gain recognition and acceptance (Golant, 1984, 1997; Lieberman, 1991).

AGE SEGREGATION

While some segments of the older population view senior housing as a way to avoid the youth-oriented society and cultivate satisfying social relationships with their age peers (Golant, 1985), most older Americans (along with their family members) hold decidedly unfavorable views toward planned age-segregated residences. They may take this position for any of the following reasons:

— On reaching old age, they seek to deny their oldness and their membership in the class of the elderly. They display a dissociation pattern of age identification (Rosow, 1967), meaning that they do not want to be identified with the elderly and want to keep a distance between themselves and other older people. Not wanting to admit to their oldness, they look unfavorably on any residential setting identified as a home for the elderly.

— They view elderly housing as a manifestation of an ageist society that deals with its frail and sick old by isolating and segregating them from the young and active populace in a manner reminiscent of the American almshouses or poorhouses of the early twentieth century (Mumford, 1987). Residential enclaves for the old are thus viewed as geriatric ghettos occupied by a culture of powerless persons who have lost their individuality, freedom, and rights.

— They view their age peers who prefer living among others in their age group as warped or deviant, for they consider it normal to live with a mixture of ages (Streib, Folts, and Hilker, 1984).

— They view elderly housing as evidence that American families neglect their elder care responsibilities (Laws, 1993).

— They claim that elderly housing unfairly and unnecessarily draws public attention to an unrepresentative group of elderly citizens, those who are physically and mentally frail. As such, these alternatives reinforce the "misperception of the old as a problem group" and stigmatize rather than liberate older people from the negative effects of being labeled old (Neugarten, 1982:27).

— They view older persons living in elderly housing as a privileged group who have received more than their fair share of societal resources at the expense of more needy groups. As occupants of segregated housing, they are construed as powerful voting concentrations that discriminate against the young (Thurow, 1996).

— They view shelter arrangements designed exclusively for low-income seniors as evidence of unwarranted age discrimination, because these accommodations deny younger populations—such as families with children and young disabled persons—similar rights of occupancy.

CONSUMER CONFUSION

When a housing product has such negative connotations, developers and providers must make a special effort to overcome poor consumer awareness and inaccurate product identity (Gold, 1996). While marketing efforts have improved (Campbell, 1996), a 1995 national survey suggests that most Americans still have an incomplete understanding of this alternative (Harvard School of Public Health, 1996). It reports that among Americans aged 50 and older most at risk of needing long-term care services, 77 percent are familiar with nursing homes but only 47 percent are familiar with assisted living. This latter figure, moreover, may be deceptively high, given that many of the respondents undoubtedly held ambiguous and discrepant views about assisted living. Also, they had not planned for their future long-term care needs, with about 80 percent having never discussed the possibility of their living in a senior housing facility with a family member or a friend. The dominant impression is of a marketplace that is still relatively poorly educated about what assisted living is and its role in the long-term care system.

Such survey results, however, may confuse more than they clarify, because they imply that frail elders themselves are mainly responsible for selecting this residential option. In fact, those making or steering the residential decision are often family members or professionals. In a national survey of how occupants of assisted living learned of their present residence, 14 percent had received their information from other facility residents, 25 percent had been referred by family members, and 61 percent had been referred by physicians, hospitals, area agencies on aging, nursing homes, home health agencies, churches, and related sources (Coopers & Lybrand, 1993). Some housing providers are aware of this market reality; one of the largest for-profit assisted-living chains in the United States specifically targets the children of frail elders when marketing their facilities, recognizing that "few seniors admit themselves to personal-care facilities" (Regnier, Hamilton, and Yatabe, 1995:209).

That professionals function as the key decision makers is not surprising. A supportive shelter and care setting must often be arranged quickly, often after a hospital discharge or a home accident (Maloney, Finn, and Patterson, 1996). While professionals are now more cognizant of assisted-living facilities, "nursing homes are viewed by many as the only option for long-term care" (21). Two factors are central: first, the nursing home is viewed as the long-term care environment most likely to offer the comprehensive care needed by many hospital-discharged elders; second, hospitals often have strong organizational linkages with nursing homes either through ownership or management relationships or because health care insurance plans specify qualified potential sites of posthospital care (Kane, 1995–96). The role played by professionals and organizations as decision makers is crucial for understanding the future demand for this alternative, because it undermines the view that the increased interest in assisted living is primarily a "consumer-driven" phenomenon (Gold, 1996).

A CONFUSING PRODUCT LINE

When deciding on the feasibility of the assisted-living option, elderly consumers and their advisers confront two difficult tasks. The first is to discern the severity of physical and mental impairments that are accepted and tolerated by a facility. The second is to judge the quality of its shelter accommodations and services. Poor product definition has hindered these assessments. Housing alternatives that claim to be assisted living are now identified by many different labels. They present very different physical or architectural styles, offer varied types and levels of care and service, and use different organizational strategies to deliver their care. Professionals and advocates, for their part, do not speak consistently about what they mean by the assisted-living option. Even among the scientific and research community, studies of assisted living do more to confuse than to clarify (Hawes, Mor, and Wildfire, 1995). Nor does the future appear hopeful. According to one knowledgeable provider, "by the end of the 90s, we will see at least

30 different, well-established flavors of assisted living" (Klaassen, 1994:23). Although more choices often benefit consumers, they pay a price for this diversity, especially given their limited experience with such search and evaluation tasks. Consequently, there is so much variability in this product and so many instances of poor or inadequate quality, that the public not only is confused as to what assisted living should be (the ideal model) but also is likely to hold some very negative images about this housing product (Can your loved ones avoid a nursing home? 1995).

The absence of a standardized housing product impacts housing providers and sponsors in three ways: it reduces the potential size of their consumer base; it makes their marketing efforts more difficult and expensive; and it threatens the backing of lenders and investors who seek certainty and clarity in the products they finance (Campbell, 1996). Recognizing the importance of a standardized product, several senior citizen organizations have attempted to draft voluntary national guidelines to establish uniform quality standards. It is unclear, however, whether state governments will follow the lead of these groups. At least as of this date, these organizations could not agree among themselves (Newsfronts, 1996).

A VARIETY OF STATE REGULATIONS

The multiple identities assumed by assisted-living facilities throughout the country largely results from the strong and idiosyncratic influence that state governments have had on their development and operation. With little influence from the federal government, today's assisted-living facilities reflect their state's long-term care philosophy and regulatory practices (Mollica et al., 1995).

States differ most fundamentally in level of client impairment (that is, limitations in activities of daily living, medical and cognitive needs, and nursing supervisory demands) and in the types and duration of personal assistance and skilled nursing services allowed. Regulations in some states dictate detailed lists of health and care conditions that their assisted-living facilities can accommodate, and these standards may be different for entry into the facility and for staying on in the facility. Some states have flexible interpretations of a resident's frailty and allow their assisted-living facilities to provide a level of skilled care compatible with the traditional intermediate-care facility nursing home standard (Mollica et al., 1995). These legislative responses help account for the wide variations in admission and retention policies among states and the extent to which their assisted-living facilities offer care comparable to that found in their nursing homes.

State regulations identify who can administer nursing-related services such as catheterization, ostomy care, preparation of food and tube feedings, care of skin wounds, and oxygen administration. Through their nurse practice statutes and regulations, states differently allow licensed health personnel, such as registered nurses and licensed practitioner nurses, to delegate such services to unlicensed staff, such as nurses aides or certified nurses assistants. They also differ as to the types of care setting in which they allow nurse delegation (Kane, O'Connor, and Baker, 1995). Oregon's Nurse Practice Act is notable, for example, because nurses are allowed "to delegate nursing functions to another person if the nurse is convinced that the non-nurse can appropriately perform the function" (Fralich et al., 1995:24). Because a facility's overall service costs are so tied to the costs of performing nursing services, assisted-living facilities that can delegate nursing responsibilities to lesser qualified personnel have lower operating costs even as they serve a more frail group of occupants (Kane, O'Connor, and Baker, 1995). Consumers, for their part, must consider whether such practices jeopardize their quality of care and whether these risks outweigh the advantages of their less expensive accommodations.

States also do not have the same physical plant requirements. For example, they differently require housing providers to offer single-occupancy as opposed to shared bedroom units, unit-specific bathing facilities as opposed to shared bathroom and bathing facilities, and residential units with their own kitchenettes or with equipment for preparing and storing food (Mollica et al., 1995). These differences have special significance, because many proponents of assisted living consider the presence or absence of these physical features the basis for differentiating their product from other elderly housing options. For example, some argue that assisted-living facilities purporting to offer a social model of care should contain single-occupancy apartments and private bathroom and kitchen areas, to distinguish them from board-and-care facilities. In practice, group housing accommodations identified as assisted living may not offer these features.

For older persons with dementia, states specifically differ as to their tenant, service, supervisory, physical plant, and staffing requirements. For example, they differently allow their assisted-living facilities to accommodate confused residents (who cannot make their needs known), to permit providers to create secured units for people with dementia in settings with distinctive physical design attributes (e.g., color-coded walls, wandering paths, special alarm systems, orientation cues), and to have specially trained staff, specially programmed activities, and behavior modification strategies. State policy on this issue is obviously of major importance, given the strong latent demand for these facilities by cognitively impaired older persons (Mollica et al., 1995).

ASSISTED LIVING: A SERVICE OR A HOUSING ALTERNATIVE?

States fundamentally differ as to whether they conceive of assisted living as a set of delivered services or as a housing option with distinguishable physical infrastructure and permanent and planned in-house service programs. States taking the former view would include under the rubric of assisted living group housing that caters to more independent elderly tenants—such as, congregate housing apartments, rental retirement buildings, and board-and-care facilities—if tenants or management subcontract with an outside home care agency or community organization to deliver personal care or skilled nursing services (Mollica et al., 1995). In some instances, the home care agency itself may be physically located on the housing site.

Viewing assisted living as strictly a service alternative has several major advantages: housing operators can avoid the financial, administrative, and legal obligations and problems that accompany provision of personal care and on-site nursing services; state governments can avoid complex administrative decisions and restrict their licensing and regulatory requirements to the service provider; housing providers can obtain nursing care for their tenants without having to satisfy the licensure requirements of dedicated assisted-living facilities; and tenants who might otherwise be forced to relocate to a more institutional setting can be cared for in place.

There are, however, several potential downsides of the service alternative. Older persons (or their advisers) making the residential care decision must decide on whether this stripped-down version of assisted living offers the appropriate level of shelter and care. While there are no absolutes in this evaluation, several of the following consequences of this long-term care approach may conflict with the basic ideals of the assisted-living social model (Golant, 1995):

— Older residents may have difficulty availing themselves of unscheduled staff assistance and care because the service agency allocates only fixed and limited staff resources to the project.
— The shelter arrangement may lack the social programs, staffing, and physical design features consistent with the needs of frailer older persons, especially those with cognitive impairments as presented by Alzheimer's disease.
— The housing provider assumes a more passive administrative role because much of the care responsibility has shifted to the service provider; thus the philosophy of care reflects that of the service provider, who conceivably may subscribe to a medical model.
— The legal or ethical responsibility of the housing provider for the well-being and occupancy rights of the older occupants receiving the outside care inevitably becomes ambiguous.
— No single provider assumes total responsibility for the quality of life and quality of care of the older resident.
— Older persons may have less say over their plan of care because the service agency is accountable to government or proprietary guidelines.
— Decisions about moving to a higher level of care (such as a nursing home) may be influenced more by the service subcontractor than by the housing provider.
— In-home service delivery may be more expensive than service delivery in a dedicated assisted-living facility because it does not benefit from the economies of scale realized by caring for larger subgroups of older persons with similar service and care needs.

More generally, the idea of assisted living qua delivered services may so dilute the concept of assisted living as to make it a meaningless distinction. If assisted living is merely a service delivery strategy, are there any shelter and care arrangements that could potentially be precluded from being labeled as assisted living?

Home: The Major Competition

However unambiguously packaged and marketed the assisted-living product, it faces formidable competition from an alternative that has tremendous appeal to older Americans. Most elders cope with their physical or mental disabilities and chronic medical conditions in their conventional dwellings. They apparently find that the downsides of aging in place are more than outweighed by its advantages. Along with the disadvantages of moving, staying put is associated with having control over how and when personal care is delivered and avoiding the perceived negatives of living in any kind of living arrangement in which there are administrative controls. It is also linked to a desire (however poorly it might be articulated) to remain a "whole person" (Golant, 1984). People have complex histories, lifestyles, and social relationships. They are averse to being thrust into a residential setting in which they are simply thought of as tenants, patients, or boarders by a staff that fails to recognize their existence as persons with rich, interesting, and diverse past lives. While assisted-living facilities are ideally less guilty of superficially segmenting or homogenizing their occupants in this way, the perceived risk persists.

The propensity of frail older persons to stay put not only reduces the overall demand for assisted living, it also increases the likelihood that by the time older persons decide that they cannot cope with their physical and mental impairments, they are of such severity as to require them to seek the level of care traditionally found in the nursing home (Golant, 1992). The result is that some assisted-living facilities will miss an important market segment if they cannot accommodate a population with higher dependency levels.

HOME CARE

Even as group shelter and care alternatives for less dependent elders have become more available and increasingly attractive, it is more feasible than ever to stay put. The caregiving role of the American family—in particular, spouses and daughters—has been central. About 75 percent of the U.S. elderly population with disabilities depends exclusively on such caregiving, while 90 percent rely at least in part on this informal assistance. These percentages may even be higher in the future, given the increased representation of Hispanic, African American, and Asian groups among the elderly population and their greater propensity than white elders to deal with their frailties in a family setting (Golant, 1992).

As much care may be provided in the home as in a nursing facility. If costs are not prohibitive, there are few disabilities, chronic and postacute care conditions, problem behaviors, or nursing needs that cannot be managed. A wide array of preventive, diagnostic, therapeutic, rehabilitative, and long-term maintenance services—from washing dishes to intravenous therapy and chemotherapy—can be delivered in the home (Freeman, 1995). Most technological and biomedical equipment is sufficiently small or portable to be used in the home. For-profit and not-for-profit home- and community-based care providers are more available than ever thanks to national and state policies that have created strong economic incentives for serving the elder market. The 1980s expansion of Medicare benefits through the easing of payment and certification restrictions and the expanded Medicaid waiver coverage of home services to poor elders are examples (Kane, 1995). These policies have helped make home health care not only the fastest growing segment of health care services but also price competitive with other long-term care alternatives (Wright, 1996).

Any trends that portend a decline in the availability of informal caregivers would have important ramifications for the ability of older persons to stay in their own homes and thus would change their receptiveness to alternatives such as assisted living. It is well established, for example, that elderly individuals without kin are more likely to be institutionalized (Coughlin, McBride, and Liu, 1990). Several researchers predict that when the baby boomers reach old age they will have weaker family supports because of their higher early divorce rates and their lower birth rates than previous elderly generations. Although these may be valid fears, the current population reaching old age is made up of parents of the baby boom generation, "a group for whom childbearing was nearly universal and most families had more than one child" (Himes, 1992:S24). At least until the second decade of the twenty-first century, then, "those married with children and those unmarried with children, contain the majority of the populations and [will] increase in their share over time." Other trends, on the other hand, could counter these expectations, albeit less dramatically: the increased demands on women caregivers because of employment responsibilities and their own childrearing responsibilities, and greater geographic distances separating older persons and their family members. In the main, however, the demographics of family care do not suggest that the conventional home will, any time soon, become a less attractive setting to deliver care.

HOMEOWNERSHIP

As of 1991, a historically high 81 percent of aged 65–74 householders (heads of households) and 67 percent of 85 and older householders owned their homes. Among householders aged 55–64, the next population cohort that will enter old age, 80 percent were homeowners (Naifeh, 1993). Homeowners, in particular, have strong economic incentives to deal with their frailties in their current residences. The majority (82%) have paid off their mortgages, and their median monthly costs are only $217, representing about 29 percent of their monthly income. Among those still holding mortgages, median costs are still a relatively low $549 (U.S. Bureau of the Census, 1996). Because comparable rental units are likely to be more expensive and their current homes are still appreciating in value and are earmarked for their heirs, most older persons do not believe that they are incurring large opportunity costs by not selling their home and reinvesting its proceeds. (In 1993, the home equity of elderly homeowners aged 75 and older averaged about $83,000.) Homeowners may also perceive the costs of moving as too high relative to the shelter cost savings or benefits they would realize over their remaining lifetime (Golant, 1996; Venti and Wise, 1989). These economic considerations are apparently not counteracted by the slow-rising home prices in most markets or by the moving incentive of the capital gains tax exclusion (since May 1997, it is $250,000 for individuals and $500,000 for married couples filing joint tax returns).

Older persons also do not have to move in order to realize cash equivalents for the single largest component of their wealth. When in need of financial assistance, they can realize much of the equity in their dwellings by relying on such conventional financial instruments as second mortgages, home equity loans, or home equity line of credit loans (Hobbs, Keest, and DeWaal, 1989). While these are available to income-qualified homeowners of all ages, older persons, irrespective of their incomes, can obtain reverse mortgages marketed especially to them (Pynoos and Golant, 1996).

Older homeowners' incentive to remain in their homes is further strengthened by several public policies. Private sector offerings of reverse mortgages are encouraged by the availability of federal insurance. Older homeowners financially stressed by the cost of maintaining their homes can turn to various federal and state programs such as state-administered property tax relief and federally subsidized home repair and home energy subsidies and grants. Most need-based government programs also do not count housing wealth as a criterion for eligibility for their benefits. This is true for the Supplemental Security Income (SSI) and food stamp programs. Various home- and community-based services such as senior centers, congregate and home-delivered meals, home chore services, and home energy subsidies also are available to older homeowners irrespective of their housing wealth. The Medicaid program's asset eligibility requirements for nursing home care or for home-based services also do not count the owned home. While states are now mandated to seek recovery from the estates of a broad class of individuals who have received Medicaid reimbursements, compliance with this federal regulation still varies greatly by state.

The Cost of Assisted Living

The relatively high price consumers must pay for assisted-living accommodations considerably narrows its market appeal. Minimum monthly costs are usually more than $800 and generally average between $1,500 to $2,000 (Coopers & Lybrand, 1993). Accessing assisted-living facilities found in continuing care retirement communities additionally requires upfront minimum average entry fees of more than $22,000 (Ernst & Young, 1993). None of these costs is usually covered by private insurance or government programs. Assuming a ratio of 40 percent housing cost to consumer income, these monthly costs for an efficiency unit would by one estimate require an annual income of close to $25,000 (Newman, 1993). This may understate the real cost of occupancy to the extent that residents are charged extra (on a fee-for-service basis) for certain residential services and personal care. Wright (1996) estimates that at most only 10 percent of the total aged 75 and older population can afford assisted living and that less than 15 percent of this group are likely to seek these accommodations. Demand is also sensitive to housing prices, because the affordability of the assisted-living option may depend on prospective older consumers selling their homes. Many proponents fear that the costs of assisted living will become even higher—and the demand lower—if states impose more stringent regulatory standards requiring expensive physical plant changes or staff additions.

The market for assisted living would be greatly expanded if states made this option affordable to their poor frail elderly constituencies. In most states, the poor frail elderly without family supports are accommodated in nursing homes, board-and-care facilities, or their own homes with services funded under the Medicaid waiver program. A growing number of states have made assisted-living facilities accessible to their poor frail elders by subsidizing their service component through the use of Medicaid waivers or by offering supplements to Supplemental Security Income (Mollica et al., 1995). Whether this trend will continue is uncertain, given the prospects that Medicaid funds will become even less available, especially if they are administered as a state block grant program. Even if government subsidies can make assisted living affordable to low-income elders, the caps placed on these reimbursements may result in their occupying poorer quality accommodations than private paying residents occupy.

Unfortunately, double standards for the rich and the poor have already emerged. To accommodate low-income elders in assisted-living facilities and at the same time ensure that sufficient rental income is generated, government agencies often require low-income frail elders to share their residential units (Regnier, Hamilton, and Yatabe, 1995). (It is noteworthy that in one such instance there is still a one-year waiting list.) As another example, Sunrise Assisted Living, one of the largest chains of assisted-living facilities in the country that cater to the middle- and high-income frail elderly, accommodates select numbers of low-income residents—but primarily in double-occupancy units. The obvious question is, How many of the principals of the ideal social model of assisted living can be sacrificed without unduly destroying the worthiness of this alternative?

Assisted Living as a Substitute for Nursing Homes

If assisted-living providers could tap into the group of frail elderly consumers now served by nursing homes, they could increase their potential market share. Recent research findings are promising. One study conservatively estimates that approximately 15 percent of nursing home residents could be accommodated in lower levels of care because they need help with less than three activities of daily living, were continent, did not have substantial rehabilitation or medical needs, and did not exhibit serious behavior problems (Spector, Reschovsky, and Cohen, 1996). Comparable earlier estimates are 20–33 percent (Coopers & Lybrand, 1993).

Increasingly, at least since the early 1980s, nursing homes have served sicker and more frail older persons, while other shelter and care facilities have increasingly accommodated those dependent seniors not requiring skilled nursing care or unscheduled around-the-clock assistance (Spector, Reschovsky, and Cohen, 1996). This trend reflects an elderly population with more of the very old and changes in federal and state health care policies. Medicare's specification of diagnosis-related groups (DRGs) soon resulted in patients being discharged from hospitals "quicker and sicker." Afterward, many state Medicaid programs shifted from a flat-rate to a case-mix reimbursement strategy, offering nursing homes an incentive to provide higher-profit-margin and more complex services to elders needing subacute care and intensive rehabilitation on an inpatient basis, once the preserve of hospitals (ASHA, 1994; Price, 1996; Wiener and Skaggs, 1995). (Under flat-rate reimbursement, nursing homes were motivated to serve older persons with lighter care needs.)

This new focus also allowed nursing homes to become major participants in the Medicare (Part A) program, whereby they are reimbursed for post-hospital rehabilitation and subacute care of up to a hundred days. Third-party payers (insurance companies, health maintenance organizations, preferred provider organizations), in turn, fueled demand by having nursing homes perform these subacute and rehabilitative services at much lower costs than those charged by hospitals (ASHA, 1994; Fralich et al., 1995; Kane, 1995). Together, these policies also strengthened the nursing home referral links between hospitals and physicians. Nursing homes also began to offer specialized programming for residents with dementia in special care units "to identify a special service technology to merit a higher reimbursement under case-mix reimbursement schemes, which otherwise favored skilled nursing treatment" (Mor, Banaszak-Holl, and Zinn, 1995–96:25). The profiles of nursing home residents as more frail also resulted from other efforts by states to control their Medicaid budgets. These included more stringent preadmission screening and eligibility criteria and a greater reliance on case-managed home care.

Other policies are being implemented that are likely to ensure the continuation of this trend. There are continuing federal government efforts to curb the abuses by higher-income elders who become eligible for Medicaid nursing home beds by spending down their assets through creative accounting methods that often benefit their heirs (Moses, 1995). States are also strengthening and more rigorously enforcing their lien and estate recovery programs. By seniors (and their heirs) assuming more responsibility for the costs of long-term care, it is expected that they will be more highly motivated to look to less expensive shelter and care alternatives such as assisted living, if they do not require highly skilled nursing care.

INCREASED DEMAND

Assisted-living facilities in some states may have more difficulty than others in capturing the market of the impaired elderly. First, old habits die hard, and many health care professionals are reluctant to embrace the assisted-living alternative. Second, given that most assisted-living facilities are not government subsidized, it is unclear what percentage of this diverted nursing home population would find the assisted-living alternative affordable, even assuming liquid house assets and the possibility that the extended family will have economic incentives to bear the costs of long-term care. Third, in some states, a strong nursing home lobby will effectively stall if not prevent the assisted-living industry from encroaching on their market. Fourth, there is a danger of misrepresenting the realities of the nursing home market. Evidence comes from studies focusing specifically on the demand and occupancy patterns of nursing homes in rural areas. Coward, Horne, and Peek (1995) find that elders coping with urinary incontinence in sparsely populated and remote rural communities are more likely than their urban and suburban counterparts to enter a nursing home. They suggest that nursing homes may be overutilized in locations in which other long-term care alternatives (such as home health services and assisted-living facilities) are either costly, difficult to access, or unavailable. Alternatively, the organizational linkages between hospitals and nursing homes may be stronger in rural areas; physicians, for example, may refer their patients to nursing homes out of ignorance or because they do not perceive any other option. Yet another interpretation is that older people in some rural areas hold more favorable attitudes toward the nursing home and view it as a community resource (Rowles, Concotelli, and High, 1996).

THE FRAIL ELDERLY

Even assuming that elderly persons diverted from nursing homes would seek out assisted living, it is unclear whether most assisted-living facilities could accommodate consumers with heavy care needs. Some facilities would be thwarted by regulatory constraints, some would have inadequate staff or equipment, and others would have difficulty maintaining adequate economic returns given their higher operating costs, their need for additional capital expenditures, and their reduced monthly rent inflows and increased marketing costs resulting from their higher turnover rates.

One less-than-perfect measure of the extent that assisted-living facilities are currently accommodating very frail residents is offered by data on resident turnover and discharge patterns of assisted-living facilities in Oregon, which has more liberal skilled nursing care provisions and flexible nurse delegation statutes than the national average. Oregon's resident turnover rate (the average number of residents that annually depart from a facility) averaged 38 percent, compared with 34 percent nationally. In Oregon, residents were discharged for the following reasons: death, 35 percent; going into a nursing home, 20 percent; going into a hospital, 10 percent; going home, 15 percent; going to other supportive settings, 20 percent (Kane and Wilson, 1993). Nationally, the reasons were death, 24 percent; nursing homes, 46 percent; hospitals, 12 percent; own homes, 6 percent; other supportive housing, 12 percent (Coopers & Lybrand, 1993). Yet another national survey showed that 50 percent of the turnover in assisted-living residences was a result of residents needing more care (ASHA, 1995).

Two conclusions can be drawn. First, compared to assisted-living facilities nationwide, Oregon's assisted-living facilities are now caring for a more dependent population, as indicated by their higher turnover rate, higher death rate, and lower nursing home discharge rate. Second, even in Oregon, where state regulations allow assisted-living facilities to accommodate residents with greater nursing needs, a significant percentage inevitably require the care offered in skilled nursing homes. These conclusions warn against professionals and advocates overselling the assisted-living concept as a substitute for nursing homes. Clearly, in many states, assisted living will function only as a temporary solution. On the other hand, the Oregon statistics demonstrate the nationwide potential for larger numbers of frail residents opting for assisted living.

These findings also suggest that the assisted-living model might be inappropriate for certain older groups. Elderly persons with degenerative mental or physical conditions, for example, while initially accommodated by an assisted-living facility, may soon require full-time and unscheduled skilled nursing care. Nursing home placement might be preferable for this group if only to avoid a stressful move shortly after moving to an assisted-living facility (Golant, 1997). "Once the elderly have given up their traditional home and moved to a more supportive living environment, their fondest hope is not to move again" (D'Angelo (1996:29). Elderly persons might also benefit from a nursing home stay if they require only a short-term and protective environment that specializes in health monitoring, convalescent care, and rehabilitation, after which they can return to their homes (Kane, 1995–96).

The Social Model of Care: Can It Be Achieved in Practice?

Safety and Quality of Care versus Quality of Life

The social model of care envisioned by advocates of assisted living stands in sharp relief to the medical model practiced in most nursing homes (Baggett, 1989; Mor, Sherwood, and Gutkin, 1986). The medical model assumes that vulnerable clients "must be controlled and tightly regulated with the threat of punitive force" (Collopy, 1995:65) and that care must be provided in a setting that conforms to the building codes of a health care facility. Failing such standards, the occupants are exposed to an intolerable risk of incompetent care and harm. Such a philosophy of care necessarily demands the micromanagement of providers to ensure ethically correct practices by "setting eligibility standards, monitoring everything from medical equipment and personal care to safety, cleanliness, and other physical aspects of the care setting" (65).

Supporters of the medical, or nursing home, model argue that there is a resident vulnerability threshold above which the physical plant, staffing patterns, and heavily regulated environment of the nursing home become necessary. They express reservations about whether assisted-living facilities can accommodate physically and mentally frail older persons and still subscribe to the tenets of a social model of care. They further suggest that dependent older residents who benefit from the services and social surroundings of supportive group housing must inevitably sacrifice some rights and individual freedoms (Parmelee and Lawton, 1990).

They question whether assisted-living providers can deal with a very frail population's complex health care needs, including their use of medications, the management of their chronic physical conditions, the detection of threatening medical conditions, and the diagnosis and treatment of depression and other cognitive disorders. They argue that the quality of care has improved in nursing homes only because of increased regulations and point to the frequently reported resident abuses (for example, the improper dispensing of prescriptions) in less-regulated long-term care settings such as board-and-care facilities (U.S. General Accounting Office, 1989). They also refer to the recent example of alleged violations found by Maryland's Department of Health and Mental Hygiene in a facility owned by one of the country's largest assisted-living facility chains. These include their failure to investigate suspicious bruises and to properly administer medications and follow proper food serving procedures and residents' weight loss and other health problems (*Housing the Elderly Report*, 1996).

Moreover, they recommend that nursing homes could benefit from still more regulation because of their currently deficient staffing standards. They refer to studies showing that nursing homes have "insufficient numbers of nursing aides to provide the hands-on care as well as too few geriatrically prepared professional nurses to supervise care and provide leadership and guidance to staff" and that many lack a 24-hour, on-site, registered nurse (Maas, Buckwalter, and Specht, 1996:393). They point to evaluations that conclude that nursing homes have inadequate mental health professionals and services even with their high concentration of residents with cognitive and affective disorders (Golant, 1998; Lombardo, 1994). They emphasize that, in nursing homes with these inadequate staffing patterns, the residents have experienced high rates of medication errors, falls, hospitalization, and poor eating behaviors.

Proponents of a social model of care respond that an overly protective, supportive, and hospital-like environment produces a number of negative personal consequences. Residents have poor morale because their individual care needs are ignored, their privacy rights are violated, their activities are unnecessarily restricted, and they are often unable to fully exercise their existing functional abilities (Krause, 1987). Lawton (1985:459), for example, argues that the "environmental demands on the more competent may become reduced to the point where their skills are not sufficiently exercised." Langer (1983:285) similarly argues that "simply helping people may make them incompetent. While meaning well, it communicates to the person that he or she is not able to do whatever it is for him- or herself . . . [resulting] in feelings of incompetence and dependence." Proponents further point out that resident abuses have continued in nursing homes despite their being heavily regulated and that the staff in these facilities often neglect the emotional and social well-being of their residents.

Advocates of assisted living argue that, in return for a more normal housing environment, residents and their family members must assume greater responsibilities and risks. If residents are to maintain their dignity and personal freedom, they must be prepared to be monitored less intensively than residents in a nursing home and assume greater responsibility for their own care. Thus, it is unfair to evaluate assisted-living facilities using the same regulatory guidelines applied to nursing homes. As articulated by an Oregon administrator: "Safety is the most important value for regulators. It's the quality of life that should count most, not safety. In pursuing quality of life, I'm willing to take a lot of risk" (Mollica et al., 1992:19). Or as another expert puts it: "To achieve success, it will be necessary to set aside professional orthodoxy and the urge to provide complete protection for people with disabilities who come into our care" (Kane, 1995–96:68).

Increasing risk for the sake of improving individual freedom and morale, however, creates an ethical dilemma for providers whose background and experiences have been in the health care professions. As Colopy (1995:61) summarizes it:

> In a health care system that has traditionally made safety a hierarchy among values, how can providers recognize risk taking as a normal element in adult life, an inalienable part of being autonomous, even when one is elderly and frail? What boundaries—or better, what tolerances—should long-term care develop for the "behavioral outliers," for individuals who are sharply singular or eccentric, who persistently breach social decorum and convention? How should providers balance the right of elderly individuals to take risks with their own obligations to protect these individuals from harm—and from harming others? How should they weigh an individual's autonomy against the common good of the institutional or local community?

Not all experts, however, agree that taking a simple position on these issues is especially productive. Kane and Kane (1989:67) argue that the debate between the relative desirability of the social versus the medical model is spurious, just as is the false dichotomy between quality of life and quality of care. One necessarily follows the other. In their words, "If the quality of healthcare—either preventive, diagnostic, or therapeutic—is substandard, the effect on the client's overall well-being—that is quality of life—can be profound. Adequate healthcare leading to expected outcomes is a necessary aspect of quality of life. Too often, a salutary emphasis on psychological and social well-being is paired with a harmful de-emphasis on the importance of healthcare."

In searching for some middle ground between these positions, some state governments seeking flexible but effective ways to regulate their assisted-living facilities are embracing the idea of managed risk. This involves "negotiating an acceptable risk level between the resident and provider as a way to solve problems and to recognize individual preferences" (Gulyas, 1995:4). Managed risk requires that frail elderly residents and their family members (or legal guardians) participate to a much greater extent in decisions regarding how much and what types of care and supervision they want from a facility, how much flexibility the facility will have in implementing such a care plan, and how much input residents (and family members) will have in modifying these care and supervision practices. In the instance of bathing, for example, under what circumstances can the resident choose to bathe without staff present despite the increased risks of an accident?

Adopting such a management philosophy places new responsibilities on both housing providers and older residents (and their caregivers). Housing providers must identify the risks of not carrying out certain care or supervisory activities and the strategies that residents must follow to mitigate these risks. They must carefully communicate the possible consequences of selected care options and anticipate the varied consequences of alternative responses. Residents and their family members must decide on what care and supervision practices they are willing to forgo in return for greater resident autonomy and quality of life (Wilson, 1990; Mollika et al., 1995). Furthermore, they must subscribe to the principal—whether implied or contractual—that the facility will not be held liable for injuries resulting from this negotiated risk agreement (Magan, 1996).

In theory, a managed risk organizational style offers older persons a more humane living environment, in which they have more control over their everyday life and activities. It is unclear, however, whether housing providers are administratively willing or capable of entering into these negotiations and whether older persons and their family members are sophisticated, educated, and motivated enough to assume the risks and responsibilities inherent in this contractual relationship. Various obstacles exist. It may be unrealistic, for example, to expect older residents themselves to participate in the decision-making process if they are cognitively impaired, suffering from affective disorders, poorly educated, risk averse, or afraid of reprisals from staff or providers. It is estimated, for example, that an average of 42 percent of assisted-living residents in this country suffer from some type of cognitive impairment (Coopers & Lybrand, 1993). Many family members will also have difficulty with these negotiations. The very reason that they resigned themselves to placing their older family member in an assisted-living facility was because they felt incapable (either because they were emotionally stressed or lacked care expertise) to continue to make caregiving decisions (Yee, Capitman, and Sciegai, 1993). Older persons without a family member acting on their behalf will have the additional difficulty of selecting a caring and thoughtful surrogate decision maker who might eventually have to act in the resident's best interests. Housing providers for their part may view such agreements as excessively complex (except in very small projects), cumbersome to administer, and opening them up to liability claims. These legal uncertainties may also deter the participation of appointed guardians or case managers.

The Social Well-Being of Assisted-Living Residents

Residents in assisted-living facilities, benefiting from a less structured environment and more autonomy, are believed to enjoy warmer and closer interpersonal relations than residents in nursing homes (Timko and Moos, 1991). It is thus paradoxical that this more favorable social and recreational environment may be threatened in those assisted-living facilities that, true to a social model of care, allow their residents to age in place even as they experience declines in their physical and cognitive abilities. In such settings, there is a concern that the quality of life of the less frail residents will deteriorate as a result of their having to interact daily with age peers more vulnerable than themselves. Thus, the issue arises of whether it is more desirable to physically separate the residential accommodations and common (activity) areas (e.g., dining rooms) of elders with different levels of impairment—or even to demand that the more frail residents depart from the facility.

Many operators fear that if they deny an admission or seek a discharge based on physical disability or if they segregate residents by care level, they will be guilty of violating the Fair Housing Amendments Act of 1988 (FHAA) (Gamzon, 1995). The act, which applies to programs offering long-term lodging, was amended to prevent discrimination against persons with disabilities (and families with children). FHAA requires housing providers to make reasonable modifications and accommodations to disabled persons upon request (Edelstein, 1995).

Yet there is considerable evidence suggesting that older persons do not enjoy sharing space with those more frail than themselves, especially when these disabilities are overt, apparent, irreversible, and affect the image of the facility (Golant, 1992). Their emotional well-being suffers because they are continually reminded of their own vulnerability, even as they seek to delay this reality. One study of four nursing homes shows, for example, that cognitively intact elderly persons expressed considerable dissatisfaction with sharing either their private or public spaces (common areas) with cognitively impaired persons. The study found a "significant trend for 'excess' depression/demoralization related to dissatisfaction with the environment due to commingling with the cognitively and/or behaviorally impaired" (Teresi, Holmes, and Monaco, 1993:357). In such mixed social situations, the more independent residents may actively discriminate against their frail neighbors by either avoidance or open hostility. The more frail residents in turn may be reluctant to initiate social relationships with those more independent than themselves (Hooyman and Lustbader, 1986; Sheehan, 1992).

Facilities that attempt to serve without differentiation a broad mix of both more active and more frail residents are criticized for other reasons. Very frail residents may enjoy less appropriate leisure and recreational events because a facility's organized activities are geared to the more independent residents. Unable to live up to the more active norms of activity, they feel a strong sense of discomfort (Gubrium, 1973). These more vulnerable older persons "may experience the negative effects of a too-demanding environment, with reductions in their self-initiated activity to below the level found for similarly impaired residents in less demanding environments" (Lemke and Moos, 1989:S146). Conversely, more competent or "high functioning residents [will be] more active in settings where other residents are active, functionally able, and have more social resources and where autonomy is greater" (S146). Problems have also arisen when an assisted-living facility attempts to accommodate both younger and older frail residents. Older persons have suffered both physical and mental abuse as a result of sharing their living situations with young mentally impaired residents (Golant, 1995).

While many studies have reached similar conclusions, not all research agrees (Levesque, Cossette, and Potvin, 1993). Housing providers themselves differ. Some argue that mixing primarily creates problems because of public sexuality displays (Keren Brown Wilson, April 1996, personal communication). Others argue that the social and care advantages of having a separate floor increase when residents have discernible dementia problems, "with wandering behavior that compromises safely, disruptive dining behavior, conversation difficulties, and abusive or violent outbursts" (Regnier, Hamilton, and Yatabe, 1995:213). On the other hand, in at least one assisted-living facility, residents themselves view the segregation of residents by frailty in the dining room areas as unnecessary (Regnier, Hamilton, and Yatabe, 1995). Moreover, some providers argue that segregating all residents with dementia—irrespective of its stage—may exacerbate the course of the disease for persons with early-stage Alzheimer's. They suggest that the less confused residents—who might otherwise be with cognitively intact residents—imitate the behavior of the more confused (Mollika et al., 1995).

Defenders of the rights of both young and old cognitively impaired persons argue for their right to live in a normal setting where they will benefit from the role models of alert residents and that elderly residents' behavior can be modified by teaching them to tolerate and understand the needs and problems of confused residents (Levesque, Cossette, and Potvin, 1993). They further argue that the introduction of appropriate mental health services into projects containing the cognitively impaired will alleviate the tensions and increase the cooperation between the two groups (U.S. General Accounting Office, 1992).

Most social and psychological theory questions the utility of such mixed living arrangements. Bowker (1982) argues that the integration of demented residents with nondemented residents creates a dehumanized environment. Social exchange theory predicts that more frequent and successful social relationships occur among persons with homogeneous social and psychological attributes (Blau, 1964; Keith, 1980), because they allow for a relatively equal flow of support between persons with mutual needs and interests (Rook, 1987). Age identification theory suggests that many older persons avoid exchanges that force them to deal with the prospects of their vulnerability and that threaten their self-concept (Rosow, 1967). And human stress theory (Lazarus and Folkman, 1984) suggests that "the presence of demented peers can be seen as a potential stressor for alert residents, with the resulting disturbance and negative emotional reactions" (Levesque, Cossette, and Potvin, 1993:521). Finally, the presence of disabled persons—whether young or old—appears inconsistent with older residents' sense of social community (McMillan and Chavis, 1986).

The Medicalization of Assisted-Living Facilities

Even as the social model of care is central to ideal portrayals of the assisted-living facility, "an alarming number of newly constructed for-profit and nonprofit sponsors have embraced the medical model." Care is often provided in the wing or floor of medical-like facilities that "are so similar to nursing settings that it is hard for residents, visitors, and staff to distinguish them from institutional arrangements" (Regnier, Hamilton, and Yatabe, 1995:16). Several trends warn of the possibility that an increasing share of assisted-living facilities will look, feel, and operate more like a medical than a housing facility. These include the demographic aging of the older population; the changing consumer market for nursing homes; the expansion of managed care organizations; the increased efforts to make assisted-living facilities affordable to poor frail elders; and the decline in the availability of board-and-care facilities. Together, these developments suggest that assisted-living facilities will be catering to a more physically and cognitively frail elderly population, who will be perceived by state governments and health care providers as requiring more medically oriented supervision and care. This perception will result in the imposition of regulatory standards not unlike those now applied to nursing homes.

FUTURE DEMOGRAPHICS

Between now and the year 2020 the fastest growing group of elders will be over age 85. The U.S. Bureau of the Census conservatively projects that between 1990 and 2020 this age group will more than double, from 3 to 7 million, or by 130 percent. The population aged 75–84 will also increase significantly, but more slowly, from 10.0 to 15.5 million, or by 55 percent (U.S. Bureau of the Census, 1996). Persons in these older age brackets will constitute the most important market for assisted living. They primarily comprise women without living spouses whose children are themselves old and thus cannot be relied on to perform caregiving duties (Doty, 1992; Maloney, Finn, and Patterson, 1996). These very old are at greater risk of having physical or mental impairments demanding more intensive, hands-on, and unscheduled personal, nursing, and medical care not easily provided in home settings or in group settings that do not provide personal care and some nursing services. Whether assisted-living facilities can accommodate this more frail group of elders and still remain true to their social model of care is problematic.

THE EVOLVING NURSING HOME

As nursing homes move toward serving only the most dependent population of elders, the assisted-living market is likely to be composed increasingly of more seriously impaired elder consumers. Housing providers responding to these changing dependency profiles will in turn be motivated to make changes in their physical plant, staffing, and organization patterns.

These responses, however, may de facto push many assisted-living providers into running their facilities more like health care centers than "homes with services." States, in turn, will be pressured by an increasingly better educated and more cynical and vigilant public to ensure that their regulatory frameworks offer protection to this more vulnerable group. This will lead to their treating these facilities more like institutions than group residence alternatives.

It is also to be expected that nursing homes, mostly chain operated or owned and operated by large hospital and health care corporations, will seek to obtain a piece of this changing assisted-living market by creating new, freestanding, assisted-living facilities or by adding new wings to their facilities. It is problematic whether these accommodations will more resemble a social or a medical shelter and care model (Burton, 1994; Coopers & Lybrand, 1993). On this issue, Fralich et al. (1995:29) question: "How can policy makers be sure that life in a wing of a building is measurably different from the nursing home section? Can staff be trained to value safety in the nursing home section and resident autonomy, independence, and decision making in the assisted-living section? Can the building design be modified to accommodate the residential design of assisted living?"

There is, on the other hand, a slow but growing movement known as the Eden's Alternative that calls for the physical and organizational transformation of nursing homes to make them more resemble homes than hospitals. This raises the prospect that long-term shelter and care facilities in the future will constitute some hybrid version of both today's nursing home and the "ideal" assisted-living facility.

THE EXPANDING MANAGED HEALTH CARE DELIVERY SYSTEM

Only a relatively small percentage of frail elders are currently enrolled in Medicaid and Medicare risk-managed care programs (Horvath and Kaye, 1995), but many experts expect that the managed care organizational model (such as the HMO) will be adopted more widely, as both state governments and corporations feel pressured to reduce their health and long-term care cost burdens (Gold, 1996).

As the managed care organizational model becomes more prevalent, some argue that for assisted-living facilities to compete successfully for market share, they will have to become part of a health care organization that offers "the complete continuum of care within a specified geographic region" (Gold, 1996:25). This will increasingly occur as distinctions between acute, subacute, and long-term care become blurred. Managed care organizations will seek to contract with health care providers that offer the full range of acute and long-term care services because they will find it more cost-effective to deal with only one corporate entity than with separate providers. It will also reflect increased demands by both consumers and professionals to reduce fragmentation of care delivery and allow for "one-stop shopping for their health and long-term care needs" (Benson, 1996:31).

These developments will force assisted-living facilities that seek a stable supply of consumers to become part of both horizontally and vertically integrated health and long-term care networks. Such collaborations may be especially necessary for very small freestanding assisted-living facilities.

Horizontal linkages will be achieved by their acquiring, merging, or establishing alliances with other assisted-living providers to achieve a larger critical mass of facilities that have more bargaining and negotiating clout to secure more favorable managed care contracts. Vertical linkages will be created by otherwise dissimilar providers—hospitals, subacute centers, home care agencies, adult day centers, and nursing homes—creating new partnerships. Such integrated delivery systems will be based on a variety of ownership and contractual relationships, ranging from formal mergers and acquisitions to less formal joint ventures, affiliations, and alliances (Hessler and Price, 1995). Some obvious relationships will involve hospitals owning subacute centers, home care agencies, and assisted-living facilities and hospitals placing home health services on the site of a congregate housing or assisted-living facility. This latter arrangement not only brings in new home health and pharmacy revenues but also creates a direct patient referral source for hospital admissions (Meiches, 1996).

There is one caveat. Not all experts believe that assisted-living facilities will generally become part of such vertical and horizontal linkages. Some, for example, like Fitch bond rating service (Price, 1996), believe that the impact of the managed care trend on assisted-living facilities to be overrated, because the bulk of the care in assisted-living residences—long-term custodial or personal care—will not be covered under most managed care contracts. Rather, the portion of care likely to be covered will include the 10–15 percent of posthospitalization care covered by Medicare, including subacute care and some home care services. These observers note that until third-party payers—HMOs, Medicaid and Medicare, insurance companies—become major funding sources for occupants in assisted-living facilities, especially market-rate facilities, the influence of the managed care model will remain weak (Howell, 1996).

In any case, it is not inevitable that the managed care model will be antagonistic to the social model of assisted living. Economic realities in fact may make it good business to avoid an institutional care orientation because assisted-living facilities operating under a social model may be less expensive to operate. Nonetheless, there are two reasons to expect a stronger medical model influence.

First, the actors having the strongest negotiating clout in the formation and operation of managed care networks are likely to emerge from the health care industry—namely, the large hospital and nursing home chains. While the chains look favorably on assisted-living facilities as a relatively low-cost, long-term care alternative, their backgrounds and operating styles will lead them to view the ideal assisted-living facility as a wing of a nursing home or as an added-on home health care agency (Kane and Wilson, 1993). That is, they are more likely to conceive of assisted living as an "integrated part of the health delivery system" than as a "housing alternative for the elderly" (Gold, 1996:23).

Second, a stronger medical model orientation may be driven by distrustful consumer groups seeking better guarantees of the quality of care offered under their managed care coverage. Alert to this increasing public scrutiny, managed care organizations are likely to look with disfavor on assisted-living facilities linked with reports of resident accidents or poor care. Given the inherent resident risks associated with a social model of care, these managed care organizations are likely to demand considerable accountability from their members regarding their quality of care safeguards. Assisted-living facilities may consequently feel compelled to impose a much more regimented organizational style, revolving around structure and process criteria (e.g., staffing requirements) rather than performance-based criteria (i.e., care outcomes). Comparable consequences may be generated by large nursing home chains that pressure their state regulatory agencies to scrutinize the care offered in assisted-living facilities with no less vigor than they pursue the nursing home industry.

LOW-INCOME CONSUMERS

Paradoxically, the medicalizing of assisted living may be hastened by these facilities becoming increasingly affordable to the poor frail elderly population through federal and state government subsidies. A key issue is whether a state's regulatory philosophy will change as assisted-living facilities become occupied by higher percentages of poor persons. The appearance, if not the reality, of provider abuses will become more apparent because these income-poor elders are more likely to be poorly educated and thus more vulnerable (Duggar and associates, 1994). Given that state governments are often risk averse, it is unclear if they will be willing to fiscally support this long-term care alternative without receiving stronger quality and safety assurances (Kane and Wilson, 1993).

Such a prospect poses yet another threat to assisted-living facilities operating under the social model. Doubters of this scenario are reminded of how professionals and advocates view the unregulated or poorly regulated board-and-care industry—the haven of frail poor persons (U.S. General Accounting Office, 1989)—or of how they have reacted to the prospects of removing nursing homes from the regulatory authority of the federal government and placing them under state oversight. The reaction of the executive director of the National Citizens' Coalition for Nursing Home Reform is typical: "Any proposal that would wipe out federal nursing home reforms spells a national tragedy. . . . Federal standards assure taxpayers accountability for their hard-earned dollars and give families and friends of nursing home residents the security that loved ones are safe and receiving decent, appropriate care" (*Aging Network News*, 1995:4).

THE DEMISE OF BOARD-AND-CARE FACILITIES

As the health care industry and managed care organizations become prominent players in the assisted-living industry, small mom-and-pop board-and-care facilities may be one of the fatalities. This category of senior housing, which also accommodates a frail elderly population, is not simple to distinguish from assisted-living facilities (Golant, 1992). Although these facilities are generally occupied by poorer residents and usually lack single-occupancy units and the many physical design features and amenities of high-end assisted-living facilities, they have many of its other ideal attributes (Hawes, Mor, and Wildfire, 1995). They are small in scale, have a homelike ambiance, have simple organizational environments, and often tailor their care to meet the individual needs of their residents (Kalymun, 1992).

What often distinguishes board-and-care facilities are their operators. They are typically owned and managed by poorly remunerated, middle-aged women or married couples who live on the premises and who are responsible for all shelter and care aspects. Although many have professional care qualifications related to earlier occupations, the majority have not been trained as administrators, nurses, or caregivers. Simply put, board-and-care operators are concerned and well-intentioned amateurs. They are "unaffiliated" and "socially marginal" workers who "run their homes in the unmarked, marginal territory between family and formal institution. . . . Being an underground service-delivery system . . . they are not organized, case-managed, and funded by a single agency, instead dealing with haphazard and sometimes overlapping interventions from a variety of agencies and groups" (Morgan, Eckert, and Lyon, 1995:117). In short, the board-and-care operator is unlikely to be viewed as a legitimate player in the rapidly evolving long-term care network, which is increasingly dominated by corporate- and chain-operated housing and health care providers. Not surprisingly, for-profit providers of assisted living have been quick to distance themselves from this option.

State governments in turn have a love-hate relationship with their board-and-care providers. On the one hand, these facilities have accommodated poor and frail older persons who might otherwise have ended up in costly Medicaid nursing home beds. On the other hand, budget constraints have prevented states from adequately regulating these facilities, and states have been embarrassed by widely publicized reports of poor-quality care and resident abuses.

The growth of the assisted-living facility option—an option favorably viewed by private, nonprofit, and public sectors alike and run by professional operators—offers state governments an opportunity to phase out their subsidized board-and-care option. A possible scenario is for state governments to shift their fiscal support—Supplemental Security Income state supplements and Medicaid waiver support—from board-and-care facilities to operators of assisted-living facilities. Assuming an average of five residents per board-and-care facility and sixty residents per assisted-living facility, subsidizing one assisted-living facility would allow the closure of twelve board-and-care facilities. The demise of the small board-and-care operator would mimic the fate of other mom-and-pop establishments, such as the small drugstore or grocery store. Like these other establishments, surviving board-and-care facilities will probably be high-end or specialty operations that attract a high-income elderly constituency seeking a very homelike, upscale, caring, and personalized supportive environment.

Final Thoughts

The professionally administered assisted-living facility, as distinguished from the mom-and-pop board-and-care facility, constitutes an important and attractive, long-term care, residential-like alternative for older persons in need of a more protective environment, personal assistance, and some nursing care. Future demand for this alternative will remain steady, and assisted-living providers—especially the larger chains and corporations—are likely to capture some of the board-and-care and nursing home market. Older Americans and their family members will increasingly become aware of this alternative, as assisted-living providers improve their marketing techniques, as case managers and health care professionals become more aware of its strengths and cost-effectiveness, and as nursing homes increasingly serve only the most dependent elderly in need of subacute, rehabilitative, and dementia care.

Even with the less institutional appearance and operation of assisted-living facilities, however, their overall appeal to older Americans will be limited by their identity as age-segregated group housing, their confusing image, their relatively high cost, and the strong attraction of the home as a place to deal with frailty. Inadequate market research will inevitably lead providers in some locations to misjudge the size of their consumer market, the significance of their competition, or the dependency profiles of prospective occupants. In some states it is also likely that unwieldy and overly stringent regulatory standards will drive up operating costs and prices, further reducing the size of the market. Financial failures will occur, but they will not be as numerous or widespread as those afflicting congregate housing operators in the 1980s.

The forces underlying the growth and acceptance of the assisted-living alternative, however, are unlikely to result in its emerging as a uniform product. The assisted-living facility will reflect local values and market realities. Consequently, consumers considering the appropriateness of this alternative will have to judge carefully how well it accommodates their shelter and care needs. If this shelter and care option does become homogenized, it will be less because of nationally imposed regulatory and quality assurance standards than because of the strong and pervasive managed care model. Driven by its own administrative, cost, and liability concerns, the managed care industry will impose its own philosophy of care on the assisted-living facility, as just one of many components of its vertically linked acute, subacute, and long-term care network. This may unfortunately produce assisted-living facilities that more resemble nursing homes than the ideal social model so passionately advocated by its proponents.

The social model of care may also be threatened, however, by its own ideals. Well-intended efforts to accommodate more physically and mentally dependent residents may have the effect of degrading the living environment of more independent occupants. Likewise, seeking to create a more humane and less institutional environment may increase both the real and perceived risk of inappropriate resident care, leading some states to impose more stringent regulations, which will move the assisted-living facility closer to a medical model of care.

The most critical unknown, however, is not whether the ideal assisted-living model will exist. It will. The question is whether it will be available to only a relatively small group of high-income elderly consumers or whether it will also be accessible to the majority of low- and middle-income frail elderly seeking a true alternative to today's nursing home.

References

AARP. 1990. *Understanding Senior Housing for the 1990s.* Washington, D.C.: American Association of Retired Persons.

Aging Network News. 1995. 13:4.

ASHA. 1994. *Seniors Housing: The Market-Driven Solution*. Washington, D.C.: American Seniors Housing Association.

——. 1995. *The State of Seniors Housing, 1994*. Washington, D.C.: American Seniors Housing Association.

Baggett, S. A. 1989. *Residential Care for the Elderly: Critical Issues in Public Policy*. New York: Greenwood.

Benson, W. 1996. Health care '96: A diversified, humane approach. *Assisted Living Today* 3:31–35.

Blau, P. 1964. *Exchange and Power in Social Life*. New York: Wiley.

Bowker, L. H. 1982. *Humanizing Institutions for the Aged*. Lexington, Mass.: Lexington Books.

Burton, J. 1994. The evolution of nursing homes into comprehensive geriatric centers: A perspective. *Journal of the American Geriatrics Society* 42:769–96.

Campbell, W. 1996. Seniors housing finance. In L. Vitt and J. Siegenthaler, eds., *Encyclopedia of Financial Gerontology*. Westport, Conn.: Greenwood.

Can your loved ones avoid a nursing home? The promise and pitfalls of assisted living for the elderly. 1995. *Consumer Reports* 60:656–60.

Collopy, B. 1995. Home versus nursing home: Getting beyond the differences. In E. Olson, E. Chichin, and L. Libow, eds., *Controversies in Ethics in Long-term Care*. New York: Springer.

Coopers & Lybrand. 1993. *An Overview of the Assisted Living Industry*. Fairfax, Va.: Assisted Living Federation of America.

Coughlin, T., T. McBride, and K. Liu. 1990. Determinants of transitory and permanent nursing home admissions. *Medical Care* 28:616–31.

Coward, R., C. Horne, and C. Peek. 1995. Predicting nursing home admissions among incontinent older adults: A comparison of residential differences across six years. *Gerontologist* 35:732–43.

D'Angelo, H., Jr. 1996. Caring in place. *Assisted Living Today* 3:29–31.

Doty, P. 1992. The oldest old and the use of institutional long-term care from an international perspective. In R. Suzman, D. Willis, and K. Manton, eds., *The Oldest Old*. New York: Oxford University Press.

Duggar, M., and associates. 1994. *The Unfinished Business of Learning*. Tallahassee: Florida Council on Aging.

Edelstein, S. 1995. *Fair Housing Laws and Group Residences for Frail Older Persons*. Washington, D.C.: American Association of Retired Persons.

Ernst & Young. 1993. *Continuing Care Retirement Communities: An Industry in Action*. Vol. 1. Washington, D.C.: American Association of Homes and Services for the Aging.

Fralich, J., et al. 1995. *Reducing the Cost of Institutional Care: Downsizing, Diversion, Closing, and Conversion of Nursing Homes*. Portland, Maine: National Academy for State Health Policy.

Freeman, L. 1995. Home-sweet-home health care. *Monthly Labor Review* 118:3–11.

Gamzon, M. 1995. Senior housing comes of age. *Contemporary Long-term Care* 18:46–51.

Golant, S. 1984. *A Place to Grow: The Meaning of Environment in Old Age*. New York: Columbia University Press.

——. 1985. In defense of age-segregated housing. *Aging* 348:22–26.

——. 1992. *Housing America's Elderly: Many Possibilities, Few Choices*. Newbury Park, Calif.: Sage.

——. 1995. The desirability of housing occupied exclusively by older Americans. In *Expanding Housing Choices for Older People: Proceedings of American Association of Retired Persons White House Conference on Aging Mini-Conference*. Washington, D.C.: American Association of Retired Persons.

——. 1996. Homeownership. In L. Vitt and J. Siegenthaler, eds., *Encyclopedia of Financial Gerontology*. Westport, Conn.: Greenwood.

―――. 1997. Changing an older person's shelter and care setting: A model to explain personal and environmental outcomes. In R. Scheidt and P. Windley, eds., *Environment and Aging Theory: A Focus on Housing*. New York: Greenwood.

―――. 1998. Accommodating older persons with mental disorders: How important is the shelter and care context? *Journal of Geriatric Psychiatry* 31:7–35.

Gold, D. 1996. Managed care is coming: Is assisted living ready? *Assisted Living Today* 3:20–27.

Gubrium, J. 1973. *The Myth of the Golden Years*. Springfield, Ill.: Charles C. Thomas.

Gulyas, R. 1995. *AAHSA's Position on Assisted Living*. Washington, D.C.: American Association of Homes and Services for the Aging.

Hambrook, A. 1990. Assisted living takes hold in the 90s. *Retirement Housing Report* 4:10–11.

Harvard School of Public Health and Louis Harris & Associates. 1996. *Long-term Care Awareness Survey*. Annapolis, Md.: National Investment Conference.

Hawes, C., V. Mor, J. Wildfire, et al. 1995. *Analysis of the Effect of Regulation on the Quality of Care in Board and Care Homes: Executive Summary*. Research Triangle Park, N.C.: Research Triangle Institute and Brown University.

Hessler, F., and J. Price. 1995. Strategic capital planning in a changing health care environment. *Capital* (Fall/Winter).

Himes, C. 1992. Future caregivers: Projected family structures of older persons. *Journal of Gerontology: Social Sciences* 47:S17–26.

Hobbs, R., K. Keest, and I. DeWaal. 1989. *Consumer Problems with Home Equity Scams, Second Mortgages, and Home Equity Lines of Credit*. Washington, D.C.: American Association of Retired Persons.

Hooyman, N., and W. Lustbader. 1986. *Taking Care: Supporting Older People and Their Families*. New York: Free Press.

Horvath, J., and N. Kaye. 1995. *Medicaid Managed Care: A Guide for States*. 2d ed. Portland, Maine: National Academy for State Health Policy.

Housing the Elderly Report. 1996. (June).

Howell, J. 1996. Trend watching. *Assisted Living Today* 4:33–38.

Kalymun, M. 1992. Board and care versus assisted living: Ascertaining the similarities and differences. *Adult Residential Care Journal* 6:35–44.

Kane, R. 1995. Expanding the home care concept: Blurring distinctions among home care, institutional care, and other long-term care services. *Milbank Quarterly* 73:161–86.

―――. 1995–96. Transforming care institutions for the frail elderly: Out of one shall be many. *Generations* 19:62–68.

Kane, R., C. O'Connor, and M. Baker. 1995. *Delegation of Nursing Activities: Implications for Patterns of Long-term Care*. Washington, D.C.: American Association of Retired Persons.

Kane, R., and R. Kane. 1989. Reflections on quality control. *Generations* 13:63–68.

Kane, R., and K. Wilson. 1993. *Assisted Living in the United States: A New Paradigm for Residential Care for Frail Older Persons?* Washington, D.C.: American Association of Retired Persons.

Keith, J. 1980. Old age and community creation. In C. Fry, ed., *Aging in Culture and Society: Comparative Viewpoints and Strategies*. New York: Praeger.

Klaassen, P. 1994. Editorial. *Assisted Living Today* 1:3.

Krause, N. 1987. Understanding the stress process: Linking social support with locus of control beliefs. *Journal of Gerontology* 42:589–93.

Langer, E. 1983. *The Psychology of Control*. Beverly Hills, Calif.: Sage.

Laws, G. 1993. The land of old age: Society's changing attitudes towards urban built environments for elderly people. *Annals of the Association of American Geographers* 83:672–93.

Lawton, M. 1985. Housing and living environments of older people. In R. Binstock and

E. Shanas, eds., *Handbook of Aging and the Social Sciences*, 2d ed. New York: Van Nostrand Reinhold.

Lazarus, R., and S. Folkman. 1984. *Stress, Appraisal, and Coping.* New York: Springer.

Lemke, S., and R. Moos. 1989. Personal and environmental determinants of activity involvement among elderly residents of congregate facilities. *Journal of Gerontology: Social Sciences* 44:S139–48.

Levesque, L., S. Cossette, and L. Potvin. 1993. Why alert residents are more or less willing to cohabitate with cognitively impaired peers: An exploratory model. *Gerontologist* 33:514–22.

Lieberman, M. 1991. Relocation of the frail elderly. In J. Birren, J. Lubben, J. Rowe, and D. Deutchman, eds., *The Concept and Measurement of Quality of Life in the Frail Elderly.* New York: Academic.

Lombardo, N. 1994. *Barriers to Mental Health Services for Nursing Home Residents.* Washington, D.C.: American Association of Retired Persons.

Maas, M., K. Buckwalter, and J. Specht. 1996. Nursing staff and quality of care in nursing homes. In G. Wunderlich, F. Sloan, and C. Davis, eds., *Nursing Staff in Hospitals and Nursing Homes: Is It Adequate?* Washington, D.C.: National Academy Press.

McMillan, D., and D. Chavis. 1986. Sense of community: A definition and theory. *Journal of Community Psychology* 14:6–23.

Magan, G. 1996. Autonomy and risk pose tough decisions for consumers, providers, and regulators. *AARP Housing Report* (Spring): 6–11.

Maloney, S., J. Finn, and K. Patterson. 1996. Making decisions about long-term care: Views from professions. *Perspective on Aging* 25:20–23.

Meiches, D. 1996. Partnership allows hospital to finance project without additional debt. *Capital* (Spring/Summer): 10–11.

Mollica, R., R. Ladd, S. Dietsche, K. Wilson, and B. Ryther. 1992. *Building Assisted Living for the Elderly into Public Long-term Care Policy: A Guide for States.* Portland, Maine: National Academy for State Health Policy.

Mollica, R., K. Wilson, B. Ryther, and H. Lamarch. 1995. *Guide to Assisted Living and State Policy.* Washington, D.C.: National Academy for State Health Policy.

Mor, V., J. Banaszak-Holl, and J. Zinn. 1995–96. The trend toward specialization in nursing care facilities. *Generations* 19:24–29.

Mor, V., S. Sherwood, and C. Gutkin. 1986. A national study of residential care for the aged. *Gerontologist* 26:405–17.

Morgan, L., J. Eckert, and S. Lyon. 1995. *Small Board-and-Care Homes: Residential Care in Transition.* Baltimore: Johns Hopkins University Press.

Moses, S. 1995. *The Magic Bullet: How to Pay for Universal Long-term Care.* Seattle: LTC, Inc.

Mumford, L. 1987. For older people—not segregation but integration. In J. Hancock, ed., *Housing the Elderly.* New Brunswick: Rutgers University Press.

Naifeh, M. 1993. *Housing of the Elderly, 1991.* Current Housing Reports, Series H123/93-1. Washington, D.C.: Government Printing Office.

Neugarten, B. 1982. Policy for the 1980s: Age or need entitlement? In B. Neugarten, ed., *Age or Need: Public Policies for Older Persons.* Beverly Hills, Calif.: Sage.

Newman, S. 1993. Comment on Donald L. Redfoot's long-term care reform and the role of housing finance. *Housing Policy Debate* 4:551–63.

Newsfronts. 1996. Split spawns second assisted-living quality initiative. *Contemporary Long-term Care* 19:15–16.

Parmelee, P., and M. Lawton. 1990. The design of special environments for the aged. In J. Birren and K. Schaie, eds., *Handbook of the Psychology of Aging*, 3d ed. San Diego: Academic.

Price, J. 1996. Key strategies from the proprietary long-term care market. *Capital* (Fall/Winter): 14–15.

Pynoos, J., and S. Golant. 1996. Housing and living arrangements for the elderly. In R.

Binstock and L. George, eds., *Handbook of Aging and the Social Sciences*. 4th ed. New York: Academic.

Regnier, V., J. Hamilton, and S. Yatabe. 1995. *Assisted Living for the Aged and Frail: Innovations in Design, Management, and Financing*. New York: Columbia University Press.

Rook, K. 1987. Reciprocity of social exchange and social satisfaction among older women. *Journal of Personality and Social Psychology* 52:145–54.

Rosow, I. 1967. *Social Integration of the Aged*. New York: Free Press.

Rowles, G., J. Concotelli, and D. High. 1996. Community integration of a rural nursing home. *Journal of Applied Gerontology* 15:188–201.

Sheehan, N. 1992. *Successful Administration in Senior Housing*. Newbury Park, Calif.: Sage.

Spector, W., J. Reschovsky, and J. Cohen. 1996. Appropriate placement of nursing home residents in lower levels of care. *Milbank Quarterly* 74:139–60.

Streib, G., W. Folts, and M. Hilker. 1984. *Old Homes — New Families: Shared Living for the Elderly*. New York: Columbia University Press.

Teresi, J., D. Holmes, and C. Monaco. 1993. An evaluation of the effects of commingling cognitively and noncognitively impaired individuals in long-term care facilities. *Gerontologist* 33:350–58.

Thurow, L. 1996. The birth of a revolutionary class. *New York Times Magazine*, May 19, 46–47.

Timko, C., and R. Moos. 1991. A typology of social climates in group residential facilities for older people. *Journal of Gerontology: Social Sciences* 46:S160–69.

U.S. Bureau of the Census. 1996. *Special Studies: 65+ in the United States*. Current Population Reports P23–190. Washington, D.C.: Government Printing Office.

U.S. General Accounting Office. 1989. *Board and Care: Insufficient Assurance that Residents Needs Are Being Met*. Washington, D.C.: General Accounting Office.

———. 1992. *Public Housing: Housing Persons with Mental Disabilities with the Elderly*. Washington, D.C.: General Accounting Office.

Venti, S., and D. Wise. 1989. Aging, moving, and housing wealth. In D. Wise, ed., *The Economics of Aging*. Chicago: University of Chicago Press.

Wiener, J., and J. Skaggs. 1995. *Current Approaches to Integrating Acute and Long-term Care Financing and Services*. Washington, D.C.: American Association of Retired Persons.

Wilson, K. 1990. Assisted living: The merger of housing and long-term care services. Duke University Center for the Study of Aging and Human Development.

Wright, S. 1996. Retirement and assisted living as a lower price option for seniors no longer true. *Retirement Community Business* 5:17, 27.

Yee, D., J. Capitman, and M. Sciegai. 1993. *Phase 1: Ensuring Resident-centered Care in Assisted Living*. Waltham, Mass.: Institute for Health Policy, Brandeis University.

PART II

ATTRIBUTES OF PLACE AND BEHAVIORS OF PEOPLE

CHAPTER 4

Gerontopia
A Place to Grow Old and Die

RUTH BRENT

*When I am old, I will dwell
at the windowsill.
Near a family genealogy—
photos, pillows, and pearls.*

*Recall history as nostalgia;
sweeten knowledge that was
    suppressed;
regenerate legend for the hereafter.
The lessons of life are best remembered
while rocking in a creaking rocking
    chair.*

*Telling folktales, swaying back and forth.
Life is simple, life is predictable.
From past to present, from present to
    past.
I know this place, I call it home.*

*When death comes close, I still
want to dwell at the windowsill.*

*Too weak to chew an apple,
a knowing caregiver scrapes the pulp
with the round of a spoon to feed.
Like mother scraped, when I was sick,
like I scraped for my babies, before
    teeth.*

*Respiration labored,
words slurred,
caregivers take a feverish hand.*

*The illumination now darker,
oxygen more scarce.*

*Begin and end in the horizontal bed.
Alpha and omega: birth and death.
Glorious and savage rites.
And the capricious globe whirls.*

*I know this place—where death comes,
my eyes will close. My last home.*

Entangled in plastic tubes and life support machinery in her hospital bed, my dying friend Amanda uttered, "I want to go home." She said it over and over, "I want to go home." We all know what she meant. Instead of being in touch with our own shrouded impulses and honoring her wishes, we allowed the staff in a subacute care wing to move her to an antiseptic-smelling, slick-surfaced private room, where she received medical care and a chimerical promise of a cure. A team of physicians and nursing staff administered life-sustaining treatments of artificial feeding and mechanical ventilation for what lung cancer had not yet destroyed. The nightmarish days stretched to weeks and then to two and a half months. The awful reality, which none of us verbalized but all of us understood, was that the hour was too late to purge this assault. It was too late to unplug the network of cords, halt the treatments, help her into a car, make a 45-minute drive, and ease her into her own bed—where she wanted to die.

Like Amanda, the great majority of people fail to leave life in a way they choose and, instead, are victimized by a spiritual malaise in an alienating environment. In too many cases, the setting in which one dies neglects the wishes of a dying person, and the greatest dignity to be found in death is the dignity of the life that preceded it (Nuland, 1994).

The places we want to live are characterized by the highly qualitative notions of dignity, individuality, independence, privacy, and familiarity. These are therapeutic goals that scholars (e.g., Wilson, 1990; Regnier and Pynoos, 1992) identify in assisted-living arrangements. They recognize a broad range of considerations for judging the responsiveness of the environment to the needs of very old people in assisted living (Regnier, Hamilton, and Yatabe, 1995:24). These positive characteristics are experienced in the context of people's lives and, therefore, are those that assisted-living developers attempt to emulate and to translate in the sociophysical environment of their settings.

We are much more timid in identifying the characteristics of the place in which life meets death. This chapter goes beyond identifying therapeutic goals; it describes how environmental attributes and the larger milieu make a difference in the places in which people live *and* die. The physical, social, cultural, clinical, and phenomenological context is considered the total milieu (Rowles and Ohta, 1983). Kastenbaum (1983) may have been among the first to ask: Can the clinical milieu be therapeutic? How can holistic care occur in a fragmented system?

We may call a place to grow old *gerontopia*. The word is coined from the Greek words *geron*, referring to old age, and *topia*, meaning a place. To understand the environmental qualities of gerontopias in their ultimate application, one must begin with them in the raw—in the events and scenes experienced by eye, ear, nose, and fingertips. Listening to personal stories and reading through humanistic literature on aging leads to a heightened sensitivity to the environmental contexts of people's lives. Ordinary people, sharing their truths in their places of residence during the last chapter of their lives, teach us that most of us want to age in place. Moreover, common citizens can stir the general public and legislators to realize that places in which people die should have the same attributes as places in which people grow old. Even in hospitals and hospice care facilities, people desire dignity, meaning, and serenity. Residential, assisted-care settings, or gerontopias, that incorporate therapeutic needs should especially strive to meet these emotional and ideological needs.

This chapter draws from diverse sources. It listens to the voices of frail elders and explores the places they grow old and die, a task that requires more discernment than formulating doctrinaire design guidelines. The role of place is interpreted here as it intersects with the themes of aging, autonomy, and architecture. The emphasis is on integrating these themes to make advancements in assisted living that promote sustainable and poetic habitats imbued with meaning and cultural symbols—human-scale settings that are symbiotic with medical technology but not driven by it. A portfolio of scenarios, based on real-life vignettes, illustrates attributes that assisted-living arrangements attempt to interpret and to imitate. The characters in the stories live in various locations: a hospital, a subacute care unit, a private home, the home of an adult child, a nursing home, a "granny cottage," a freestanding assisted-living facility, a special care unit, and a continuing care retirement community.

Science, Stories, and Transcending Dwellings

Studies of people and place relationships have generated a rich literature that bridges social science, philosophy, architecture, cultural geography, and planning. Environment and behavior researchers often follow a systematic social science method coupled with environmental design premises; that is, purposeful decisions made in the design programming process, in which all important needs are accounted for, have a predictable relationship with the resulting building and thier users. To some extent, this process is based on the scientific perspective of positivism-objectivism, which implies reductionism. Positivism assumes that the real world is measurable. Objectivism implies that there is a world that can be studied separately from ourselves. And reductionism presupposes that the best way to study the world is by examining its discrete, elemental parts.

Environmental design scholars often embrace a science-based perspective grounded in confirmation, refutation, and refinement, and from this viewpoint, researchers can contribute to a cumulative knowledge base. Rapoport (1990), for instance, explains that any design becomes a set of hypotheses to be evaluated in terms of whether the objectives have been met. Rational theories derived from hypotheses are commonly used in the post-occupancy evaluation of assisted-living facilities: there is an explicit definition of a system, a decomposition of the system into its constituent parts, a study of the mutual interactions and mechanisms of these parts, and a re-assembly of the whole at a higher level of conceptual abstraction and understanding (465). Nonetheless, the application of science-based research to improving long-term care settings is incomplete. Although social scientists such as Etzioni (1982) have analyzed social problems and concluded that there is a need for greater community belonging, what seems to be missing in the social science approach is active intervention that promotes this sense of belonging. The social science perspective is just one way to study places and to gain insight into the improvement of residences. Alternative viewpoints outside the realm of science appeal to experience or to a stream-of-consciousness telling of life stories. Naturalized epistemology, for example, lacks the aspiration to certify or to prove, yet it can enrich our understanding. Holistic, transactional, hermeneutic, and phenomenological approaches, to name a few examples, focus on the nature of subjective experience and reality.

Humanism emphasizes human welfare and dignity and is optimistic about the powers of unaided human understanding. Humanists encourage the study of diversity among elders: "Every life is different from any that has gone before it, and so is every death. The uniqueness of each of us extends even to the way we die" (Nuland, 1994:3). Goethe taught us that one vantage point has but a single validity and truth: "We see the world one way from a plain, another way from the heights of a promontory, another from the glacier fields of the primary mountains. We see, from one of these points, a larger piece of world than from the others; but that is all, and we cannot say that we see more truly from any one than from the rest" (Goethe, 1875).

Historically, stories are told, among other reasons, to celebrate and to grapple with individual preferences of place. Multiple humanistic perspectives regarding residences of elders can be patched together to understand place, age, and death, to learn from common persons' stories of joy, comfort, and fear. Every farmer, mechanic, entrepreneur, or homemaker teaches us about habitat. Each person comprehends and interprets the many-sided dimensions of place. The master architect Louis Kahn mused: "You need contact with a tremendous sweep of singularities to realize that in commonality lies the seeds of understanding, of comprehension. That is the time to talk to a common farmer, who has attachments like you have except that he has not found the same things that you have, and doesn't understand these things because his work is different and his course of life was different" (quoted in Wurman, 1986:146).

A dwelling is more involving and emotional than simply a curbside residential address: its proprietary values demand an interconnectedness between it and the person who lives there. This claim of turf gives meaning to one's life and tells others who one is. Norberg-Schulz elaborates on the meaning of dwelling: It is "something more than having a roof over our head and a certain number of square meters at our disposal. First, it means to meet others for exchange of products, ideas and feelings, that is, to experience life as a multitude of possibilities. Second, it means to come to an agreement with others, that is, to accept a set of common values. Finally, it means to be oneself, in the sense of having a small chosen world of our own" (1985:7).

Our dwellings can be astounding and wise. When we are young, new places we inhabit are strange and foreign but waiting to be filled with personal ideas and energy. When we are old, we need places already filled with our own ideas because they remind us of who we were; they evoke memories and keep us alive. Our dwellings, then, possess our identities and communicate messages about our personalities and lifestyles. They are intimate places holding special objects, social rituals, secret and safe territories, and benchmarks of growth. They can contribute to deliberate reverie. If one is sensitive to the spiritual nature of the architecture in which one grows old, one derives an imprint of place.

For us to learn from the ordinary and to transcend to the inspirational, symbolic, enriching, and emotionally significant, we must explore places. The common entities of dwelling we experience are the internal and external components of our material world. Entities are experienced through the senses—touching texture, seeing light, hearing harmonies, and smelling aromas. Entities of dwelling allow realistic encounters through form, function, and space (Markus, 1993). Going beyond function, Louis Kahn embraced the transcending aspect, believing that all architecture is spiritual and poetic and that the architect should design beyond the accommodation of functional needs: "Never build for needs! A space evokes its use. It transcends need. If it doesn't do that, then it has failed. . . . A painting is made to be sensed for its motivation beyond seeing, just as space is made to inspire use" (Wurman, 1986:186).

Achieving the transcending quality in architecture to fulfill a sense of home is more complex than specifying the icons of home. Transplanting design motifs, such as Greek columns, fireplaces, chandeliers, and bric-a-brac, unnerves any designer with an appreciation for the material world; carelessness in transplanting design motifs annuls the original intent. Norberg-Schulz articulates this danger as a "relapse into superficial historicism" (1985:135). Getting past the superficial, en masse, specification of archetypes and construction of an architectural vanguard, altruistic designers and family members seek to provide meaning in settings. They seek to embrace self-actualization.

Because elders are mentors and sages who deserve our love, admiration, and gratitude, we would like to provide them with an ideal home; we expect this loyalty from children. Writers Lydia Sigourney and Nathaniel Willis note the prominence and respect we pay to old persons by granting them the best specimens of a home: "The best armchair, by the fireside, the privileged room, with its warmest curtains and freshest flowers, the preference and first place in all groups and scenes in which age can mingle—such is the proper frame and setting for this priceless picture in a home" (cited in Cole, 1992:142). Adult children feel guilty if their parents are institutionalized in settings of lower value than that which they think their parents deserve. Schneiderman (1996) argues that Americans are motivated by a sovereignty of guilt when they are forced to make difficult decisions. Accordingly, adult children may delay relocating parents in nursing homes because of their feelings of guilt.

Vignettes of Gerontopia

The following vignettes are based on real-life stories. They describe, explain, and interpret the evocative personal impressions, dimensions, and processes of a milieu within which aging and dying occur. Understanding the attributes of gerontopia can advance the quality of future assisted-living settings.

Bewildered, Frail, and Out of Place

Living in a charming three-story frame house, Bill had a gallery of memories. He had lived here with his young bride, worked as an automotive mechanic, raised two daughters, cared for his wife until her death, and grew old. He was a kind, good-natured man who rarely complained. After his wife's death, Bill lived modestly and in solitude for another eight years. His days were purposeful: he planted his vegetable and flower gardens and on his wife's birthday, on Memorial Day, and on religious holidays, he trimmed his wife's grave. The adjoining flat portion would be his own final resting place.

Thanks to Meals-on-Wheels and regular visits from family, friends, and neighbors, Bill continued to age in the house where he had lived with his wife for fifty years. Then, on a drizzly October day, he collapsed with a stroke and required hospitalization. When he returned to the house after his seizure, he was unable to maintain his regular lifestyle—he forgot to nourish and clothe himself; he had lost strength and balance. Disorientated and unstable, he one evening fell to the floor and blacked out. His memory declined.

Thus, Bill relinquished his house and joined one of his daughters in her home, where his condition worsened. Over a period of a year, his well-intentioned daughter wore out from arising four times a night to help him to the bathroom. "Even with Depends," she confessed to me in exasperation, "he couldn't keep himself clean. . . . He had a loose stool, and I had to wipe him . . . or he'd get it all over the bathroom, himself, under his nails. . . . I couldn't possibly leave him, and I was going crazy."

Episodes of passing out took him to the hospital another six times. Eventually, Bill's doctor intervened and convinced his daughter to take him to the local nursing home. "That's when things really tumbled downhill fast," his daughter reflected. "He didn't want to go to the nursing home, but in this small town, we didn't have any other choice. In the nursing home, we tried to talk to him, but he would fall asleep in the middle of his sentence," she sighed. "You know, I think they gave him too many drugs, and he became depressed." He drifted into a state of ennui.

"The real turn of events happened when the staff moved him to a room with a stranger who had been in an accident. The man was paralyzed and really sick and got all kinds of medical treatments and life-support systems. He moaned throughout the day and night; the smell of urine was horrible. I tried to have Dad moved, but they were out of rooms. Being in that room was a real disaster. Within a week," she divulged, wiping a tear from her eye, "Dad was dead."

While some places can help confused older people, the wrong place dissolves an individual's social fabric and personal independence. One's feelings about places are key to remembering one's life courses and to strengthening the self for continuing independence (Rubinstein and Parmelee, 1992). In Bill's case, being in an unfamiliar setting with a very sick stranger in severe pain appeared to be more than Bill could handle. The alien medical environment lacked connection to his past; it seemed to make him more isolated, fatigued, confused, and depressed. His ability to adjust to the threatening, foreign place degenerated.

The experience of place has a potent, though subliminal, impact on our psyche as we travel along the journey of life. While the nursing home had its clinical and therapeutic components, for Bill it was essentially no milieu at all. As Kastenbaum (1983) taught, "Residents are suspended in a floating world that bears little relationship to their previous lives and in which most of their deepest thoughts, feelings, and values are irrelevant" (6).

Memories with Glass Plates, Wooden Rockers, and a Stone Barn

As we age, our biological self declines and becomes a threat to our stability. With age comes new vulnerabilities and new disabilities—interfering with the ability to age in place. Of those chronic diseases, the loss of memory is what many of us fear the most. Memory keeps us productive, balanced, and oriented in the places that give us meaning.

In *Swann's Way*, Proust describes the importance of place in our lives. For Proust, the experience and memory of place goes beyond the mental; it involves the experience of memory through the body:

> Its memory, the composite memory of its ribs, its knees, its shoulder-blades, offered it a whole series of rooms in which it had at one time or another slept; while the unseen walls, shifting and adapting themselves to the shape of each successive room that it remembered, whirled round it in the dark. And even before my brain, lingering in cogitation over when things had happened and what they had looked like, had reassembled the circumstances sufficiently to identify the room, it, my body, would recall from each room in succession the style of the bed, the position of the doors, the angle at which the daylight came in at the windows, whether there was a passage outside. (1928:5)

Memory is an active, creative process that makes sense of both the personal and the collective past. Reminiscence is connected to place and is both enigmatic and therapeutic—as in Mildred's story.

Mildred twinkled at the garden club, at the lodge, at the fair board. She attended all high school reunions and many estate sales. Auctions allowed her to add to her prized collection of antique linens, kitchen equipment, furniture, dishes, and animal figures. She maintained a separation, however, between her public life and her intimate private domain. Never entertaining at home, she protected her privacy and the collections that served as her glass menagerie.

As a wife and mother and now widow, she lived in the three-story farmhouse that her father had homesteaded. She was petite, bore a "widow's hump," a sign of osteoporosis, and walked slowly and bent over. At the fairgrounds, she drove an electric golf cart. On her way back from the grounds one day, she made a turn too fast, fell to the pavement, and fractured her hip. After a brief hospitalization, and unable to return to her farmhouse with its numerous stairs and awkward bathroom, Mildred voluntarily moved to an assisted-living facility, where she received daily assistance with bathing, toileting, and walking. The most valued pieces of her collections followed her to her new home: her mother's antique bed, a dresser, and two rocking chairs. She also brought pillows, dishes, sewing baskets, and photographs, including those of the historic stone barn on the homestead. For the next four years, she kept her home, with its mountains of treasures, and her red Dodge locked. Osteoporosis, declining strength, and cancer, requiring extensive treatments and hospitalizations, brought on depression. Mildred felt the loss of her figure, her womanhood, her financial resources, her friends, and her previous roles. She was mad that she was going to die and terrified of pain. Eventually, with an estimated six months of life remaining, a physician made the referral for hospice care.

The hospice nurse helped Mildred go beyond a sense of hopelessness to acceptance. The hospice nurse assisted in pain management, talked with Mildred about unfinished business, and encouraged her to enjoy life. As she became more weak and less verbal, her gnarled fingers and fleshless hands reached out to hold the hands of her son. In a barely audible voice, she asked him to take her home for the last time.

Preparations for the pilgrimage included a good night's sleep, a nourishing breakfast, and pain medication. They drove in the old Dodge as close as possible to the farmhouse, and she eased herself cautiously from the car. A gust of wind rustled across her balding head. Standing arm-in-arm with her son, she heard a rooster crow, smelled the freshly cut hay, and saw the nearly unchanged house where she had lived as a farm girl and rural matriarch.

In this milieu, Mildred had enjoyed place identification with strong community sentiment. Her homestead enveloped, traced, and became her life story. Community identity was derived through biographical experience with a locale, transforming the local landscape into an extension of self by imbuing it with the personal meanings of life experiences (Hummon, 1992:258). The homestead served as an important sign, or locus, of self, of emotional commitment, of affiliation. Her space had been transformed into place as it acquired definition and meaning (Tuan, 1977:36), and her sense of place gave her a powerful foundation as she traveled along a personal journey of life. "Old places and old persons in their turn, when spirit dwells in them, have an intrinsic vitality of which youth is incapable; precisely the balance and wisdom that comes from long perspectives and broad foundations" (Santayana, quoted in Seldes, 1996).

Mildred picked a blossom of Queen Anne's lace, the only flower she really knew, and she feebly pretended to pump water from the dried-up cistern. Inside the house, in the living room, she imagined her childhood self, framed by the annual Christmas tree and what once had been a wooden mantlepiece, reciting Bible verses. Her son and grandchildren had been positioned to recite at this same place, except that a porch door had replaced the mantlepiece. She slowly walked to the dining room, where the draperies were torn and the light bulbs burned out. Sunlight penetrated two double-hung windows, and a certain decaying odor permeated the air. Memories returned of how her father lay dying for months in a hospital bed beneath these windows. Here at his bedside, among the same crumbling furniture, her leukemia-stricken father taught her how to tie a string knot and play cat's cradle. She remembered her exhausted mother feeding her father and the sounds of his suffering. And she recalled how her mother tearfully folded and tucked her wedding dress under his deathbed pillow. Mildred looked around once more and calmly uttered, "Time to go." Several days later, she died peacefully in her sleep.

Hospice workers are familiar with the phenomenon of place memories taking on momentous importance or spiritual illuminations for dying patients. Memories keep dying persons alive and help them die. Hospice programs, therefore, encourage patients to take a last look; they encourage place reminiscence. Andre, Brookman, and Livingston (1996) cite a case of a hospice worker driving a patient 250 miles to watch the ocean for the last time. In another case, the site was an old furnace where the patient's father had worked. "For mythical thinking the relation between what a thing 'is' and the place in which it is situated is never purely external and accidental; the place is itself a part of the thing's being, and the place confers very specific inner ties upon the thing" (Cassirer, 1955:92).

The self-history of a person's inner ties are marked by persistent recollections: lighting candles on a birthday cake in a childhood home; offering a toast, with a spouse, over a glass of wine at the lodge; sleeping on embroidered pillowcases. Imposing furniture, modest paperweights, photographs, painted dishes, pocketed stones from a family homestead, these are all tangible testaments of life and memory. But although the objects of place may be tangible, the powerful force in spirit of place is subjective and elusive. The meaning of place, in the broad and profound context of the meaning of life, deserves to be the focus. As we age, we experience changes in our physical and emotional selves, and we attribute meaning to a concrete, physical place in which those changes occur. Interpretations of place strive for clarity, accuracy, and comprehension. A family genealogy, for example, may be grasped by cataloguing place, events, and progeny. Mildred's house, stone barn, red Dodge, favorite dishes, and photographs of family reunions were anchors. The philosopher Bachelard writes about the philosophic connection with objects: "Objects that are cherished in this way really are born of an intimate light, and they attain to a higher degree of reality than indifferent objects, or those that are defined by geometric reality. For they produce a new reality of being, and they take their place not only in an order but in a community of order. From one object in a room to another, housewifely care weaves the ties that unite a very ancient past to the new epoch. The housewife awakens furniture that was asleep" (1994:68).

The individualism of place acknowledges daunting changes in who we are. Furthermore, throughout the aging process, place falls on a epistolary continuum from stimulating to peaceful, debilitating to aligning. A habitat is both a private sanctuary and a public throng; it ranges from romantic to rational, natural to high tech, simple to extravagant—and birth to death. Rich in both meaning and myth, place is linked to epochal and minute events. Place is bound to the people whom we become. "We shape our buildings, and our buildings shape us," Winston Churchill noted.

An Abiding Abode

David lived in an ignoble house above his shop in a small Missouri town. Here, he owned and operated multiple businesses for 60 of his 82 years: farm machinery and automotive sales; excavating, hauling, and construction services; real estate speculation; and rental management. The oldest child in a third-generation German family, he was in his youth dapper, with a quick step. In midlife, David was thought of as a cranky curmudgeon. Strong willed and low on sentiment, he adjusted to inconvenience but rebelled against hardship. While he tolerated a colostomy for fifteen years, he complained profusely over a revoked driver's license.

In his late 70s and unable to negotiate stairs, he moved essential items close at hand, adapted his quarters, and maintained a place to reside, work, and dream. In his situation, idiosyncratic adaptations were needed to help him remain in his own dwelling. He customized his chair with chunky foam-rubber cushions; he outfitted his nearby walker with hand-stitched muslin pockets for a cordless phone, paper, and pens. He pulled himself up flights of stairs using cabinet handles he screwed into the walls; he walked with his workers to plumbing jobs and then, sitting on a wooden box, watched and directed their work to his level of perfection.

When David became an octogenarian, he slowed his canter and slouched his shoulders, but kept the bullheaded clarity, volume, and cadence of his words. Parts of his body became rigid and fixed and other parts became soft and flaccid. With assistance in doing his laundry, shopping, cleaning, and secretarial tasks, he maintained his indomitable spirit and lifestyle. He still dressed himself, irrigated his colostomy daily, meticulously sliced vegetables for a salad, and kept his business enterprises alive. His age was expressed in the time it took him to perform these daily tasks, in his increasing stubbornness and determination, and in his clumsy walk. David adamantly refused to have institutional handrails installed in the bathroom; he braced himself with strategically placed furniture. He declined the use of a wheelchair, except one rented from a shopping mall by the hour.

Although the number of steps he could manage gradually decreased, he continued to make his forays between bed, bathroom, and kitchen table. At the kitchen table, he sipped his white coffee and snipped columns from the local newspaper. The linoleum beneath his chair blackened with wear. Here, he did his "book work," answered the phone, and watched the clock as he directed his workers and mused on new money-making projects. As he gazed out his window, he ruminated on the properties he wanted to buy, the buildings he wanted to build, the deals he wanted to make, and the legal wills he wanted to check.

Relatives and friends told David he should liquidate properties so he could rest, but he would retort, "I'll retire when I'm in the grave!" His lifestyle was a tour de force until he had trouble irrigating himself because of an intestinal blockage. Still belligerent and in control, he called for an ambulance and agreed to emergency surgery. The next day, although severely weakened by the surgery, and with a voice barely audible, he still gave out a message of unemotional strength. When his daughter telephoned, expressing her love for him, he did not reciprocate the words because it would have been to admit his death. Unsentimentally, he only said good-bye, meaning only that the telephone conversation was ended. Yet, on this night, he died in his sleep.

Bachelard characterizes dreaming as a household activity:

If I were asked to name the chief benefit of the house, I should say: the house shelters daydreaming, the house protects the dreamer, the house allows one to dream in peace. . . . The values that belong to daydreaming mark humanity in its depths. Daydreaming even has a privilege of autovalorization. It derives direct pleasure from its own being. . . . Therefore, the places in which we have *experienced daydreaming* reconstitute themselves in a new daydream, and it is because our memories of former home-places are relived as daydreams that these home-places of the past remain in us for all time. (1994:6)

Where David chose to live, up until his concluding hours, was neither clinical nor therapeutic. It was home. For most elders, this place is most preferred. A true home provides autonomy to the greatest degree and in a sense that is prized. David epitomized freedom of will, self-rule, self-determination, and individuality. He valued his hold on the small circumference of his living space, he adapted his shrinking space, and he retained his control with fanaticism. Self-reliance defines individual worth (Agich, 1993).

Crossing Thresholds

When Samantha's memory started to deteriorate, so did her self-reliance. She had orientation and spatial problems, an inability to complete complex tasks, and was agitated. A gregarious and talkative person, she became more forgetful and unable to handle the daily managerial operations of a college sorority, where she served as house mother. Realizing the gravity of her disease, her family moved her to a special care unit designed for persons with dementia.

Over time, Samantha became more confused, phobic, and incontinent. Her previous friendly character reversed to asocial behaviors and enfeeblement. She caused havoc by wandering into residents' unlocked rooms, pulling clothes from closets and dumping them in the trash, and trying to remove the trash can from the premises. She tormented those who were unknown to her and those who were trespassing in her territory. She screamed to make outsiders leave. Her capers were tolerated when they merely annoyed but were rebuked when they frightened others.

Samantha lived in a private room, and she routinely walked in a secured enclosed courtyard. The door to her room became an illuminated vertical landmark with her name and a large photograph of herself in her 30s. A tall aviary with iridescent yellow canaries served as another landmark on her walks. The staff provided a pile of clothing for rummaging and disposal, eliminated the bathroom mirror, simplified storage areas, increased lighting, and eliminated noises. Her dwelling was safe and secure, maintaining links with her past. Nonetheless, Samantha had crossed significant thresholds from the sorority to the special care unit, and she required increased assistance with orientation.

For many days, her daughter kept vigil by Samantha's side. Samantha began to look haggard, her limbs became decrepit and her body emaciated. During the late stages of Alzheimer's disease, the erstwhile sorority mother crumpled. Unaware of time, space, and events, her stupor worsened. Dressing, feeding, bodily functions, keeping air passages free from phlegm, all hastened her dependency.

During the distortion of Samantha's personality and the anguish of dying, the requirements of the milieu were those of satisfying the needs of both residents and caregivers. Family members congregated at Samantha's bedside, held hands, and prayed. They ate their meals with her, sang favorite hymns, and napped by her side. From the balcony where Samantha's bed was wheeled, they watched the leaves of the maple trees along the river bluffs turn from green to red to brown. Samantha's deathbed environment allowed family members to mourn throughout the long, agonizing process of death. Multiple chairs and makeshift sleeping arrangements supported the family's watchfulness. Right at dusk, with her exhausted relatives nearby, Samantha died.

Residents of special care units are blessed if they live their last days "in place." In many special care units, residents are moved to skilled nursing care in the final stages of dementia. Samantha was fortunate to have died peacefully, with loving relatives nearby, in a facility that helped her family in the grieving process. Furthermore, the facility allowed for cultural and social diversity among patients and relatives. While Samantha's family prayed and sang hymns in her room, other rooms accommodated quiet meditation, fresh flowers, poetry reading, photograph montages, and the burning of incense.

Pampered Lodging in a Landscaped Granny Cottage

Pearl's family constructed a cottage adjacent to their 1930s Tudor dwelling for Pearl's new home. They celebrated her 85th birthday in this cottage, just before doctors predicted she had six months to live. Pearl's past life revolved around her husband and children; now she turned to her family for help. Her eyes lost their luster and acquired a gray ring around the cornea. She grew white hair, a swollen abdomen, and an elaborate branching network of blue and purple varicose veins.

Pearl easily maneuvered with a walker and a wheelchair. Her cottage had no stairs, had an easily accessible bedroom and bathroom, and a functional and accessible kitchen. A gingham blue-and-white fringed cloth draped the round dining table; blue towels and blue scented soaps decorated a roll-in shower stall. There were unmatched bulging bureaus, pillow-crowded upholstered chairs, and a paper-stuffed secretary. Shelving encircled the rooms holding first editions of Faulkner, Twain, Dickinson, and Melville; framed family photographs; collections of porcelain figurines, coral, and shells from international junkets with her late husband. The cottage could have supported elaborate medical technology or a hospital bed, but none was present; her family rigged a simple five-dollar doorbell to ring in her daughter's upstairs bedroom.

Selected for its good view, the living space nestled in a grove of birch trees. Large windows with orientations to the north, east, and south allowed a view of changing daylight. Whether seated or lying in bed, Pearl could watch the mail carrier traveling door to door, neighbors gardening in their yards, and great-grandchildren returning from school. The landscape seemed to soothe her in an almost magical way. Gardens grew, blossomed, bore fruit, and shriveled. "The garden, with its well-watered trees and pruned plants, represents the reassuring compromise of life contained—an oasis in the desert, a clearing in the forest, a sequestered spot in the city. It is a piece of the natural world which man encloses in order to hold out alien presences and to cultivate desirable plants" (Lutwack, 1984:48).

Pearl's milieu was reminiscent of village life or of small towns and hamlets where people share their dwellings and take care of one another. In village life, people help one another recover from crises and maintained family structures; volunteer household caregivers serve as therapists, with sensitivity, empathy, and affection. Pearl's home adjoined her daughter's residence without violating the privacy of family members. Although Pearl knew this arrangement was her last, it reassured her because it resembled her life-long dwelling. For over forty years, she had lived with the same braided wool rugs, heirloom dishes, patchwork quilt made of her grandmother's dresses, bedroom set, alarm clock, and cross-stitched towels. When Pearl's condition rapidly unraveled, the family moved a low cot to her side. At 6 o'clock in the morning, she died. For several hours after her death, Pearl lay in her bed while grandchildren and great-grandchildren were called to her side. There, they delivered farewells and grappled with life's greatest mysteries—love and death. At her death, Pearl was with her loved ones, her books, her belongings in familiar surroundings. Her place permitted autonomy in dying.

Stylish, Sensory, and Safe

Sadie, a violinist in a major orchestra, was talented and kind, a trait displayed during an international guest performance of Brahms' violin concerto. When the star's violin string broke in the fourth movement, Sadie held out her own instrument to swap, and the concerto continued to its grand finale. Sadie's marriage to a wealthy entrepreneur provided a privileged life of sophistication, affluence, and philanthropy.

Gradually, Sadie's musical career slowed because of complications with arthritis, and Sadie's daughter encouraged her mother to move to a one-bedroom, catered, independent-living apartment in an exclusive neighborhood. The first visit to the premier senior community, long before Sadie's move, was memorable. They walked past an entourage of professionals: the chauffeur at his limousine in the circle drive, the cheerful door attendant greeting them in the vestibule. Sadie met the concierge, who took messages and delivered packages, and she engaged in conversation with the stately gentleman in a handsome suit at the front desk, a specialist in what the Romans call *arte di arrangiarsi*—the art of finessing problems. Past the jungle-sized plants and massive-scaled art by internationally recognized artists was a six-story atrium with marble surfaces, oriental rugs, Chippendale furniture, and brass chandeliers. Off the atrium was an intimate sitting room with a grand piano and a gas fireplace. A proscenium theater might present politicians giving campaign speeches, poets reading their verses, and schoolchildren performing. As a flute played in the background, residents meandered through a mall equipped with gift shop, a full-service bank, a greenhouse, an art studio, a dance studio, a restaurant, and a bar. Along the restaurant's kitchen and loading area, an infrequently traveled, circuitous pathway led from the atrium to the assisted-living and skilled nursing home facilities.

After she moved to her apartment in the senior community, Sadie began to notice changes in herself. Her one-time blond hair faded to a silver gray, her feet shuffled when she walked, and her shrinking stature showed weak-ening skeletal musculature. Yet, as a member of a city's elite, Sadie tried to dress in fashionable name-brand suits and accessories.

Windows had views to gardens and funneled outdoor breezes of fresh air to the inside. Sunshine poured through windows, doors, and skylights to ori-ent shadows like a sundial; green plants flourished like an exotic rain forest. Sadie would sit in her comfortable living room chair and engage in a psy-chotherapeutic monologue with her bright-feathered parrot. Nearby were the memorabilia, trophies, and silver trays that were musical awards or ac-knowledgments of community service—and her silent violin. Like her inter-national friends in neighboring apartments, Sadie carried out her own do-mestic and religious rituals. Each morning she made her bed and tended to her bird; at 4 o'clock in the afternoon, on the third Wednesday of each month, she used her good silver for afternoon Bible study and tea with neigh-boring ladies.

Cushioned and safe, her home flaunted vanguard technology. One of the safety features was an unobtrusive, electronic sensor that indicated when the toilet was flushed. A toilet not flushed for 12 hours turned on a light in the main office; when this happened, a staff member would go to the room to check on the resident. On one spring day in May, the light came on for Sadie's room. After washing dishes from her afternoon tea, Sadie had had a stroke; she lay sprawled on the floor unconscious for several hours. The event pre-cipitated a move to the adjoining assisted-living facility.

Somewhat smaller in size, her new residence allowed her to bring only a sampling of her household and her violin. This environment was attuned to safety: chair moldings served as handrails, fire doors were tucked into al-coves, and bathroom fixtures allowed for accessibility. Living areas invited music listening; intersecting axis nodes invited gatherings. Here were freshly cut flowers to smell and a small fluffy dog to pet. Moreover, like the consol-ing power of beauty from poets and painters, the architectural beauty of place inspired and motivated. But the environment could not compensate for Sadie's declining health.

Sobered by her failing health, increased pain, and the loss of close friends, Sadie talked openly with her daughter of death. Mirroring the views of six-teenth-century French essayist Michel de Montaigne, Sadie saw her life as part of the changing universe and was ready to give her place to others as they had done for her. Grateful for what her wealth had provided, she knew she had lived her life fully. As she offered her violin to a stranger so many years before, she contributed her space in life to a replacement she would never know. At first resisting her mother's giving up, Sadie's daughter eventu-ally resigned herself to her mother's imminent death. Old age is as insoluble as it is inevitable; the natural limits of an individual's life permit little tamper-ing (Nuland, 1994:71,72).

Shortly after the July Fourth holiday, Sadie, weakened by a cold and fever, died from pneumonia. In her final hours, she made additional contributions to charities that would invest in educating young aspiring musicians. Curled up in bed, with scholarship applications beside her, she fell asleep and swiftly glided to her new destination.

At her death, Sadie was living in a normal milieu. Her domicile was a sample of the larger world functioning as normal by virtue of special planning and enrichments. Not clinical or curative, it possessed a low-profile professional presence.

Salient Themes

Designers are often stymied in creating meaning for the residents of the places they design. The increasing change rate of persons living in the facilities, the diversity of ethnospecific and culture-specific rituals, the variation in resident personalities, conflicts among customer groups, and the seclusion of the deathbed lead to this bewilderment. Designers are more educated in creating environments than in helping residents find meaning in them.

While unforeseen consequences and interpretations create more questions than answers in designing ideal gerontopias, the voices of elders may be translated to related themes. Perhaps the most important advice derived from these stories is to advocate and invest in settings that continuously promote personal autonomy and dignity until death. It is feasible to design assisted-living settings with these forward-looking intentions.

Personal Autonomy

Personal autonomy emerges as a dominant attribute in these case studies; it signals a valued consequential investment. The terms *control*, *choice*, and *personal autonomy* are used in the literature interchangeably and are fundamental aspects of residential environments. Alternatively, a resident's pleading to go home is a disturbing cry for autonomy; too often, it is one that is futile. While autonomy has diverse expressions, the concept continues to prevail as an overarching goal. The vignettes demonstrate that autonomy is integral to one's personality: it can mean keeping an excessive number of personal possessions, traveling, supervising workmen, being able to eat and sleep at will, keeping pets, and entertaining ladies at tea.

For providers who wish to nurture autonomy, the challenge is to treat residents as human beings, to consider "old people as people" (Keith, 1982). Respecting stories of residents' former lifestyles and homes is just the first step. It needs to be followed by interpreting these stories and creating individual supports in each one's environment. Autonomy is unique and varied. When autonomy is experienced, it perhaps indicates the achievement of other positive therapeutic goals. If it is not experienced, many other needs and wants are abandoned.

Dignity in Domicile 'til Death

The milieu in which to grow old and the milieu in which to die have essentially the same goals. When we look in the mirror, we see an old person; inside, however, we feel we are still young. We are the same person, with all the same attributes, when we are young as when we are old. Without a clear division between being young and being old, the place where we grow old and the place where we die should also be without separation—even though we do not choose or control our place of death.

A close connection exists between care of elders and the philosophy of death and dying. Dignified and caring treatment attends to placeness, as described in the following:

My death, as I picture it, occurs in my own bedroom, not a hospital room. The surroundings are comfortable and familiar. It seems foolish to me to consider the decor of the room. Nevertheless that's what pops into my mind first. This I believe reflects my desire to die content. The bed, higher than the average, has a beautiful floral spread with matching sheets and lace pillow cases. The carpet, drapes, and wallpaper are softly colored and create an open and fresh feeling. The atmosphere in the room will be accented by the weather outside. The season is midspring, a sunny morning with a light, warm breeze and birds singing outside. The importance of the type of day to me signifies a sense of freedom or the lifting of burden. (Kastenbaum, 1992:9)

Kastenbaum explains that the deathbed has both an actual physical location and an indeterminate location but that the comforting placeness quality of the deathbed really matters. The physical connection to place is heard in statements: "I want to die in the place I made to live"; "I want to die where I am in the midst of life." Transcendent place—a place that evokes a positive feeling—is more intangible. Transcendence may also be related to an individual's faith: place contributes to a belief in the passage to an afterlife, or a heavenly home.

While designers are taught to listen to users, few clients articulate their needs and desires. Standing at the edge of a precipice, we are uncertain of well-defined goals and without resolution (Levinson and Levinson, 1996). We are ill prepared to accept mortality and defeat in realistic terms. We avoid the question, Where do you want to dwell at death? The separation between life and death is incomprehensible and formidable. About the time that Vincent van Gogh painted *Starry Night*, he mused on the difficulty of comparing the travels on earth and the travels following the stars in the sky: "Why, I ask myself, shouldn't the shining dots of the sky be as accessible as the black dots on the map of France? Just as we take the train to Tarascon or Rouen, we take death to reach a star. One thing undoubtedly true in this reasoning is that we cannot get to a star while we are alive, any more than we can take a train when we are dead" (Cole, 1992:250). Literature often gives us our images of the deathbed. Edgar Allan Poe, for example, offers lines about feeling "out of Space—out of Time." In contrast, the Egyptians of antiquity developed and practiced an explicit death system. The *Book of the Dead* is considered an effort to locate death within the scope of the culture. The Egyptian system offers the reassurance of bridging the chasm between the living and the dead through the care of the dead (Kastenbaum and Aisenberg, 1972).

While we cannot control where we will be when we die, we can control where we will grow old and might attempt to make the place in which we grow old the place of our death. It is possible that this last place can meet medical needs and still be sensitive to the essentials of living. Michel de Montaigne advised, "It is uncertain where death awaits us: let us await it everywhere. Premeditation of death is premeditation of freedom" (Schatzki and Natter, 1996:93). The quality of placeness at a deathbed can be sought in the dwellings that precede it. Succinctly, the choice of the place in which one breathes one's last breath should be governed by the individual's idea of a dignified death.

At this time, assisted living is underpromoted for aging in place, including death; annual resident turnover in assisted living is at 40–50 percent (Moore, 1996). Because the place in which we want to die is likely to have the same environmental attributes of the place in which we want to live, we should be designing for both the living and the dying. This means bringing to the dwelling the services and the necessary methods to control pain as needed and desired; and it means maximizing personal autonomy and incorporating home- and community-based services in the package of managed care.

Assisted living complements long-term care options by materializing individual dignity characteristics. Presuming that assisted living can fulfill positive environmental attributes, these settings may also be places where older people want to die. While assisted living can be integral to the development of an extended pathway of care, it has yet to be experienced at this optimal level. Many facilities fail to offer a place in which frail elders can live to the end of their lives. Needless impediments include contraining building codes, lack of ancillary services, and confusing reimbursement systems. Until these impediments are addressed, assisted living is beyond the means of most frail elders.

Denouement and Final Thoughts

As the denouement of a play results from what has gone before, the vignettes and themes in this chapter lead to an exposition of where we might want to grow old and die. Gerontopias are not in the lists of most livable cities or best vacation hotels; they are described in idiosyncratic impressions and individual imaginations. I hesitate to make recommendations, because the prototypical milieu is to some degree ineffable. A metaphysical poetry exists when an individual experiences delight of place. For most residents, a setting's spaciousness, sunlight, furnishings, and esthetics may enhance a facility. At some point, however, the importance of the concrete physicality is superseded by personal perceptions.

Bachelard's philosophy highlights the personal images of things rather than the physical things themselves. Bachelard would not condone design guidelines, specifications, or the purchase of things; rather, he would promote better understanding of individuals and their backgrounds. Similarly, for a designer to purchase and install vintage memorabilia from a flea market and call them "homelike accessories" disturbs a resident's intimate meditation. Silk flowers, plants, and trees, along with broken typewriters and stuffed animals, give an illusion of home to outsiders like a theater set gives an illusion of place to an audience. A resident's home is hardly a stage. Meaningless knickknacks and extrinsic decorations may be as disrupting to a habitation as a decor that is soporific, anonymous, and enervating. The critical challenge for the designer is to provide user-oriented design emphasizing resident and family involvement, which encourages residents to bring their own personal interpretations. User-oriented design is crucial in both creating and experiencing a milieu.

Helping residents feel a sense of belonging to a community begins with understanding them as individuals. Each writer, merchant, housewife, laborer, symphony conductor, and farmer has his or her own definition of meaningful inhabitation. A writer claims her spiritual meditation place at a quiet seat by a western windowsill; a merchant might want an outdoor bench to straddle as he watches truck deliveries; a housewife might wish to perch at a kitchen table to smell yeast bread baking. Places reflect our culture and ethnic heritage. As these places become more personal, our lives become unique. For example, while the sounds of a train may make some people nostalgic, they may be an annoyance to others. A laborer may be captured by country western music, an orchestra conductor by a symphony, a farmer by the rooster's crow. Therefore, preferences and images are individually fostered.

In the final hours of life, some would say that personal images and interpretations of comforting placeness are far more precious than the physical place itself. At our final destination in our journey of life, snapshot images and interpretations really matter. The images of making a house a home are indelible and precious. Perhaps this high value on connectedness is one reason we grieve the erosion of memory. Because of this, designers labor to use therapeutic environments as stimuli for maintaining memory. The work of a designer is to help residents focus on achieving personal images and interpretations of comforting placeness.

Caring about individual impressions of place parallels patient-focused care, which means listening to the voices of elders, supporting personal autonomy, and maneuvering pathways within an integrated health care model in a larger health care system. In addition, patient-focused care means respecting the wishes of the person. Patient-focused care, one might conclude, should be user oriented. The assisted-living residential option, with its concomitant personal care and catered living, requires the involvement of its residents in its creation. Ultimately, architects, interior designers, physicians, health providers, family members, and enablers will accept that the real designers are the dwellers themselves. Our purpose is to honor a dweller's needs, wants, and choices.

> How can earthly designers create a sense of place
> so it is felt in the heart and soul?
> The designer inside each of us creates and constructs.
> To say that another can create this union is
> to say that another can create religious belief.
>
> For some, the awe, feeling, and emotion are proof enough
> that links exist between the universe and us,
> between earth and being.
> Belief in this unifying chain is championed in life,
> comforting at death.

References

Agich, G. 1993. *Autonomy and Long-term Care.* New York: Oxford University Press.

Andre, D., P. Brookman, and J. Livingston. 1996. *Hospice: A Photographic Inquiry.* New York: Little, Brown.

Bachelard, G. 1994. *The Poetics of Space.* Boston: Beacon. Published in French under the title *La poetique de l'espace.* 1958. Presses Universitaires de France.

Cassirer, E. 1955. *The Philosophy of Symbolic Forms*. New Haven: Yale University Press.

Cole, T. 1992. *The Journey of Life: A Cultural History of Aging in America*. Cambridge: Cambridge University Press.

Etzioni, A. 1982. *An Immodest Agenda: Rebuilding America before the Twenty-first Century*. New York: McGraw-Hill.

Goethe, J. von. 1875. *Conversations of Goethe with Eckermann and Soret*. Translated by John Oxenford. London: George Bell and Sons.

Hummon, D. 1992. Community attachment: Local sentiment and sense of place. In I. Altman and S. Low, eds., *Place Attachment: Human Behavior and Environment*. New York: Plenum.

Kastenbaum, R. 1983. Can the clinical milieu be therapeutic? In G. Rowles and R. Ohta, eds., *Aging and Milieu: Environmental Perspectives on Growing Old*. New York: Academic.

———. 1992. *The Psychology of Death*. 2d ed. New York: Springer.

Kastenbaum, R., and R. Aisenberg. 1972. *The Psychology of Death*. New York: Springer.

Keith, J. 1982. *Old People as People: Social and Cultural Influences on Aging and Old Age*. Boston: Little, Brown.

Levinson, D., and J. Levinson. 1996. *The Seasons of a Woman's Life*. New York: Knopf.

Lutwack, L. 1984. *The Role of Place in Literature*. Syracuse: Syracuse University Press.

Markus, T. 1993. Buildings as social objects. In B. Farmer and H. Louw, eds., *Companion to Contemporary Architectural Thought*. New York: Routledge.

Moore, J. 1996. *Assisted Living: Pure and Simple Development and Operating Strategies*. Fort Worth: More Diversified Services.

Norberg-Schulz, C. 1985 (reprinted in 1993). *The Concept of Dwelling: On the Way to Figurative Architecture*. New York: Rizzoli.

Nuland, S. 1994. *How We Die: Reflections on Life's Final Chapter*. New York: Knopf.

Proust, M. 1928. *Remembrance of Things Past*. Vol. 1, *Swann's Way*. Translated by C. K. Scott Moncrieff. New York: Modern Library.

Rapoport, A. 1990. *History and Precedent in Environmental Design*. New York: Plenum.

Regnier, V., J. Hamilton, and S. Yatabe. 1995. *Assisted Living for the Aged and Frail: Innovations in Design, Management, and Financing*. New York: Columbia University Press.

Regnier, V., and J. Pynoos. 1992. Environmental interventions for cognitively impaired older persons. In J. Birren, B. Sloane, and G. Cohen, eds., *Handbook of Mental Health and Aging*. 2d ed. New York: Academic.

Rowles, G., and R. Ohta, eds. 1983. *Aging and Milieu: Environmental Perspectives on Growing Old*. New York: Academic.

Rubinstein, R., and P. Parmelee. 1992. Attachment to place and representation of the life course by the elderly. In I. Altman and S. Low, eds., *Place Attachment: Human Behavior and Environment*. New York: Plenum.

Schatzki, T., and W. Natter, eds. 1996. *The Social and Political Body*. New York: Guilford.

Schneiderman, S. 1996. *Saving Face: America and the Politics of Shame*. New York: Knopf.

Seldes, G. 1996. *The Great Thoughts*. New York: Ballantine.

Tuan, Y. 1977. *Space and Place: The Perspective of Experience*. Minneapolis: University of Minnesota Press.

Wilson, K. 1990. Assisted living: The merger of housing and long term services. *Long Term Care Advances* (Duke University Center for the Study of Aging and Human Development) 1.

Wurman, R. 1986. *What Will Be Has Always Been*. New York: Rizzoli.

CHAPTER 5

Personal Rituals

Identity, Attachment to Place, and Community Solidarity

LEON A. PASTALAN
JANICE E. BARNES

Memories are the fabric of life. . . .
Dusting, packing or storage optional.

Memories are tag-a-longs that move with you,
never far away in your mind.

Some travel in photo albums or on wax to be
spun again and again leaving musical
footprints in the corners of your soul.

Some live pressed between yellowed pages or
tied with silk ribbons for your eyes only.

But the very best travel safest in your
heart and come to your lodging not as
baggage but as the trimmings that make your
chosen dwelling place a HOME.

Gwen Powers, 1995

Whenever the subject of residential environments for older adults arises, particularly as it relates to purpose-built retirement facilities, one of the first questions raised is, How much like home is it? Research suggests that the need for a home is a fundamental human imperative that, among other things, provides a locus of order and control in a world of uncertainty. Home imparts a sense of identity, security, and belonging. To be at home is to know where you are; it means to inhabit a secure center and to be oriented in space (Pastalan et al., 1993). We inhabit home day after day, slowly developing a sense of familiarity with the environment to the degree that it becomes predictable, taken for granted, and comfortable.

Assisted living has in the past several years become one of the most active and popular retirement housing options. It is still in the process of defining itself, and the regulatory machinery has not yet imposed an institutional straitjacket on its many variations. During this period of experimentation, it is hoped that, whatever variations emerge, the residential model as opposed to the medical model will prevail. It is crucial, therefore, to recognize that to fully implement the residential model it must establish a homelike ambiance. To develop such a homelike ambiance exhaustive efforts must be made to transfer as many attributes of home to an assisted-living setting as possible. A central theme of this chapter is that one of the most important attributes of home is the personalization of the activities of daily life, or personal rituals.

Dining, visiting, reading, bathing, sleeping, watching television, and so forth take place as a matter of routine. These activities of daily life orient us in space and time. They are not embodied in a house or a certain building but in our personal experience and behavior, and therefore these behaviors and experiences must be transferable from one place to another if identity and attachment to place is to occur. These behaviors and experiences are manifested in the form of personal rituals and act as important life-centering activities. If these activities are allowed to autonomously take root in the retirement facility, they will serve as the essential building blocks for a real community of residents, staff, and management to emerge and sustain itself. A reciprocity takes place when the community understands and supports the autonomous personalization of life's daily activities on the part of the resident and when the resident in turn gives a commitment to the community to maintain group solidarity.

Personal Rituals and Adaptation to Life Changes

The life-centering activities called personal rituals help give meaning to our daily lives; yet ironically most of us pay scant attention to these activities and attach no great significance to them. Their importance is perceived only after they have been altered or eliminated due to a change in our personal lives. These changes are usually the result of major life events such as illness, the death of spouse, or a change in our housing or living arrangements.

Life change, no matter whether it is positive or negative, is disruptive. It is clear that consequences of disruption are greater if the change is negative; and the more negative the change, the more profound the consequences. As people age, particularly beyond the seventh decade of life, serious negative changes such as death of a spouse, incapacitating illness, loss of income, and changes in housing and living arrangements significantly impact their lives. As people develop an attachment to place, special meanings and rituals evolve as part of the daily activities in that setting. These rituals connect people to their environment through their physical motor actions and by the meaningfulness of the activities themselves. These are not merely activities of daily living, although they may be interwoven with daily life activities. Personal rituals are highly personalized routines and seem to anchor a person to a particular place. Seamon (1979), for instance, reports an example of a personal ritual that denotes the kind of activity that roots a person to his or her own time-space routine.

> My mother and father lock the doors to their house every night before retiring. Usually, my father does it, but then my mother rechecks to make sure he hasn't forgotten. My father has a regular routine. He goes to the outer porch door, flips on the yard light, checks the outdoor thermometer, shuts off the light, locks the porch door, then comes in, locks the inner door which comes into the kitchen. Then about fifteen minutes later my mother gets ready for bed, and she checks the door, too. In the morning, my mother gets up first. As soon as she's downstairs, she unlocks both doors and looks out to see what the weather is like (82).

Adjustment to residential environments entails developing rituals for everyday survival. These rituals may be integrated with activities of family and social interaction, like those of greeting and parting, but may also be individually prescribed ways of doing things in the kitchen, workshop, or other domestic spaces (Saile, 1985). Individual behavior patterns have a prescribed content of some combination of components, which may include time, place, artifacts, spatial orientation, object and task, kinesthetic relationships, interaction with others, and sequence of events. Typically, the ritualized activities are habitual, involving specific behaviors that have become internalized.

Defining Personal Rituals

Personal rituals are not the same as rituals performed around significant events, such as family gatherings, holidays, or birthdays nor in special places such as churches. These socially oriented rituals are related to shared traditions whose major purpose may be transformation, reaffirmation, or renewal (Saile, 1985). For example, researchers studying family rituals in autobiographies find at least one-third of the descriptions deal with religious activities, holidays, and anniversaries, family recreation, and homecoming (Bossard and Boll, 1950). Personal rituals do not reflect common rules or shared traditions, they are personal and individual. Seamon (1979) comes close to our meaning of personal rituals when he suggests that "people at home do not have to think about what they are doing all the time, they can just do things and be themselves." He cites an example of "smooth routines," or routines that contribute to a feeling of comfort and control. "My mother knows the exact location if everything in our house. She has a place for everything. She doesn't have to figure out where a particular thing is; she goes to it automatically. I'll need some string, for example, and she'll go immediately to the right drawer. I'd have to check a few places before I'd find it—if I did then" (79).

Typically, when one moves from home to a new situation, such as an assisted-living facility, giving up one's home of long duration constitutes a break in the continuity of the "smooth routine." Thus, change signifies more than giving up one's home; a heretofore unrecognized consequence of the disruption is the negative impact it has on the ritualized activities that one relies on in the performance of daily life activities—unique, individual patterns of action that are routinely performed and that have a predictable outcome. Rituals help to give meaning to individuals in terms of who they are, where they are, what they do, and why they do it. When people become frail or otherwise unable to enact their ritualized activities, the consistency and continuity of daily life is disrupted. These individualized rituals are the glue that bonds people to a place called home. Being deprived of ritual actions creates enormous difficulties in sustaining a sense of place and a sense of self. An appropriate environmental and psychosocial context in which to situate individualized rituals is necessary to maintain or improve the quality of life for the aging individual.

The Importance of Personal Rituals

When time, place, and circumstances change and those rituals can no longer be performed in the established manner, there is diminution of self. When these losses accumulate and pervade one's entire spectrum of daily life activities, as often happens in residential retirement facilities, there may be profound loss of identity, self-esteem, and relationship to place and community. An example of a personal ritual is the application of makeup. The time and location are very specific and very individual. Perhaps the mirror must be well lighted, the products laid out methodically, and the makeup applied in a prescribed manner. If the physical setting is changed, or if these elements are not in their place and as a consequence cannot be used in the established manner, there is a disruption in the ritual. Cooking is another example, wherein using the bowls and pans, dishes and silverware and table-cloths of one's grandmother or mother is a personal ritual that exceeds the needs of daily nutrition. It is the generational link that is vital; it supplies the visual and tactile relationship to those no longer present and serves to remind each family member of who they are and where they are.

Personalizing Daily Life Activities

It is not so much daily activities per se that are of central concern as the manner in which each person routinely goes about performing these activities in a set time and place. Each individual has a singular set of routine behaviors or rituals. For instance, a woman who lived alone had a fixed morning ritual regarding the making and drinking of tea. She would first put a pan of water on the stove to boil. The pan had a family history. It had been used to warm baby bottles when she was an infant. When she went off to college, she was given the pan, after her father replaced the chipped knob on its lid. She also had a variety of cups given to her by family and friends, and these too had special meaning. Each morning she would choose one of these cups and pour in the hot tea. She would then take the tea into the bathroom and set it on the counter of the sink while she took a shower. After her shower, the tea would have cooled sufficiently to drink.

When the woman moved to a place with two roommates, she discontinued the ritual. First, all three roommates used the same bathroom, so there was little time for cooling the tea. Second, there was no counter on the bathroom sink and therefore no place to put her cup. Thus, a change to a shared residence and a design feature of that shared residence (lack of a bathroom counter) disrupted an important ritual. While this example does not constitute a severe break in the self-definition of an individual, many such disruptions that might aggregate during a major life event, such as relocation into a retirement facility, may in fact create a personal identity crisis.

Environments, Personal Rituals, and Spatial Relationships

Spatial relationships establish connections between physical space and the rituals of the individual. An examination of such relationships in four settings—hotels, rental vacation homes, shared residences, and reserved seating—reveals subtle nuances of individual and environmental interactions. Each of these settings represents a different level of "ownership," or ability to personalize and differentiate spatial relationships.

Hotels

As an environmental type, hotels are loaded with symbolic gestures addressing the issue of "home" for hotel guests. The cleaning staff thoroughly removes any traces of the previous occupant; the welcoming staff tries to nurture the incoming guest; and the concierge is charged with seeing to every possible need. As the cleaning staff takes glasses, linens, and trash away, the former occupant's residue is removed. Fresh linens, clean glasses with "sanitation cues" of paper or plastic coverings, new rolls of tissue, new bars of soap, and new information packets replace the used ones in a ritualistic preparation for the next occupant. The welcoming staff guarantees that your room will be satisfactory and waits to provide other articles such as irons, pillows, or extra towels.

Thus, hotel operators try to achieve a global "home essence" while allowing for efficient "cleansing." The guest is left with a scripted homelike environment that may frustrate personal rituals or completely suspend them. In the attempt to cover every base, the hotel designers, in simulating "home," attempt to create a space in which the individual may carry out familiar personal rituals or act out alternate rituals. Frustration may result when the ritual is not accommodated, such as when the hangers in the closet are permanently connected to the clothes bar. After a pause, a new technique of hanging clothing emerges, but the pause generates recognition of the difference in spatial relationships. Also, the guest may be frustrated upon realizing that the furniture is bolted to the floor. Minor modifications that make the room more like "back home" may be impossible to accommodate. Through these and other conditions that cause occupants to recognize the transitional nature of the spatial relationship, hotels remain arguably the least accommodating places of occupancy.

Vacation Rental Housing

While not as continually attentive in staffing, vacation rental housing is more accommodating as ritualistic space because there are more opportunities for user-initiated changes. Units are sold based on the ability of the individual to imagine an adaptation of personal ritual. Advertisements attempt to illustrate a typical family image in the unit, either through the placement of objects that may reflect a particular lifestyle or through a film of a make-believe family using the space. After renting the vacation housing, users attempt to graft personal rituals to the new space, sometimes forcibly or sometimes comfortably, because of the unfamiliar spatial relationship and lack of favorite objects. It is surprising to examine the adaptation of the rental unit to the familiar ritual of the individual. Furniture may be moved, for example, in an attempt to personalize the unit. Failure to achieve such "ownership" through personalization results in a cargo transfer of sorts. The user, unwilling in subsequent vacations to attempt afresh the ownership ritual, carries from home to the rental unit objects that carry the necessary stamp of personalization. Pillows and silverware typically serve as symbols for the home-based ritual.

Shared Residences

Shared residences include those shared by friends, relatives, and domestic partners as well as assisted-living environments and other living accommodations. Within this category, levels of proximity vary with the type of relationship, and rules for interaction are the by-product. For example, apartment roommate rules differ from couple rules, which differ from family home rules. Rules are the negotiation of personal ritual in a communal environment. In an apartment shared by friends, rules for phone calls, visitors, quiet time, and territory play critical roles. Rules are generally nonnegotiable and are devised to preserve domestic tranquillity. Violation of these rules results in turmoil in the apartment, and negotiation for resolution often leads to additional conflict. In an apartment shared by domestic partners, however, rules may be more negotiable. Role-playing occurs, as each partner assumes a level of cooperation; domestic trouble may result when partners do not voice concern over level of participation (e.g., who does the dishes). Rules about personal space may not be recognized by the other partner and often have to be restated. The issue of proximity may destabilize individual identity and result in household conflict. In the same manner, in retirement centers, individual identity is often overlooked, and the rituals and rules formerly observed by the individual may be violated by staff and management. This violation results in a critical loss of identity of self and alienation from place and community.

Reserved Seating

Reserved seating creates a heightened awareness of personal ritual that is less apparent in any other physical place. On the airplane, bus, or train, individuals engage fastidiously in the affected behaviors of personal ritual. Expressive rituals of eating, sleeping, viewing, reading, and covering occupy seemingly endless minutes of forced contact. To satisfy personal needs in vehicles that are less adaptable to change, such as airplanes, personal controls are available for air, light, and communication. Conversely, the airplane seat is sized to serve the average individual and so by its very nature reduces individuality. Any deviation results in a less optimum fit. An above-average-sized person finds that any movement may be the source of physical contact with the stranger: rubbing elbows, bumping knees, breathing into the face of the sleeping stranger. When areas of personal demarcation are reduced to the two-inch width of a shared armrest, these points of contact are continual. To further complicate the situation, airplane seats recline into the lap of the passenger behind, encroaching on another personal space. Even the accommodation of the telephone is situated to force shared space. Individuals negotiate these proximal dislocations of spatial relationship by affecting behavior that clearly signals the need to be left alone (e.g, covering the body with the provided blanket, staring resolutely out the window or down the aisle, reading with utter concentration, or sleeping).

This type of behavior may also be observed in traditional retirement facilities, which reduce the individual's control so much that the resident is forced to affect control through the same types of isolation behavior. As lack of control increases, affectations increase as well. When the place is more amenable to individual control, affectations are not as necessary, and mechanisms to support these affectations often are not provided.

Summary

Due to the short-term or temporary nature of occupancy ownership of environmental settings such as hotels, vacation rental housing, and transportation conveyances, personal rituals are often suspended, changed, or adapted. It is only when a person occupies a more permanent environment that personal rituals may be drastically impacted. Thus, not only the type of environment but also the temporality of the environment influences personal rituals. In much the same way, a person may be more willing to suspend the need for privacy for a short time in an acute health care setting such as a hospital but would without a doubt be unwilling to give up privacy prerogatives in a more permanent residential setting.

The examples of the hotel, the vacation rental housing, the shared residence, and the reserved seat considered in terms of temporality reveal the critical nature of personal ritual in an individual's adaptation to environment. It may be argued that the business traveler who frequently uses hotels and airplanes develops personal rituals for these particular environments. For example, the traveler may have a strategy for dealing with unfamiliar hotel rooms, including bringing a family photo, an alarm clock, or a journal to accommodate personal rituals. As well, the traveler may use airplanes so often that the seating limitation becomes familiar and the process of working in the seat becomes standardized. It may also be argued that vacation rental housing in the form of a time-share is the site of alternate family rituals. A family that uses the same time-share over several years establishes routines for dealing with environmental change, such as alternative meal preparation techniques. Therefore, approaching the study of personal ritual requires an acknowledgment of not only the type of environment but also the temporal quality of the environment.

Personal behavior reveals the role of ritual in daily life. As each person strives to achieve some set goal, habits and rituals entwine to affect the process. Personal ritual is the web of personal habits, daily activities, and public and private roles, which vary with each individual and thus must be evaluated on an individual level. This web is analogous to the spider web: each fiber connects to a larger whole, remaining integral while retaining the fingerprint of a particular entity; it is not a blueprint to produce an identical web. Although spider webs are structurally similarly, the patterns, like personal rituals, remain unique.

The Safety Net of Ritual Experience

The daily activities of home and work create a type of safety net of ritual experience. This net, or web, of interconnected activities reinforces a physical environmental experience that is intimately tied to a social experience of public and private realms. As the atmosphere of the physical environment changes—for example, when children leave home or when people retire—the time frame for the occupation of spaces or spatial allocation changes. The home divides into places to ignore and places to occupy. The range of home shifts as outside commitments change. The actual home may also change as people retire and move to smaller homes. Cooking and cleaning time may vary as well, as the aging population discriminates less against a social code and more against an internal code, an inverse proportion along the life span of the individual. Cleaning rituals such as laundry Monday (or as it is known in Louisiana, red beans and rice day) may alter as home commitments lessen. People may continue to observe the day that the tasks were once performed and the food that was prepared on that day, as in the example above, or they may continue to perform the actual tasks.

"Housework is the conventional cleaning, ordering, saving, and discarding common to almost everyone who lives without servants. Housework, though obviously integrated into the economic scheme of advanced societies, is akin to ritual. The wiping of dust from windowsills, the stacking of dishes, the pushing of cross-axial lines of dirt across the floor with a broom are repeated actions that contribute to a sense of salvation, preserving both the physical order of the house and the personal order of the dweller" (Ingersoll, 1987). In a culture that values the cleaning ritual and that creates validation through a list of chores accomplished, any radical shift in these rituals may be traumatic.

Residential Change and the Dreaded Three Rs

Perhaps one of the biggest challenges that the management and staff of assisted-living facilities face is the adjustment of residents moving from their private homes. When residents move, they face those dreaded three Rs: reduce, reorder, and replace.

Typically, relocatees must reduce their personal possessions, since they cannot bring everything with them to their new locale. Difficult choices must be made among the artifacts linked to a lifetime of memories. Moving from a ten-room house, for instance, to a one-bedroom apartment necessitates drastic reduction choices. It is also a reminder that one's life space is being reduced. Reordering one's schedule of life's daily activities and one's lifestyle in general includes changing priorities regarding, for example, what to wear, what to do, and where to go. Replacement has many meanings. For example, one replaces one's familiar home environment with another, old friends with new friends, and familiar fixtures, furniture, and room configurations with others. Any and all of these changes impact seriously how, when, where, and under what circumstances one's personal rituals are performed (Bourestom and Pastalan, 1975).

The Reciprocity of Personal and Social Rituals

The rituals related to activities of daily living help to preserve both the physical order of home and the personal order of the resident. Mead (1973), in her discussion of social rituals, claims that social ritual is a type of guarantee or security for both the participant and the social group. In fact, a genuine social crisis occurs when the social group loses its rituals. Without rituals, the continuity of group identity begins to break down.

There is a critical link between personal rituals and the social group or community. For our purposes, let us consider the social group to be a residential retirement community composed of residents, staff, and management. For the community to be viable, the residents, staff, and management must reflect a commitment to community solidarity. On the other hand, the community, particularly the staff and management, must understand and be sympathetic with the individual's need to autonomously perform his or her rituals as a way of maintaining individual identity and establishing an attachment to place.

A reciprocal relationship exists between the social cohesion of the group and the degree to which personal rituals are performed with group understanding and support. If personal rituals cannot be individualized in activities of daily life due to staff or management rules, then the sense of the physical order of home and the personal order of the resident is compromised, and alienation from the social group occurs. Since personal rituals are so closely tied to a sense of identity and an attachment to place, the resident's commitment to the group is deeply affected. Hence, participation in group solidarity rituals, such as cultural or recreational activities or the obeisance to community rules, breaks down. Individual and group morale is low, and in Mead's words, "the group/community is in social crisis" (94–96).

This perspective helps explain why some retirement communities have low morale or a lack of solidarity and why the residents are alienated and have little commitment to or personal investment in their community. For a community to have solidarity, there must be a mutual exchange between the individual and the group. The core of this exchange is that the group gives to the individual the necessary personal autonomy regarding activities of daily life and that the individual gives a commitment to the group for maintaining group cohesion.

Conclusion

We hope that the preceding discussion provides new perspectives on the connections between and among personal rituals, self-identity, attachment to place, and community solidarity. Nonetheless, it is unrealistic to expect most group homes to be true, normal homes. Age segregation itself sets such places apart from the norm. Assisted living by its definition strives to deliver managed personal and health care services in a group setting that is residential in character. As such, it should nurture the needs of personal rituals to retain a meaningful definition of independence, self, and place in the face of radically different conditions and processes. By fostering a greater appreciation and understanding among families, significant others, and caregivers of the need to maintain rituals important to older residents, their quality of life will be preserved or enhanced.

We suggest to researchers and practitioners that further study of personal ritual is important to gain greater insights on age-related matters of environment and behavior, since personal rituals are actions to which every person of every age may relate.

References

Bossard, J., and E. Boll. 1950. *Ritual in Family Living: A Contemporary Study.* Philadelphia: University of Pennsylvania Press.

Bourestom, N., and L. Pastalan. 1975. *Forced Relocation: Setting, Staff and Patient Effects: Final Report.* Ann Arbor: Institute of Gerontology, University of Michigan.

Ingersoll, R. 1987. Housework: Understanding the rituals of home. *CRIT* 19:38–42.

Mead, M. 1973. Ritual and social crisis. In J. Shaughnessy, ed., *The Roots of Ritual.* Grand Rapids, Mich.: Eerdmans.

Pastalan, L. 1976. *Report on Pennsylvania Nursing Home Preparation for Relocation Program.* Ann Arbor: University of Michigan Institute of Gerontology.

Pastalan, L., V. Jones, B. Schwarz, R. Sekulski, and L. Struble. 1993. *Homelike Attributes of Dementia Special Care Units.* Ann Arbor: University of Michigan College of Architecture and Urban Planning.

Saile, D. 1985. The ritual establishment of home. In I. Altman and C. Werner, eds., *Home Environments, Human Behavior, and Environment: Advances in Theory and Research.* Vol. 8. New York: Plenum.

Seamon, D. 1979. *A Geography of the Lifeworld.* New York: St. Martin's.

CHAPTER 6

Integrating Cultural Heritage into Assisted-Living Environments

URIEL COHEN
KEITH DIAZ MOORE

The recent renaissance in cultural identity illuminates the significance of cultural identity for one's positive self-image. Self-identity, self-worth, along with feelings of dignity and respect, are defining characteristics of an elder's image. A great deal of the personal identity and continuity of the self is grounded in one's cultural background. Therefore, culturally experienced phenomena provide what are often overlooked resources for creating therapeutic programs and meaningful environments for an aging society. These environments are particularly important for persons with early- and middle-stage dementia, who are often found in assisted-living facilities. The challenges in this domain include

— The thoughtful integration of culturally relevant phenomena with the latest research-based information about environments for older persons.
— The need to overcome the tendency of both designers and their clients to use imitations of shapes, forms, geometries, and decorations as an appropriate expression of culture.
— Developing for caregivers a richer inventory of environmental opportunities and activities, which reach beyond conventional cultural expressions.

This chapter employs illustrations from several case studies and focuses on a conceptual framework that facilitates discussion about the transaction between the unique needs of elderly persons and culturally responsive environmental design. It addresses the need, and presents tentative approaches, for a more thoughtful consideration of schemata behind the physical expression: the spatial organization of the environment and its responsiveness to lifestyle, social structure, daily activities, and rituals (as well as other factors), all of which hold meaning and significance to those particular users. It suggests the use of experiential—rather than abstract—cultural phenomena that reinforce and are integratable with aging-related therapeutic goals and concerns.

The Context: Moving toward Individualized Care and More Responsive Environments

Much of the research about older persons and their environments addresses universal issues of aging, such as decline in health, loss of spouse, and shrinking economic resources and their effects on housing and living environments. The common solutions typically reflect the attitude that older persons form a homogeneous group. However, this is certainly not the case in the United States, where the demography of older people is becoming increasingly heterogeneous. In the upcoming years, older persons moving into assisted-living facilities will increasingly have culturally diverse backgrounds. Part of the current trend toward individualized care responds to this cultural uniqueness and illustrates how discredited the generalizations about universal aging issues have become.

The Disconnection of Elderly Persons and Their Environment

Individualized care represents a paradigm shift toward a resident-centered model, away from the medical model of care (Rader, 1995). In the medical model, facilities "seem to concentrate on keeping the patient alive and managing behavior as expediently as possible"(Ohta and Ohta, 1988:805). Within this model, elderly residents are typically viewed as a homogeneous group—"the patients"—sharing similar losses in competency, such as visual acuity, dexterity, and cognitive capacity. The care environment reflects this view, focusing on the distribution of uniform services, with each room and each floor identical.

For residents in many congregate settings, daily existence centers on physical needs and has little resemblance to their former life in the community. Institutionalized life is organized by routines and schedules that meet institutional imperatives while providing few opportunities to exercise choice and experience activities taken for granted in the "outside" world. Rader argues that this medical model results in limited dignity and reduced normality of life for individual residents.

The costs of the medical model and its homogenization of residents are quite clear. Alienation and withdrawal from one's environment is a well-documented phenomenon in the typical institutional nursing home (Langer and Rodin, 1976; Küller, 1988). This feeling of disconnection is common in many long-term care settings. Transplanted into unfamiliar surroundings, many times against their will, elderly persons feel a separation from their social network and a disconnection from their past. These feelings result in the institutionalized elderly perceiving themselves as having a severe lack of control over their lives. Abeles (1991:297) observes that "those with little sense of control may be more likely than others to adopt the 'sick role,' to 'prematurely' withdraw from various daily activities, and to exhibit 'excess' disability." Time becomes regimented according to staff schedules rather than the residents' own personal rhythms. Events become routine and empty, disconnected from the past and the future. This rigid regimentation, together with patients' lack of control and autonomy, results in less independent, more poorly adjusted, and less engaged individuals.

Toward Individualized Care in Assisted-Living Environments

Individualized care, conversely, begins with the premise that it is critical for caregivers to build a relationship with their residents in order to know them as unique individuals, understand their behaviors, and thus be able to provide individualized interventions. This model is characterized by a process of discovery that includes the review of the life history of residents in addition to the more traditional measures of personal, physical, emotional, and mental status. The care programs that result, therefore, differ from resident to resident. It is in this movement toward individualized care that assisted living lies. Assisted living remains ill defined but usually revolves around the concept of the provision of housing and services in response to *individual needs* and to do so in a way that maximizes *independence and dignity*. Wilson

(1990) articulates four underlying concepts of the assisted-living philosophy: creating a place of one's own, serving the unique individual, sharing responsibility, and allowing resident choice and control. All four of these points parallel the goals and desires of individualized care.

The homogenized perspective of the elderly has resulted in ineffectual, sterile environments. Yet the current trend toward individualized care presents a daunting task for architects and care providers alike. While each room may certainly be designed to afford personalization (see latter discussion on culturally significant design enablers), the entire organizational and physical environments of the facility must attempt to be responsive to the needs of the group. If individualized care is the emerging paradigm, a reasonable question is, How can one conceptualize meaningful environmental interventions that would enhance self-identity and residents' quality of life in a group setting?

Cultural Heritage as a Therapeutic Resource

Every individual is a part of a particular culture, occupying a unique position within his or her social world and possessing a unique history. Culture is an integral part of self-definition and manifests in the goal-directed actions of the individual. These actions are delimited by the expectations of the social organization of which that person is a part. This highlights the importance for care professionals to create culturally meaningful experiences but also challenges environmental designers to create spaces that can adequately support and enhance such experiences. According to Henderson (1994), the cost of not addressing such cultural factors or, even worse, not understanding and not using them in a positive way, includes potential maladaptive behavior, such as disruptive verbal communication (e.g., unfamiliar language), and nonverbal communication (e.g., inappropriate touching or speaking distance). These behaviors may contribute toward a spiral into depression, disengagement, and overall loss of self-esteem. Yet culture is a global and abstract term; to design for culture is a demanding task, which most designers and care providers cannot operationalize. What is needed is a working definition and a conceptual approach for culture that can serve as a basis for the decision-making process.

Defining Culture

One of the earliest definitions of the modern usage of the term *culture* is attributed to Sir Edward Taylor (1871), who wrote that culture is "that complex whole which includes knowledge, belief, art, morals, law, language and any other capabilities and habits acquired by man [sic] as a member of society." In the context of congregate living or care environments, culture can be described as the social baggage that clients bring with them—all bundled in terms of their life experience. According to Boyle and Andrews (1995:12), there are four basic characteristics of culture:

1. Culture is *learned* from birth through the processes of language acquisition and socialization. From society's viewpoint, socialization is the way culture is transmitted and the individual is fitted into the group's organized way of life.

2. Culture is *shared* by all members of the same cultural group; in fact, it is the

sharing of cultural beliefs and patterns that binds people under one identity as a group (even though this is not always a conscious process).

3. Culture is an *adaptation* to specific conditions related to environmental and technical factors and to the availability of natural resources.
4. Culture is a *dynamic*, ever-changing process.

To these four should be added a fifth:

5. Although culture is a universal phenomena attributed to larger groups (e.g., Native Americans), its manifested expressions are always group-specific, where the group is identified by a smaller common denominator (e.g., the Oneida of Wisconsin).

Thus culture, as a concept, needs to be pared down to manageable parts, to concrete and potentially observable manifestations such as social networks, roles, and institutions. Rapoport (1990) provides a framework for subdividing culture into four "expressions": worldview, values, lifestyle, and activities. Rapoport argues that the conceptualization of lifestyle is particularly useful for the study of environments and leads to activities and systems of activities. The rationale for this is that the characteristics that distinguish subcultural groups are more immediate and more tangible than those that differentiate entirely different societies (e.g., recently immigrated Russian Jews share little with native New York City elderly Jews and may have more in common with first-generation, non-Jewish, elderly Americans of Slavic origin).

Lifestyle groupings are especially appropriate as means to operationalize culture when cultural pluralism exists. In such heterogeneity, cultures mix and become multifarious. However, there remains a core of cultural uniqueness within each lifestyle group, whether that be in terms of values, social norms, or the like. According to Rapoport, lifestyles determine how residential settings are utilized and what activities will occur there. Activities and settings are interconnected phenomena related to lifestyle membership. The specificities of activities, and particularly their more latent aspects (i.e., their meaning), vary from culture to culture and from lifestyle to lifestyle, and they begin to explain the diversity of environments that serve humankind.

The implications of culture being group-specific are clear. The environmental expressions of cultural heritage are not generalizable to large classes of persons; rather, they respond to specific lifestyle needs. For instance, the environment created for retired farmers in Oklahoma should be distinguishable from that created for urban dwellers in Manhattan. Therefore, the organizational and physical environments of housing for older persons *need to be as congruent as possible with the experiential needs and desires of the residents* for whom the care facility is home.

The Significance of Material and Social Culture

While physical, social, and organizational environments do not determine an individual's quality of life, together they certainly have a substantial impact upon people, particularly upon those with reduced competence. Such reduced competence increases the criticality of the environment, which must be especially supportive of the needs and activities of the residents. Therefore, culturally experienced phenomena can provide often overlooked resources for creating therapeutic programs and meaningful environments for older persons.

The person's material and social heritage provide the sources, reference points, and background on which activities can be built. In defining those reference points, both the scale of group membership and the temporal dimensions are factors in establishing the "audience" for particular environmental interventions. In terms of scale, humans are inherently social animals and associate themselves with group membership at several levels of aggregation. For example, dairy farmers may associate themselves with their neighboring farmers, the farmers that belong to their local co-op, all farmers in the state, and dairy farmers in general. Each of these groups contain within them expected cultural norms as interpreted by a particular farmer. Thus, culture is a collective term, incorporating references to properties of groups at a multiplicity of scales. Rowles (1984), discussing the sociocultural milieu of the rural elderly, vividly illustrates the lifestyle and value systems in his case study but acknowledges that such systems are not universal but, rather, are aspects of a particular subculture within a larger cultural system.

Cultural norms are not static but evolving, and therefore they involve a temporal component. Different generations have different life experiences, and what is appropriate for one generation may be viewed differently a generation or two removed. The most immediate ramification of this can be seen in the phenomenon of ageism, wherein one individual tries to force others into particular behaviors based on their age. Beliefs, social customs, and manners evolve through time; in the context of assisted-living facilities, staff will have different cultural expectations than will the residents. When designing the social, physical, and organizational aspects of assisted-living environments for the elderly, residents and staff actively need to integrate the concepts and expectations of the residents' culture, as defined in terms of scale and time, with therapeutic goals aimed at successful aging. A study examining a number of special care units suggests that when the physical, social, and organizational environments are structured to meet the needs of a specific population, there is a noticeable improvement in the quality of life of residents coupled with a decrease in the amount of maladaptive behavior (Mace, 1993). The question becomes how to define this "specific population." The concept of lifestyle helps target those organizational and physical interventions that would be appropriate for a specific audience with a given material culture and social heritage.

Integrating Cultural Heritage into the Environment: Problems and Challenges

Mace and other researchers argue that the purpose of special care environments for dementia is to focus interventions that are appropriate to a specific population. These populations, unfortunately, remain typically defined in clinical-medical terms. Yet, with the movement toward special care environments for older persons gaining currency, the door is open to a more socially meaningful interpretation. However, even contemporary and innovative settings that attempt more socially based programming use only a

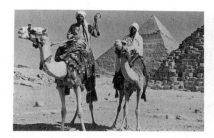

FIGURE 6.1. The pyramids in Giza (left) and a contemporary health clinic in Cairo, Egypt (right)

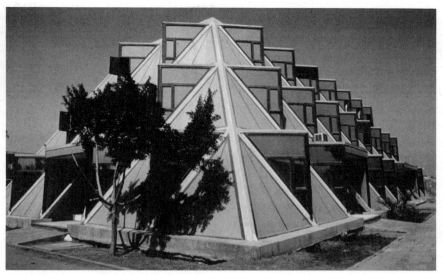

limited and unimaginative range of cultural, religious, and ethnic expressions.

Several problems contribute to the underdeveloped state of this domain. Foremost is the lack of a conceptual framework, or theory, that describes, explains, and organizes knowledge about applied cultural heritage in the context of assisted living and other care environments for older persons. As a result, care-providing organizations lack the tools to operationalize cultural heritage into programs, activities, and environments. What is typically practiced is limited to a few obvious areas of application—religious practices and rituals, celebration of holidays, and the like. While these cultural expressions are important and useful, they represent only a part of a much larger and richer expanse of untapped potential. Because of the limited input from clients and care providers, designers of environments for older persons also suffer from a lack of conceptual and substantive guidance. Architects' natural tendency is to focus on symbolic and abstract aspects of building form. Their interpretations of cultural phenomena are often either too abstract or, conversely, too literal. The pyramids in Giza, for example, served as the inspiration for a contemporary health clinic in Cairo, Egypt (see figure 6.1). However, field evaluations indicate that the clinic fails to convey any cultural message to its users and appears to be operationally dysfunctional, primarily because of its arbitrary, vacuous architecture (Schramm, 1996). As Rapoport (1983) comments in regard to designers operating in an applied-cultural context: "Imitation leads to inappropriate results because it typically involves superficial appearance . . . shape, geometry, decoration . . . rather than the principles behind the physical expression, the spatial organization and its relation to lifestyle and social structure" (251).

Toward a Conceptual Framework: A Convergence of Therapeutic Goals and Culturally Based Interventions

A Conceptual Framework for Therapeutic Environments

Throughout this chapter, it is suggested that culture provides untapped resources for creating activities and environments that reinforce and are integratable with aging-related therapeutic goals and concerns. Relating therapeutic goals to environmental design principles has become commonplace in the aging-environment literature (e.g., Calkins, 1988; Wilson, 1990; Regnier, Hamilton, and Yatabe, 1995). Cohen and Weisman (1991) present a conceptual framework for environments for people with dementia, which Regnier and colleagues extend to assisted living environments in general (see figure 6.2). This framework conceptualizes the environment into three components: the social, the physical, and the organizational. The relationships between the individual and the environment are transactional in nature. In other words, the environmental experience of the individual involves a continuing mutual reciprocity between person and environment. The framework assumes that the nature and needs of residents define therapeutic goals, which in turn help shape the physical setting directly; the therapeutic goals also influence the physical setting indirectly through their relationships with the social and organizational contexts.

Therapeutic Goals: Focusing on Continuity of the Self

Cohen and Weisman (1991) developed a list of resident-based therapeutic goals that respond to critical issues, symptoms, and concerns of people with cognitive impairments and their caregivers:

— Maximum safety and security
— Maximum awareness and orientation
— Support of functional abilities
— Facilitation of social contact
— Provision of privacy
— Provision of opportunities for personal control
— Regulation of stimulation
— Provision of continuity of the self

Arguably, all of these goals apply to gerontological environments in general, as is illustrated by Regnier and colleagues in their principles for assisted-living housing. The goals are intentionally expressed in broad and abstract language. "One cannot make specific planning or design decisions on the basis of broad statements regarding 'preservation of dignity' or 'maximizing independence'" (Cohen and Weisman, 1991:29). The intention is for the goals to highlight the desired relationships between residents and the environments they occupy.

There is a recognition of the importance that the sociocultural context plays in the environmental experience of older persons in congregate living environments (figure 6.2). Rather than viewing the social context as passively defined by the therapeutic goals, here it is suggested that the social context is a significant player in understanding and developing those therapeutic goals. An important but latent quality of self is membership in a social group. Canter (1988:7) asserts "that the actions which an individual performs are structured by the possibilities made available through the role structure of which that individual is a part." This has direct implications for deepening the understanding of these therapeutic goals, because it widens

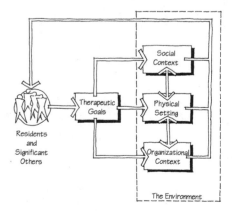

FIGURE 6.2. *A conceptual framework of therapeutic environments for older persons*
SOURCE: *Adapted from Cohen and Weisman, 1991:2*

the vision from the individual to include the cultural context in which that person acts. Continuity of the self thus can be expanded as a concept to focus not solely on individual people but also on their sociocultural identity.

A Conceptual Framework for Culturally Responsive Environments

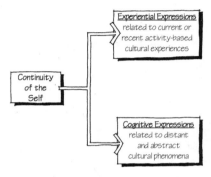

FIGURE 6.3. *The two primary expressions of continuity of self*

Continuity of the self becomes a primary therapeutic goal with implications for each of the others. It requires the provisions for continuity of a familiar lifestyle and the use of residents' life experience: childhood, education, religion, community, family, work, social relations, ethnicity, language, and whatever else defines a person. As a therapeutic goal, continuity of the self addresses the continuity between the residents' past and present lives and their past and present selves. A very simplified division of the universe of cultural expressions groups them into two categories: *cognitive expressions*, which require abstract thinking and involves remote phenomenon (e.g., the use of symbolism); and *experiential expressions*, which are tangible and related to activity-based cultural experiences (see figure 6.3).

Cognitive expressions of cultural phenomena typically employ symbolic and abstract material. Examples include a high school building formed in the shape of a turtle on an Indian reservation (depicting the clan of the turtle, which has a special meaning to the local Indian nation), or the Confederate flag hung in a community center in a southern community. The commonality among these and countless other possible cognitive expressions are their evocative potential, level of abstraction, and their passive, symbolic nature. Experiential expressions, unlike cognitive ones, involve situations in which the cultural material is tangible and perceptually accessible and contributes to engagement and interaction and typically involves activity.

Integrating Cultural Heritage in Environments for Older Persons

The role of abstract thinking, information processing, and symbolism in human life is critical. Yet, in the context of assisted-living environments for older persons, reduced cognitive capacities and other limitations on users' capabilities lead to greater emphasis on their remaining capabilities. The therapeutic goals listed above focus on interventions that stimulate interaction and engagement, aimed at the maintenance of functional independence. Many of these therapeutic goals translate into environmental interventions and solutions whose characteristics overlap with experiential expressions: environmental experiences that are perceptually and physically accessible; that involve activity, engagement, and interaction; and that are based on cultural phenomena. This approach is particularly applicable to assisted-living environments in which more than 40 percent of residents have some form of cognitive impairment (Coopers & Lybrand, 1993). Thus, experiential expressions provide a better approach for achieving continuity of the self among assisted-living residents.

Culturally Based Activities and Environments: Case Studies

Through the following case studies, we hope to demonstrate how to meaningfully address culturally significant environmental experiences. These cases are categorized into three bases for environmental interventions: ethnicity, religion, and shared life experience (see figure 6.4). These three groups are neither mutually exclusive nor exhaustive. As mentioned previously, there are different ways of parceling the universe of cultural expressions. Ethnicity, religion, and common life experience were selected for heuristic purposes, facilitating a manageable organization and analysis of the cases.

A fourth category of culturally based interventions is that of design enablers. These are open-ended solutions that facilitate and accommodate future and variable solutions by users (e.g., personalization of the individual room by its resident). While the specific expressions presented in the case studies should not be considered universally applicable, the underlying theme of sensitivity to, and meaningful use of, cultural phenomena is a powerful universal resource.

Environmental Interventions Based on Ethnicity

CASE STUDY: THE LONGHOUSES OF THE ONEIDA
The longhouse of the Oneida was used as a model for a group home for thirty-six residents on their reservation in Hobart, Wisconsin. The home has four clusters of nine residents each, with each cluster emulating the traditional organization of the Oneida domicile vernacular—the Oneida longhouse (see figure 6.5). However, the building form is not the main vehicle of the cultural message: the interior design and general planning reflect an integration of the latest research-based information about environments for older persons with the material culture and traditions of the Oneida.

Culturally Meaningful Experiences: The meaningful experiences tapped in this setting were old veteran's social smoking, the pursuit of traditional crafts, and gardening and harvesting. Each has a particular meaning for the Oneida and is therefore uniquely addressed in this design.

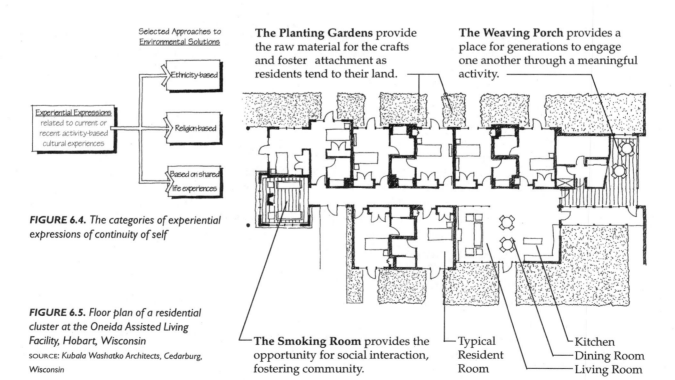

The Planting Gardens provide the raw material for the crafts and foster attachment as residents tend to their land.

The Weaving Porch provides a place for generations to engage one another through a meaningful activity.

FIGURE 6.4. The categories of experiential expressions of continuity of self

FIGURE 6.5. Floor plan of a residential cluster at the Oneida Assisted Living Facility, Hobart, Wisconsin
SOURCE: Kubala Washatko Architects, Cedarburg, Wisconsin

The Smoking Room provides the opportunity for social interaction, fostering community.

Typical Resident Room

Kitchen
Dining Room
Living Room

The smoking room: A feature of traditional Oneida Indian culture is the gathering of males to smoke, typically reflected in folklore as the sharing of the peace pipe. For this particular generation of Oneida male elders, a common historical connection is military service. As has been seen in many army movies and retold in countless family histories, smoking often served as a common social bond. The significant experience of male comradeship—here facilitated by social smoking, drinking beer, and telling tales—is addressed in the activity-setting of the smoking room. Called the fireplace lounge, the room is designed in each longhouse to offer the opportunity for social gatherings. The smoking room is the veteran's club; it fosters meaningful social interaction, resulting in a reinforced, positive notion of self.

The weaving porch and the planting gardens: The weaving porch facilitates the meeting between residents and the younger Oneida generation—who are often supervised by their grandmothers after school hours—to learn and experience a traditional craft. The skill of the craft is only part of the activity, as the entire tapestry of the experience is considered in this design. A planting garden is provided for each resident, and with it the full cycle of traditional agriculture can be experienced, from cultivating the soil, to planting the seeds, to harvesting the plants. Working in the garden promotes both socialization and self-worth, and these attributes extend also through the traditional craft of weaving. Prairie grasses from the gardens become the raw material for the woven products. Weaving is particularly meaningful for the women of the Oneida, as it has always provided an opportunity for social engagement among women.

Discussion: The smoking room and the weaving porch may in themselves be good design interventions, since they create a residential atmosphere and provide opportunities for socialization. In this particular case, the cultural experience informs the design decisions that, in the end, renders a rich and meaningful environment. All three interventions support functional ability through meaningful activity. Gardening and harvesting encourage physical exercise and outdoor activity. Engagement in traditional craft encourages digital dexterity and enhances self-esteem from a completed meaningful activity. Even social smoking helps to maintain the individual's ability to socialize. Meaningful activity settings, such as the smoking room and weaving porches, are illustrations of a creative response to selected therapeutic goals nurtured by the consideration of activity-based cultural experiences.

Environmental Interventions Based on Religion

CASE STUDY: THE HELEN BADER CENTER
The Helen Bader Center is a residential setting for twenty-four residents with early to midstage dementia of the Alzheimer's type (see figure 6.6). It is located at the Milwaukee Jewish Home. The environment is designed to facilitate the highest level of residents' independence, to respect their privacy and dignity, and to promote activities and social interaction.

A Culturally Meaningful Experience: This facility pursues, among other goals, the promotion of Jewish identity and continuity in the elderly population that it serves.

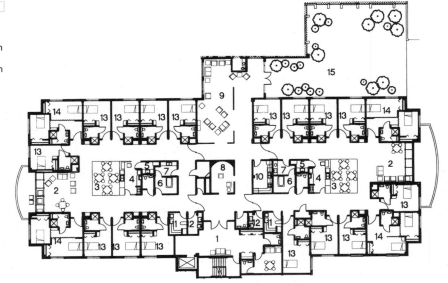

HELEN BADER CENTER

1 Lobby
2 Living Room
3 Dining Room
4 Nurishment Center
5 Med. Room
6 Bathing
7 Grooming
8 Religious Corner
9 Activity Area
10 Meat Kitchen

11 Laundry
12 Soiled Utility
13 Resident's Room (single)
14 Resident's Room (double)
15 Roof Garden

FIGURE 6.6. *Floor plan of the Helen Bader Center Special Care Unit, Helen Bader Center, Milwaukee, Wisconsin*
SOURCE: *Kahler Slater Architects*

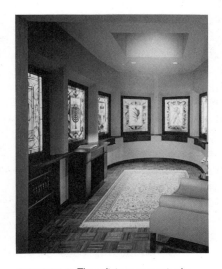

FIGURE 6.7. *The religious corner in the Helen Bader Center*

The religious corner: The religious corner is a den filled with artifacts connected with the residents' religious heritage. These artifacts are to be available as a means for engagement (e.g., candlesticks that can be used by residents in Friday-night services). The room itself is conceived as an intimate inglenook, providing an opportunity for cozy interactions of small groups (see figure 6.7).

Discussion: The overarching therapeutic goal addressed in the religious corner is to establish links to the healthy and the familiar. The plan is to provide a culturally meaningful experience of engagement with familiar religious artifacts in such a way as to facilitate simple rituals in an intimate, social atmosphere. The final design has yet to be completed. The den concept is unfortunately overshadowed by the stained glass windows depicting seven Jewish holidays. None of the books or candlesticks have yet been made available to the residents. So far, meaningful active engagement is secondary to the abstract, symbolic, and relatively sterile minishrine.

CASE STUDY: THE MILWAUKEE JEWISH HOME
The Milwaukee Jewish Home operates a continuum of care environments serving the needs of the urban Jewish community of Milwaukee. The Jewish Home offers skilled nursing and both assisted and independent-living environments in an urban neighborhood on a site overlooking Lake Michigan.

Culturally Meaningful Experiences: Two particular experiences are supported in the design of the Kosher Oasis in the Milwaukee Jewish Home: the familiar ethnic experience of socializing—or kibitzing—in the neighborhood kosher delicatessen and the religious premeal ritual of hand washing (see figures 6.8 and 6.9).

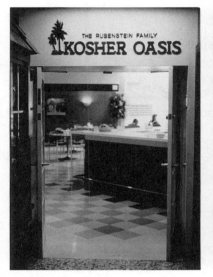

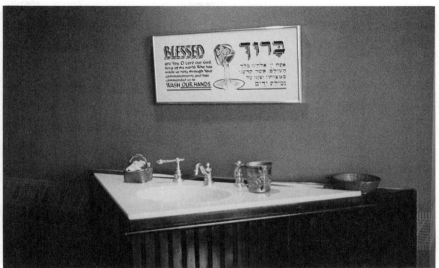

FIGURE 6.8. *Entry to the Kosher Oasis deli in the Milwaukee Jewish Home, Milwaukee, Wisconsin*
SOURCE: *Miller Meier Kenyon Cooper Architects*

FIGURE 6.9. *The handwashing sink in the Kosher Oasis deli, Milwaukee Jewish Home*

The Kosher Oasis deli and the hand-washing sink: The traditional deli functions as one of the informal social institutions in traditional Jewish neighborhoods. To be a regular at the deli, to meet friends and neighbors, and to talk over lox and bagels is common to most of the residents of the Jewish Home. Providing residents with a familiar gathering place—the neighborhood deli—facilitates socialization and independence. Residents may invite friends or family members to the Kosher Oasis in their assisted-living "neighborhood" and retain a sense of autonomy, control, and connection to community life. The Kosher Oasis incorporates the intriguing design concept of the hand-washing sink, which is available for Jewish residents and their guests to engage in the premeal ritual of hand washing. The prayer associated with the ritual is inscribed immediately above the sink. The hand-washing ritual is simple and ordinary; even partial accomplishment of this ritual can be very meaningful to a religious individual and satisfying even to a nonobservant Jew.

Discussion: The Kosher Oasis supports three therapeutic goals simultaneously by focusing on an activity common to the life experience of this given constituency. The deli maximizes autonomy and control by providing residents of the Jewish Home the ability to invite friends out for lunch, thereby providing the opportunity for socialization within the safety and security of the Jewish Home campus. The activity setting establishes links to the healthy and the familiar—the neighborhood deli. The social rules of the deli are an integral part of urban Jewish life and support the continuity of one's life experience. The overall design concept of the deli has been taken one step further through consideration of a meaningful religious ritual associated with meals. The hand-washing sink is very simple and single-purposed in supporting functional ability through the meaningful activity of premeal hand washing, a common religious ritual.

CASE STUDY: ELDERHAUS

Elderhaus, a residential facility in Stevens Point, Wisconsin, is a group home for persons with cognitive impairments. The home has two autonomous duplexes, each with eight residents. Stevens Point is home to a large concentration of first- and second-generation Polish immigrants, a community steeped in Catholicism. Catholicism, like Judaism, is a religion with many rituals and religious observances that hold great significance for devoted believers.

A Culturally Meaningful Experience: Because of the constituency being served, it was imperative that the design provide for the continuity of Catholic religious engagement. The dedicated holy place in one's home, where one engages in intimate prayer and other rituals, serves as a deeply personalized outlet for religious participation.

The Catholic shrine: In the family room of each duplex is a shrine with various religious artifacts, including crucifixes, candles, and rosaries. While some of the artifacts are solely symbolic, others, such as the candles and rosaries, promote meaningful engagement, connecting residents to their religious heritage. The shrine provides a recognizable place for this religious activity. To further encourage this cultural connection, retired nuns visit Elderhaus several times a week, providing the potential for such therapeutic religious interactions as devotions, communion, hymn singing, and one-on-one religious guidance and support. The residents also observe many of the Catholic canon laws, such as Friday abstinence from eating meat. All of these interventions promote the concept of continuity of the self in a spiritually meaningful fashion.

Discussion: Providing a place for religious observance and practice (e.g., a chapel) is not unusual in large facilities; it is less common in smaller facilities. This case study illustrates an economical yet effective implementation of an environmental solution. Two points should be noted: the importance of an activity-based connection and an environment conducive to such activity. Crucifixes and pictures of Jesus reflect the Christian heritage, but the artifacts that stimulate most residents are those that trigger a religious connection through active engagement. Many traditional Catholic residences have such shrines in which rosaries or other prayers are offered. This intervention promotes resident participation, establishes a link to the healthy and the familiar, and reinforces the individual's sense of self.

Environmental Interventions Based on Shared Life Experience

CASE STUDY: THE SEDGEWOOD COMMONS ALZHEIMER'S CARE FACILITY

The Sedgewood Commons Alzheimer's Care Facility, in Falmouth, Maine, is a home for ninety-six residents, many suffering from Alzheimer's disease and related dementias. This 46,000-square-foot facility stresses the preservation of the residents' individual identity by supporting their responsibility for the activities of everyday living. The design of the facility recreates what is meaningful about a home, attempting to draw on residents' long-

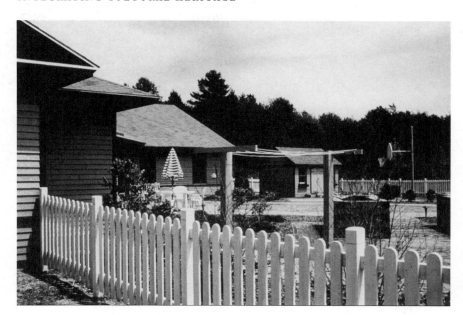

FIGURE 6.10. *Garden at Sedgewood Commons, Sedgewood Commons Alzheimer's Care Facility, Falmouth, Maine*
SOURCE: *SMRT Architects*

term memory. One main design directive was to address the positive therapeutic potential of outdoor space.

A Culturally Meaningful Experience: The outdoor yard reflects the traditional New England home garden with white picket fence bordering a tree-lined street (the walking path)(see figure 6.10). A significant part of New England life has roots in the area's English colonial era. This history has heavily influenced the rules of place in New England, where the yard symbolizes the fertility and blessing of a family. Jackson (1994) writes of the New England garden: "It was where the members of the family worked together and learned traditions and beliefs. What would otherwise have been an endless succession of chores and responsibilities was coordinated into a routine, a schedule, a calendar punctuated by celebrations and new beginnings" (123).

The New England backyard: This context sets the stage for the attractive implementation of the New England backyard at Sedgewood Commons. The patio and the lawn panel are designed for group activities. The gazebo offers a place for sheltered social interaction. Also provided are a toolshed, a wood pile, a basketball hoop, and a clothesline. These familiar elements are connected to domestic and residential New England living and provide cues for stimulating meaningful activity. One of the most successful of these interventions is the clothesline, which provides residents with a recognizable activity (see figure 6.11). The clothesline is not only therapeutic but also meaningful, as it engages residents in a necessary daily task for the "household." Other activity-based features include raised planting beds with such familiar plants as rhododendrons, azaleas, lilacs, honeysuckle, and roses that "provide colors and smells that bring us back in time and evoke memories of our past" (Hoover, 1995:7). Residents are given the opportunity to water and cultivate the garden.

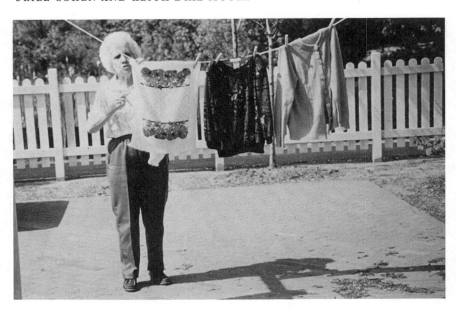

FIGURE 6.11. Clothesline at Sedgewood
Commons Alzheimer's Care Facility

Discussion: Supporting functional ability through meaningful activity and establishing links to the healthy and the familiar are two therapeutic goals addressed by outdoor activity. The tie between maintenance, or "taking care of," and the domestic experience of home should not be overlooked. Some of the most meaningful activity that we engage in are those that we consider the most routine. While availability of positive outdoor space is good design practice, these activities and environmental experiences are tailored specifically to the experience of home in New England. Because of the range of opportunities for possible engagement offered in this design, it promotes resident autonomy and control; and due to the nature of nature, the yard is constantly changing with the seasons. And the ritual character of landscape maintenance maximizes awareness and orientation.

CASE STUDY: ADARDS, TASMANIA
ADARDS is a thirty-two-person assisted-living facility for residents with dementia-related behavioral problems in Warrane, Tasmania. The design was guided by a vision of residents participating in the activities of normal living. The unit is divided into four clusters of eight residents each; meals are prepared and served within each cluster. Each cluster also has its own secured garden area, with a clothesline, an aviary, chickens, cats, and dogs.

A Culturally Meaningful Experience: In the relatively young nation of Australia, the yard still retains its historic homesteading flavor—that is, the notion of claiming possession of land. The yard is where animals are kept, plants are cultivated, and the spirit of individualism is expressed through the very act of dwelling on and with the land.

The Australian backyard: ADARDS makes a concerted effort to create an environment reminiscent of the local homestead. While this has some stylistic implications for the architecture in terms of style, the most interesting aspect of the design are the opportunities for typical domestic activities. On-site, there is a chicken coop that requires daily as well as seasonal maintenance and from which eggs must be collected on a daily basis. For those residents less able, the ceaseless chicken scratching provides a stimulating, if somewhat less engaging, visual and auditory experience of a familiar activity. ADARDS also has a vegetable garden, and some residents spend part of their day keeping the garden immaculate. The traditional Australian "barby," or barbecue, exists not solely as a symbolic ritual but also as a vehicle for active engagement in a familiar social interaction. Residents visit from one "house" to another in response to the social invitation associated with the barbecue. Tending to the barby, its smells, and its preparation all are very familiar and significant experiences in Australian life.

Discussion: ADARDS accepts residents who exhibit inappropriate behaviors prior to their admittance. The facility is therefore designed for a "troubled" population. The organizational environment aggressively promotes therapeutic activity, reflecting a belief that one way of ensuring safety and security is through establishing links to healthy and familiar activity-based experiences. This places a large burden on the staff to continuously prompt residents to take on the many tasks actually required for the facility's operation. Relying on the notion of attachment to place, the program is quite successful in promoting culturally significant therapeutic experiences. For example, the use of the barby as a recognizable setting to provide opportunities for socialization reflects the importance of experiential expressions of culture.

Environmental Intervention Based on Design Enablers

Design enablers, as their name implies, provide an opportunity for culture-based expression but, more important, enable the end user to manipulate his or her environment and make choices. Enablers allow residents to express their own personality and, thereby, the meaningful aspects of their cultural life experience. The open-ended nature of enablers make them conceptually appropriate for facilities with homogeneous populations. They provide platforms for individuals to imbue their own environments with meaningful content. Enablers are then, metaphorically speaking, the frames for resident-selected paintings. These frames can be culturally neutral, or they can, in themselves, be carriers of a cultural message.

CASE STUDY: THE JAPANESE TAKANOMA

An important place in the traditional Japanese home is the *takanoma*, or recessed alcove, which is typically located near the entry in the main room of the house (see figure 6.12). Here, pieces of art and objects of symbolic value are displayed with pride. Architecturally, three distinct features are present in a *takanoma:* a raised platform, a window to provide daylight, and a displayed object.

A Culturally Meaningful Experience: The personal display near the entry to each resident's room serves as a sign, a landmark, a personalized expression of self, and a territorial marker. The combination of mailbox, display, and formal identification provides a personalized front to resident units in a congregate living context (see figure 6.13).

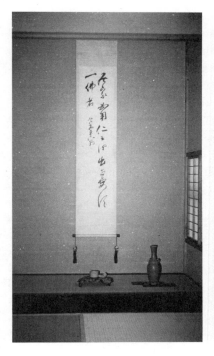

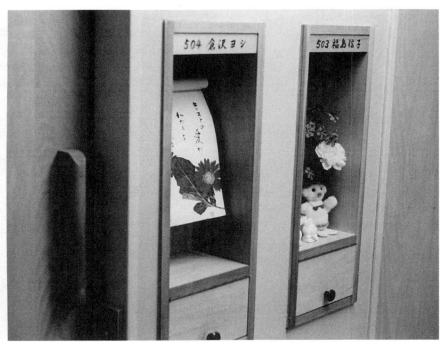

FIGURE 6.12. *A traditional Japanese* takanoma

FIGURE 6.13. *An interpretation of takanoma in a Japanese independent living environment*

Discussion: The *takanoma* is where the identity of the owning family is expressed, usually by displaying something of value and meaning. The arrangement of the art within the *takanoma* is as important as the art itself, for the composition implies the care and reverence the family has for these objects. Utilizing a *takanoma* within resident units in a Japanese assisted-living facility provides a culturally meaningful solution that maximizes awareness and orientation on behalf of residents. Resident rooms that have an exterior *takanoma* are more familiar and identifiable. The *takanoma* provides a therapeutic activity for residents, because arranging the display and maintaining the *takanoma* is a source of great pride.

CASE STUDY: WOODSIDE PLACE
In Woodside Place, an assisted-living facility in Oakmont, Pennsylvania, each resident room has a continuous, three-inch-deep, plate shelf for displaying personal items. A series of pegs below allow for items to be hung. The architectural detail of this enabler has the simplicity characteristic of Pennsylvania Dutch craftsmanship (see figure 14.6).

A Culturally Meaningful Experience: For the Pennsylvania Dutch, a good life was defined as one lived simply, filled with work and humility. The spirit of a person, or a thing for that matter, would reveal itself through its usefulness. While elegantly simple and esthetically beautiful, the Pennsylvania Dutch hat rack serves a useful purpose by affording the opportunity to hang items that otherwise might create clutter. The artistry of the piece does not come through flamboyance but rather through elegant understatement.

Discussion: While not specifically geared to Pennsylvania Dutch residents, the facility's geographic location makes Pennsylvania Dutch design part of the local vernacular. This fact adds to the familiarity this artifact may have, but the most powerful aspect of the design feature is its utility. The hat rack is an open-ended design intervention, inviting resident personalization of his or her environment. Such personalization creates an expression of social identity. A personalized environment not only says who a person is but claims territory for the person and creates a sense of autonomy and control. The opportunity for self-expression is compellingly powerful and provides residents the chance to create their own culturally meaningful statement in their room.

Conclusion

Two emerging factors provided the impetus for this chapter: the growing influence that cultural plurality will have in assisted-living environments heading into the next century and the paradigm shift toward individualized care in assisted-living environments. The goal of this chapter is to present a conceptual framework to facilitate discussion about the transaction between the unique therapeutic needs of elderly persons and culturally responsive environmental design. An individual's culture—here defined as lifestyle groups that possess commonly shared experiences—is seen as a key for a positive environmental intervention.

Kahana (1980), in her proposed notion of congruence, suggests that the morale of a person is a function not simply of the environment but also of the degree of fit between the elderly person's needs and the ability of the environment to meet those needs. Here, it is proposed that congruence, if viewed in terms of cultural significance, points out often overlooked resources for creating more therapeutic programs and more meaningful environments for older persons. As is illustrated, cultural responsiveness has implications not only for the social environment of assisted-living facilities but also for the organizational and physical environments.

It is easy to misinterpret this chapter as holding a culturally deterministic view toward intervention (i.e., farmers get rural design and urban dwellers get a high-rise). This is not what is intended. The intent is to illustrate what is possible and to demystify the process. If the conceptual framework suggested here is heeded, choices based on lifestyle will be made available. This currently is not the case. A number of assisted-living organizations are developing the same prototype facility in different states throughout the country. This is an area in which the industry can do better, and it can do so through consideration of meaningful cultural experiences in their physical and organization decision making.

The conceptual framework does suggest broader implications. Providing residents with meaningful, culturally based experiences that are congruent with their commonly shared lifestyle group and related activities implies sizing the facility appropriately to reflect the properties of that lifestyle group. To organizationally recognize the strengths and weaknesses of residents and tap into those resources appropriately would foster a more healthy and interesting social environment. Finally, like the individualized care model, this culturally responsive approach asks much more of staffs, families, and care-providing organizations. Consistent staffing, with a staff familiar with the social rules of the lifestyle group, is imperative. Outcome measures for the staff must shift from a concentration on completed tasks toward enhancing residents' quality of life.

It is hoped that this discussion fosters creative thinking by environmental designers and care providers alike and that it challenges both disciplines not only to create therapeutic environments but also to integrate those therapeutic goals with experientially based cultural phenomena in the hopes of creating better and more meaningful environments for elderly persons. A clear definition of the audience to which their assisted-living facility is targeted will facilitate more thoughtful consideration of the environmental experiences they hope to create. A focus on meaningful experiences will have direct implications on the physical, social, individual, and organizational aspects of the environment. This focus redresses the disconnection of elderly persons from their environments by integrating the vision of the assisted-living philosophy with the reality of cultural diversity in a significant way.

References

Abeles, R. 1991. Sense of control, quality of life, and frail older people. In J. Birren, J. Lubben, J. Rowe, and D. Deutchman, eds., *The Concept and Measurement of Quality of Life in the Frail Elderly.* San Diego: Academic.

Boyle, J., and M. Andrews. 1995. *Transcultural Concepts on Nursing Care.* Glenview, Ill.: Scott, Foresman.

Calkins, M. 1988. *Design for Dementia.* Owings Mills, Md.: National Health Publishing.

Canter, D. 1988. Action and place: An existential dialectic. In D. Canter, M. Krampen, and D. Stea, eds., *Environmental Perspectives.* Vol. 1, *Ethnoscapes.* Aldershot, U.K.: Avebury.

Cohen, U., and G. Weisman. 1991. *Holding on to Home: Designing Environments for People with Dementia.* Baltimore: Johns Hopkins University Press.

Coopers & Lybrand. 1993. *An Overview of the Assisted Living Industry.* Fairfax, Va.: Assisted-Living Federation of America.

Henderson, N. 1994. The culture of special care units: An anthropological perspective on ethnographic research in nursing home settings. *Alzheimer Disease and Associated Disorders* 8 (supp. 1): 410–16.

Hoover, R. 1995. Healing gardens and Alzheimer's disease. *American Journal of Alzheimer's Disease* 10:1–9.

Jackson, J. 1994. *A Sense of Place, a Sense of Time.* New Haven: Yale University Press.

Kahana, E. 1980. A congruence model of person-environment interaction. In M. Lawton, P. Windley, and T. Byerts, eds., *Aging and the Environment: Directions and Perspectives.* New York: Garland.

Küller, R. 1988. Housing for the elderly in Sweden. In D. Canter, M. Krampen, and D. Stea, eds., *Environmental Policy, Assessment, and Communication.* Vol. 2, *Ethnoscapes.* Aldershot, U.K.: Avebury.

Langer, E., and J. Rodin. 1976. The effects of choice and enhanced personal responsibility for the aged. *Journal of Personality and Social Psychology* 34:191–98.

Mace, N. 1993. Observations of dementia-specific care around the world. *American Journal of Alzheimer's Care and Related Disorders and Research* 1:1–8.

Ohta, R., and B. Ohta. 1988. Special units for Alzheimer's disease patients. *Gerontologist* 28:803–8.

Rader, J. 1995. *Individualized Dementia Care: Creative Compassionate Approaches.* New York: Springer.

Rapoport, A. 1983. Development, cultural change, and supportive design. *Habitat International* 7:249–68.

———. 1990. Systems of activities and systems of settings. In S. Kent, ed., *Domestic Architecture and the Use of Space*. Cambridge: Cambridge University Press.

Regnier, V., J. Hamilton, and S. Yatabe. 1995. *Assisted Living for the Aged and Frail: Innovations in Design, Management, and Financing*. New York: Columbia University Press.

Rowles, G. 1984. Aging in rural environments. In I. Altman, M. Lawton, and J. Wohlwill, eds., *Elderly People and the Environment*. New York: Plenum.

Schramm, U. 1996. Post-occupancy evaluation in the cross-cultural context: A field study on the performance of health care facilities in Egypt and other countries. Paper presented at the CIB-ASTM-ISO-RILEM Third International Symposium, Tel Aviv.

Wilson, K. 1990. Assisted living: The merger of housing and long-term services. In *Long-term Care Advances* (Duke University Center for the Study of Aging and Human Development), 1:208.

JOHN ZEISEL

CHAPTER 7

Life-Quality Alzheimer Care in Assisted Living

The specific brain dysfunctions of people with Alzheimer's disease and related dementias make environmental design a particularly effective treatment for the symptoms of this disease, especially when appropriately combined with operational management techniques focused on enhancing the lives of persons with dementia. By understanding and taking advantage of the interactive effects of design and operations, the effect of each design or operational effect is amplified.

Alzheimer's disease poses ethical and practical dilemmas for those who care for people with this dementia. Alzheimer's is a terminal illness, and people with the disease are in the process of dying from it. It is as if these people were told, You have only a certain time to live. If that time were two days, we would clearly treat these people as if they were dying. If that time were seventy-five years, we would clearly treat them as if they were going to live and provide them with the highest quality of life possible. But for those with Alzheimer's disease the term is closer to twelve years, so the dilemma is whether we care for these people as if they were dying or living. If we see people with Alzheimer's disease as dying, then we might make their last years as comfortable as possible in a custodial environment. If we see them as people whose lives matter, we need to treat them as whole people, providing them with the highest possible quality of life.

In this century, other diseases have posed the medical and nonmedical professions with this dilemma: diabetes, Lou Gehrig's disease, rheumatoid arthritis, manic depression, and now AIDS (Jarvik and Winograd, 1988). These diseases were once hopeless conditions, from which there was no way out. But each has become treatable with proper medication, lifestyle changes, diet, and environmental design. Alzheimer's is now at the cusp of this shift from hopeless condition to treatable disease (Zeisel and Raia, draft ms.). As this shift is taking place, caregivers need to frame a way of thinking about the quality of the lives of those with the disease and then to organize coherent treatments to maintain quality of life.

This chapter begins to address these questions. First, quality of life is defined for this population. Then treatment approaches are presented in two areas: environmental design and residence management. The chapter concludes with a discussion of interactive effects of environment and management on care that amplify the effects of each.

Quality of Life

Half a century ago, Maslow (1954, 1968) defined the components of life quality for cognitively intact people as survival, maintenance, and enhancement. For those with Alzheimer's disease a similar model can be construct-

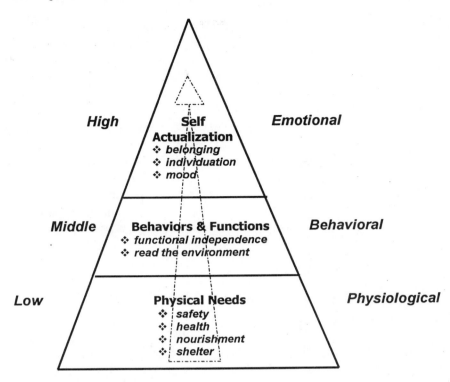

High   **Self Actualization**   *Emotional*

❖ *belonging*
❖ *individuation*
❖ *mood*

Middle   **Behaviors & Functions**   *Behavioral*

❖ *functional independence*
❖ *read the environment*

Low   **Physical Needs**   *Physiological*

❖ *safety*
❖ *health*
❖ *nourishment*
❖ *shelter*

FIGURE 7.1. *Components of life quality*

ed (see figure 7.1). Three levels of need must be met for these people to experience life quality, with the highest level representing the highest quality. The first two levels of need that caregivers must meet to provide quality of life require only brief explanation. The most basic needs are physiological: the need for safety, health, nourishment and shelter. Meeting these needs forms the basis for meeting the other sets of needs. The next are behavioral needs for appropriate functioning and use of the environment. Help is required to meet these needs because damage to the brain of people with dementia specifically affects those areas that control social behaviors, impulses, and environmental cognition.

The highest level of life quality, self-actualization, deserves explanation because popular misconception holds that people with dementias do not sense themselves the way cognitively intact people do. However, the parts of the brain that controls mood and emotion, the amygdala, is one of the last to be affected. A person's moods and emotions are therefore readily accessible to themselves and to caregivers until very late in the disease. It is difficult to maintain positive mood and emotion for this population over time, because people with Alzheimer's disease are so very sensitive. They feel negative feelings as readily as positive ones; they cannot control their anger, sadness, and anxiety. The highest goal of life-quality treatment is not only to maintain positive mood but also to maintain emotional stability around social norms (recognizing and dealing with other people) and personal norms (maintaining a sense of self).

Two treatment modalities are available to maintain the quality of life in assisted-living residences specially built for those with Alzheimer's disease and related dementias. They are environmental design and management operations. Although design and management can be analyzed separately, in life they are integrally connected. Before describing these two treatment approaches, however, it may be prudent to ask ourselves if assisted living is even an acceptable setting to care for people with dementia. Some might ask, How can those with dementia benefit from the autonomy, personal dignity, and privacy that assisted living provides? Aren't people with dementia violent, dependent, and confused? Don't people with dementia require constant surveillance?

As discussed above, even those with dementia can experience quality of life. The thesis of this chapter—namely, that it is our lack of understanding of the disease that limits the ability of people with dementia to enjoy these liberties, not their incapacities—can be demonstrated both in practice and theory. Similarly, practice and research bear out the point of view that many of the negative behaviors commonly associated with the disease are reactions to inadequate care and treatment rather than symptoms integral to the disease.

Autonomy

If people with Alzheimer's disease are in a completely safe setting, and if their families are willing to negotiate the risks of freedom with caregivers, they can enjoy autonomy as long as they do not injure themselves and others. Every person with dementia—except for those in the very end stages—has remaining skills: gardening, cooking, laughing, listening, walking, chatting, drinking coffee or tea. They can be independent and autonomous in employing their skills as long as they are protected from the dangers created by their trying to employ abilities they have lost.

Dignity

Most people with Alzheimer's disease maintain the ability to feel, express, and respond to emotion until well into the disease. Emotions include happiness, satisfaction, sadness, and pride, among others. People feeling dignity, which is linked to pride, is something that every caregiver sees daily whenever a resident successfully completes a task: getting dressed, eating, mixing a bowl of cookie dough. If we apply a narrow definition of dignity to this group, they may have very little. Applying their own expressed definition of pride to their actions, we can perceive and better understand how dignified they feel.

Privacy

When one enters the room of a person with dementia who is in an assisted-living environment, one sees a person at home. Surrounded by their own furniture and photographs of family members in their own private space, many of these residents seem well and satisfied. Only when they begin to answer questions and make conversation does their dementia strike the visitor. It is as if, shrouded in a shell of private territory, they are protected from the questions and words that make their illness so evident.

Environmental Design

A design approach composed of eight characteristics can be used to provide a quality of life through environmental design for those with Alzheimer's disease: exit control, walking paths, personal places, social spaces, healing gardens, residential features, independence, and sensory comprehensibility (see table 7.1). The eight characteristics and their sixteen associated dimensions represent environmental boundary conditions, spatial arrangements, and ambient conditions. The criteria are called environment-behavior (E-B) criteria for assisted-living residences, because they organize E-B design research information and concepts in terms of therapeutic and quality-of-life outcomes critical to residents' lives.

Exit Control

The brains of Alzheimer's patients cannot hold cognitive maps, and they frequently forget how to return home. Therefore, people with dementia

Table 7.1. Environment-Behavior (E-B) Criteria for Design

E-B Concept	Definition and Examples	Dimensions
Exit control	Boundary conditions of each special care unit; the surrounding walls, fences, doors and how they are locked or otherwise limit and allow people to come and go.	Immediacy of control, unobtrusiveness
Walking paths	Circulation space residents use for wandering and moving around.	Continuousness, wayfinding
Personal places	Spaces—primarily bedrooms—used mostly by and sometimes assigned to individuals or a limited number of residents.	Privacy, personalization
Social spaces	Sizes, relationships, and qualities of spaces used by all residents in the special care unit.	Quantity, variability
Healing gardens	Residents' access to common areas out-of-doors and the way these places support residents' needs.	Availability, supportiveness (includes safety)
Residential features	Degree to which the size of the special care unit reflects a small community and the degree to which the special care unit uses residential furnishings, design features, and personal objects.	Size, familiarity
Independence	The ways in which the facility encourages and supports residents to use their remaining faculties to carry out basic tasks and activities independently and with dignity.	Safe, prosthetic
Sensory Comprehensibility	Quality of the sensory environment—acoustic, visual, thermal, odor, and kinesthetic—in all spaces and the degree to which these conditions may confuse residents.	Management, meaningfulness

Source: Zeisel, Hyde, and Levkoff, 1994.

should only leave their homes accompanied by someone else. Doorways from a residence that open to the larger public community, therefore, need to be controlled. These residents, who spend so much time indoors, become agitated by doors with mixed messages: on the one hand, doors' windows and handles seem to invite them to go out; on the other hand, locks and key-pads prevent them going out. Exit doors that are unobtrusive, with no attracting hardware, reduce such agitation. Increasing the visibility and making more inviting any door to a secure healing garden, for example, further diverts attention from doors that exit to dangerous areas.

When exit doors need signals to indicate to staff that the door has been opened without supervision, such signals can be chosen so they do not disturb the ambiance of the residential setting: chimes, for example, rather than alarms. The less obvious the door, the signal, the handle, and the scene on the other side of the door, the greater independence the resident will have.

Walking Paths

One of the symptoms of Alzheimer's disease for certain people is the desire to walk, perhaps looking for something without knowing precisely what. While aimless wandering can be a problem for staff in a facility that has no place for this activity, a well-designed pathway can transform wandering into walking. A pathway can achieve this goal if it is interesting and does not dead-end. Such a pathway need not be circular but rather can be a thoughtful connection of corridors that pass through common areas and connect up again to corridors going in another direction. Interest along the path is important so that walkers always have some goal in sight—the next interesting picture, view, or plant. An interest at the end of the path, a social space or a fireplace, provides a place to walk to, a destination that gives purpose to the trips.

Personal Places

Because residents spend so much time together, they need places to be alone, to avoid the pressure of social interaction. Just because someone is demented does not mean that they can stand being with others 24 hours a day. Individual spaces that residents can use to get away by themselves can include private bedrooms or small, out-of-the-way, corner sitting areas in a living room or garden. Places like this can also be used by residents with visiting family members, who just need to sit together quietly. Personal places also can be decorated and furnished personally, thus creating a soothing mood that triggers positive memories.

Social Spaces

Residents in Alzheimer's assisted-living facilities spend almost all of their time in the facility and together. To satisfy their need for diversity and to reduce boredom and agitation, it is essential to have at least two if not three common spaces—dining room, kitchen, living room, foyer. The more the settings of these rooms are different from each other and interesting, the easier it is for staff to manage small familylike activities in them and for residents to feel stimulated by the differences in ambiance.

Healing Gardens

Not every residence is able to provide its residents a safe and secure outdoor area immediately adjacent to the residential area. Yet this ideal gives residents a sense of nature, weather, and plants. If nothing else, Alzheimer's residents enjoy being outdoors and are relaxed by being able to get away from the confinement they feel inside. Yet a healing garden is even more than a place to get out to; it is a sanctuary in which a basic drive to have contact with normal forces can be met.

If such an amenity is not easily provided, for example if the residential area is on an upper floor of an urban building, designers and operators need to arrange alternatives. One possibility is to have an outdoor area nearby that residents can use regularly, accompanied by staff—on grade or on a roof patio. When such an arrangement is made, the path there and back must be thought through carefully to avoid creating anxiety and a breakdown in safety.

Residential Features

Home, fireplace, front porch, and garden are residential environmental design elements that create a positive mood in residents by touching deep-seated memories. The familiarity of residential furniture, spaces, decorations, and lighting fixtures relaxes everyone in Alzheimer's facilities—residents, their families, and staff members. The size of residential features—a scale people can relate to and grasp easily—can be soothing in itself. A refrigerator, a window, a small room, a small group gathering are all familiar, understandable, and manageable elements for demented residents and everyone with whom they interact.

Independence

Details such as handrails and floors that prevent slips and falls contribute to the independence and autonomy of residents, because they support each person's ability to do things on their own. It may seem obvious that a toilet so low that it prevents an older person from rising to a standing position alone limits independence, but it does. Any nonprosthetic or unsafe design element has this effect. The safer the environment, the more likely staff members are to permit residents to move about by themselves and make independent choices.

Sensory Comprehensibility

Alzheimer's residents are not confused by everything around them. When the sounds, sights, and smells they experience are familiar, they can cope with them and enjoy them. A common myth and mistake in design for dementia care is that if everything is sedate and bland, residents will be soothed. This is not the case. Blandness can be anxiety producing if taken to an extreme. What is needed is to create enough activity to keep residents interested and to make sure that the activity provided is understandable to them. Colors are fine; wallpaper with traditional patterns is better than that with abstract patterns. A television is fine; recorded films that have few rapid changes for advertisements are more satisfying than films with random violence and loud noise. Comprehensibility comes from sensible, common-sense management.

Links to Environment-Behavior Concepts

The eight environment-behavior characteristics described above reflect basic needs that E-B research has studied in the past and, although studied with respect to the specific population of people with dementia, can be broadly generalized. Studies of people with dementia can shed light on the nature of the following basic E-B concepts among the cognitively intact.

Wayfinding

People with dementia know where they are when they are there. They know where they have been if they see it. And they know where they are going when they get there. People with dementia do not find there way as cognitively intact people do, by using a cognitive map of their surroundings that they keep in their head; rather, they move from place to place using immediate cues within their view. Spaces and objects at the end of paths, and objects along the way, seem to provide useful cues for demented people's place awareness. Is this not true for others?

Territory and Privacy

Alzheimer's patients often cannot distinguish another's room or chest of drawers from their own and as a result may enter other people's room and use other people's clothes. On the other hand, these patients seem to maintain long into the illness a sense of what is their own personal space. Such residents are calmer and more at ease in a room divided from others' sleeping areas by a territorial separation, like a wall, than in a room with several other people. Nevertheless, complete privacy is not necessarily positive for people who have spent much of their lives in bedrooms with others—sisters, brothers, husbands or wives. Perhaps society generally places more value on privacy than people really require.

Environmental and Sensory Meaning

A common misunderstanding about people with Alzheimer's disease or related dementias is that any loud noise or active visual environment is upsetting and creates anxiety, resulting in uncontrollable outbursts. Indications are, rather, that such people are not upset by stimulation as such so much as stimulation they either do not understand or know to be upsetting: rock music, random bright colors, caregivers shouting at each other, impolite strangers. Meaning is created for them by familiar surroundings, a residential feeling, kitchen smells, music they can remember. Do we sufficiently understand the way people create meaning in their lives?

Residential Quality and Archetypal Spaces

To provide familiar surroundings for people with dementia, many operators and designers of care residences try to include such residential features as kitchens, laundries, fireplaces, front porches, and backyards. While one hypothesis is that such design elements remind people of where they used to live, another is that these elements tap into profound and deep memories of archetypal spaces. What is the role of archetypal spaces in each of our lives?

Personalization

People who have Alzheimer's disease may not remember a relative's name or what happened moments before, but they do sense good feelings that come from old memories. Being able to live in an environment furnished and decorated with their own belongings increases a sense of belonging and reduces inappropriate behaviors. For this reason, being placed in a nursing home before another medical condition requires it is likely to increase their mental and physical decline. What does such awareness tell us about the importance of personalization for others?

Healing Gardens

We know that nature and the out-of-doors has healing qualities for everyone. Many people with Alzheimer's disease exhibit special behaviors late in the afternoon, behaviors called sundowning. At that time of day, many patients begin to get exceptionally agitated and say they want to go home. It is getting dark, and they may remember that at the end of the day they usually left work, school, a friend's house to go home. Being out-of-doors in a safe and secure garden where they can feel free gives them the opportunity to sense the seasons, the weather, the time of day in ways that are reported to reduce sundowning and help them sleep. How does nature impact the health of each of us?

Operations Management

The way staff and organizations provide care in assisted-living and other settings is also important for people with dementia. The approach presented here is called an individual-organization (I-O) approach, because both the individual's needs and the organization's responsibilities are considered equally. Focusing on the needs and the dignity of the individual with dementia is essential to successful caregiving, especially in community and group settings; and without careful management by the organization that provides the context for caregivers, caregivers will be unable to provide the needed individualized care. This organizational approach is composed of eight criteria: personhood, purpose, adaptability, staff suitability, life richness, family responsiveness, real-worldness, and responsibility (see table 7.2).

Personhood

Residents of facilities for people with Alzheimer's disease are unique individuals with their own character, personality, and needs. Each is still a person; having Alzheimer's disease does not make people the same. Each person's reactions to having the disease is different, requiring thorough diagnosis and care planning that is responsive to his or her own personality, strengths, and weaknesses. If staff members try to standardize care without regard to such differences, they run the risk of infringing on residents' dignity and exacerbating their catastrophic reactions.

Purpose

When care provided in assisted-living and other facilities for persons with Alzheimer's disease is organized around clear and cohesive principles, caregiving staff and family are empowered to work together to implement creative solutions. When a facility's statement of purpose is reflected in its day-to-day practices, staff and family members can consciously work together to achieve common goals. Because staff and family members make up the

Table 7.2. Individual-Organization (I-O) Operational Criteria

I-O Concept	Definition/Examples	Dimensions
Personhood	Care approaches by which caregivers focus their attention in every interaction on each individual's personal style and dignity; the degree to which care planning meetings and other attempts to plan residents' lives lead to individualization of residents.	Diagnosis and care planning, responsiveness to individual differences
Purpose	Shared philosophy of goals and care, provides unity and cohesion to caregiver teams in a residence and influences the way others perceive the residence.	Cohesive statement of purpose, consistency with practice
Adaptability	Approaches that support each caregiver's ability to make sound decisions that meet the needs of residents no matter whose job it might be to perform particular tasks.	Empowered employee teams, permeable ("fuzzy") job boundaries
Staff suitability	Staff characteristics and their natural orientation to serve older and demented residents; staff training in how to care for people with Alzheimer's disease.	Empathy, Alzheimer's training
Richness of Life	Coordinated personal care, health care, and planned activities that respond to residents' personal histories and styles; the daily rhythm and seamlessness of these linked activities throughout the day, evening, and night.	Meaningful life coordination, nonepisodic duration
Family responsiveness	The way in which caregivers in the residence relate to residents' family members; how even family members who may be upset and disruptive are supported and welcomed onto the caregiving team.	Support for family in transition, family on caregiving team
Real-worldness	The degree to which the life of residents reflects the world they knew and know through normal events and contact with the surrounding community.	Normalization, community contact
Responsibility	Operational responsibility taken seriously, focusing on financial soundness to be able to respond to changing needs of individuals, families, and the residence.	Sound business practices, responsiveness to changing resident and family needs

whole world that residents know, this leads to a sense of calm and comfort among residents.

Adaptability

The needs of individuals with Alzheimer's disease differ over time and differ from person to person. What is appropriate care for one person one day is different from appropriate care for that person the next and for another person the same day. Relations between a particular staff member and a resident may differ at different times of day. To respond adequately to residents' needs, caregivers must be empowered to work in teams to support one another throughout the day and night and to carry out a broad range of tasks. Only if this is done can the entire organization exhibit the flexibility and adaptability to respond to the shifting character of dementia.

Staff Suitability

Not everyone is a good caregiver for people with Alzheimer's disease. It takes a person with extreme patience, flexibility, self-assurance, and empathy. In addition, because appropriate reactions to a demented person's behavior are sometimes anti-intuitive, special training in dementia symptoms and behaviors and in appropriate care approaches is needed to help staff members recognize reactions to the disease and how to respond. The more empathetic caregivers are and the more solid caregivers' grounding is in their disciplines, the more flexible and creative they will be in their jobs.

Richness of Life

The central characteristic of a life-quality model of Alzheimer care is a robust activities program that lasts from morning until night—and during the night for those residents who sleep fitfully. Not only must such an activity program be structured to reflect the diurnal rhythms of residents' past lifestyles, they must also treat each activity of daily living as the opportunity for a structured and fulfilling individual or group activity. The structure of the day, the timeliness of each element of daily life, and the meaningfulness of each activity contributes to the well-being of residents.

Family Responsiveness

A person's dementia affects not only that person but also members of her or his entire family: they deny, they grieve, they support, they pay, they fear, they question. To effectively respond to the disease and its symptoms, a therapeutic setting for the person must therefore also support and integrate the family into care planning. Family members need to be invited to be part of the caregiving team so they can bring their familiarity with the person into the care equation. But also, family members' response to the disease must be supported, especially when they are in crisis and possibly responding inappropriately.

Real-Worldness

Demented residents in assisted-living residences have a natural tendency to remove themselves from and be removed from the world around them. Engaging in everyday, real-life activities, such as reading a newspaper or shopping in a local store, connects residents to the real world just as do visits from family members. Real-world contact with environments, institutions, and people who live and work in the surrounding community contributes to residents' skills and well-being. Connectedness to life in the real world connects residents to the memories and feelings that sustain them.

Responsibility

When families move demented residents into special care residences, they do so with a trust and belief in the stability of that residence and the organization it is a part of. They entrust that organization with the health, safety, and welfare of their family members, expecting the residence to provide service that is nonabusive, to communicate with them, and to manage financial matters in a way that ensures continued quality care, innovation, and growth. The organization is expected to have adequate commitment to and resources available for the programs necessary to provide the quality of care residents and families expect.

Design and Management Interactions

Environmental elements are interdependent with operational interventions in their effect. A particular design may influence residents directly: a disguised door will not be noticed easily, and residents will be less likely to find it, push on it, and get upset because it is locked. More likely, the environmental design element influences both residents and caregivers as well as their interaction. Exits, for example, prevent residents from walking away from the safety of the residence and perhaps getting lost. They also reduce the anxiety of staff members, who are justifiably concerned with resident safety. Knowing that residents are safe, even without constant surveillance, provides opportunities for staff to enable demented residents to use their environment freely and independently. Environment and management interact (see table 7.3). A line could connect each of the eight environmental characteristics to each of the eight management principles, and each would represent an important opportunity for enhanced functioning in an Alzheimer's assisted-living community.

Residential scale, interior decor, furnishings, and spatial organization provide residents with familiar and relaxing surroundings, cueing residents as to the appropriate behaviors in those places. These characteristics also provide staff with cues as to their appropriate behaviors; for example, a residential living room setting gives staff members the idea that they ought to treat residents politely there and not use it to perform medical or other procedures. Although staff offices located with doors overlooking living room, dining room, and foyer make it difficult for staff to focus on individual tasks, they also provide opportunities for unobtrusive surveillance, reducing the need to hire staff to control residents. Outdoor areas that residents can walk into whenever they like and that are safe and understandable give residents a sense of the seasons, weather, and time of day. Contact with nature reduces residents' anxiety and helps them sleep. Such outdoor areas also reduce staff stress, enabling staff members to focus on quality-of-life issues. As these examples show, environment and management interact at the individual, group, and organizational levels. Exploring these interactions more systematically by looking at the environmental elements individually indicate

Table 7.3. Environment and Management Interactions and Mutual Support

Environment	Management
Exit control	Personhood
Walking paths	Purpose
Personal places	Adaptability
Social spaces	Staff suitability
Healing gardens	Life richness
Residential features	Family responsiveness
Independence	Real-worldness
Sensory comprehensibility	Responsibility

how they can be used to treat families and to enable staff to provide service to residents.

Exit Control

Doors to the outside are locked on the inside with keypads, coded so that residents cannot use them to open the doors. From the outside, these doors are easily opened by either pressing a button or using the code. From the inside, doors provide full safety for residents; from the outside, they provide easy family and community access. Inside, the doors are disguised by low light, by their similarity to other doors, and by a lack of special hardware and signs. On the outside, doors look as normal as possible.

The effects of these design elements on care management and on other participants in the caregiving process are many. Residents are safe from the dangers of an incomprehensible world outside the residence. Staff members, knowing that residents are safe, can spend less time guaranteeing safety and more time managing the quality of life within the residence. If an individual resident walks away from an activity, staff members do not have to run after them. Family members are also more at ease, knowing their relatives are safe inside a nurturing setting and that they can come and go their own pace. Because many family members have lived a long time with their sick relative, have worried, have not slept, have not had a choice of when to interact, this freedom is a great relief. Having free choice of access also improves the relationship between relatives and residents. Exit control, then, contributes directly to the management goals of responsibility, personhood, and family involvement.

Walking Paths

Walking paths transform aimless wandering into purposeful behavior by providing natural destinations, such as social spaces at the ends of corridors, and a sense of place, by the installation of wall objects that hold residents' interest. This transformation in observed behavior in turn affects the perception that caregivers hold of people with dementia. Instead of seeing residents as "wanderers," caregivers see them as people who are moving from one destination to another. This perceived transformation in behavior changes the mental label that caregivers assign to residents, eventually changing the way caregivers treat residents. Mental labels such as "wanderer," "incontinent," "unable to complete ADLs alone" influence caregivers interactions with residents.

Several sociological phenomena are being played out simultaneously. Labeling is a way of dehumanizing people. If a caregiver says of a resident, "Oh, that's just another wanderer lost in the garden; there is nothing I can do to change the situation," it may become a self-fulfilling prophesy: if a caregiver worries always that a certain resident will get lost, the caregiver will behave in such a way to almost guarantee that the resident gets lost. People with dementia behave lost when they are expected to behave lost (learned helplessness). When environmental design reverses these interactively destructive behaviors, caregivers begin to perceive of and treat residents as people, and residents respond by acting as people.

Correctly designed walking paths contribute to residents' richness of life, as well, if we define richness as the continuity and meaningfulness of activities throughout the day. If residents wander away from a group activity with no destination, they are perceived as moving into a no-man's-land of meaningless activity; and responsible caregivers feel the need either to bring them back to the activity or in some other way to distract them from wandering. A resident who walks away from an activity is not disrupting the richness of his or her life if everyone sees walking as a meaningful activity with purpose and interest along the way.

Personal Places

Bedrooms, as well as isolated chairs in living rooms and benches in a healing garden where residents and family can feel a bit separate, can be claimed as personal places. These places allow residents to be by themselves without being lost. People with Alzheimer's disease, like people with no cognitive deficits, need to be by themselves sometimes. Just because a person is demented, it does not mean that he or she can spend all day with the same group of people without conflict, agitation, and the need to be alone. At work, we take breaks; at camp, kids take naps; at home, we hide behind the newspaper or sit in front of the TV to shut others out. The difference is that those with dementia have lost that part of the brain that helps them control their impulses. If they get upset, they express it, while those who are more "normal" have learned to keep it to themselves. Both situations are helped by having a place to go by oneself to cool down. Thus, private places contribute to residents' individual dignity and personhood. Staff members who understand this will escort a resident to some private place—often their bedroom—when they foresee a resident's need to defuse.

Private places also reinforce family members' participation in Alzheimer's residences. Family members feel more relaxed coming to a resident's "home" when they come into a small apartment they or the resident personally furnished with furniture and mementos of the resident's past. Family members can also feel more comfortable taking part in social activities in common areas, because they see these common areas as an extension of the resident's home as well.

Social Spaces

These spaces are cues to appropriate behavior for residents, staff, visitors, and family. Hired caregivers in a small four-person group home in Edmonton, Alberta, Canada, report that, in this setting, they see themselves more as guests than as hired staff. Family members, if not cued to supportive and relaxing interaction by appropriately designed social spaces, are likely to treat their relative as a patient to be visited briefly then left to the total care of others. If they realize that both they and their relative know the conventions appropriate to various social spaces in a residence, families are more likely to participate fully in the life of the residence.

Visitors in institutional settings tend to shy away from addressing and even making eye contact with patients sitting alone in a sterile dayroom. But in a living room, dining room, or garden, visitors are likely to greet residents and ask them how they feel or even make polite conversation, contributing to the richness of residents' lives. The more varied the social spaces are, the more varied will be residents' interaction with these other participants in their lives, which contributes not only to their personhood but also to their connectedness to the real world. Visitors read the environment and know that they need to connect to residents, not avoid them.

Healing Gardens

Gardens contribute to residents' lives both spiritually and practically. There is no way we can measure the importance to people's spirits of feeling sunshine and snow, of planting flowers and watching birds, of seeing the shadows mark the passing of the day. What we do hear from caregivers is that people with dementia are less agitated in the evening and sleep better if they have been outdoors.

An open and inviting door to a healing garden from a living room gives residents the feeling that they are not cooped up and tends to reduce elopement attempts from residences. Staff are likely to feel better about the care they give when they too realize that a garden gives residents a place to get out and feel free. Without outdoor activities such as gardening, raking, shoveling snow, walking on the grass, examining leaves, picking flowers, the richness of every resident's life is diminished. Healing garden activities are not conventionally "learned" activities that can be forgotten but rather are deeply rooted archetypal ones that touch profound and continually meaningful memories.

Family members are also moved by healing gardens. They feel better about their having housed a loved one in a setting with access to the out-of-doors; they too feel better walking in the sunlight with a relative than sitting in an enclosed room. In some residences, family members are invited to inaugurate a planting plan with plants brought from residents' own gardens at their homes. Whether or not a resident recognizes the plants, the symbolism is healing for family members in their grieving process.

Residential Features

Providing a homelike environment is another major treatment modality. To residents with Alzheimer's disease this means a great deal: it links their present environment to their past environment. Five participants with cognitive deficits in a day center in Vancouver were asked, What does home mean to you? (Zeisel and Baldwin, forthcoming). As their responses show, memories of home are deeply related to their entire lives, from the places they have lived to the people they have lived with:

—A calm atmosphere
—My son and daughter
—Being by myself; my husband is no longer
—Clean
—People who run it are very nice people
—A four-bedroom brick house
—Roomy
—One of the first to have a radio in town; a wooden radio with a bump
—I rode a horse to school and back
—A two-story house
—The house was green; no, it wasn't
—Lots of fruit trees: apple, pear, and cherry

—A pond in the bottom of the field
—There was a butcher shop in the front, and we killed the animals in the back
—I like the kitchen best; it's homier
—My mother played the piano in the living room
—If someone bothered me I said, "I have to go home"
—I had a brown-colored house
—The smell of home-made bread
—We had an attic in our house; I liked to look out the attic window and wave hello
—In our attic we had clothes my mother brought from Scotland in 1903
—I went to sewing class; made all the kids clothes and then my own
—I sewed up all the flies in my husband's underpants as a joke; he got the point eventually
—Our sewing machine was upstairs in a long hall
—My sewing machine was on the upper floor near a bay window; we got a lot of light there
—My machine was a "Seamstress" with a treadle
—After I got married I moved to a house with a living room, dining room, two bedrooms, and a basement
—Once I had children I moved again
—In our kitchen we had a big stove, two cupboards next to the door, and a table for six people
—A garden was OK then, but it's too much hard work now
—I live in a bungalow
—It's hard to get around in a large building

Residential features are understood by residents as cues to appropriate behavior in those spaces. A kitchen cues eating, cooking, and washing up; a dining room cues eating; a living room cues sitting together and talking; a fireplace cues sitting alone or together, feeling warm; a garden patio cues enjoying the sun. Each of these spaces also represents an archetypal feeling and experience that people may never lose, because it is so deeply rooted in our being: warmth, food, sun, company.

Residents are not the only ones who receive cues about how to act in residential spaces. Staff members receive and act on these cues as well. In institutional settings with little character to common rooms, staff need instructions as to what to do in each space: the dayroom, the nurses' station, the activity room. They need less training to know what to do with residents in a kitchen, living room, or garden. When family members are present in the residence, and even when they are not, staff act more like residents' family members than as caregivers, because they are in a home—if not at home. And daily life routines—continuous and seamless—take place naturally in such residential places.

Independence

In focus group interviews with resident assistants in Alzheimer's special care nursing units, we asked for examples of supports for independence (Zeisel et al., forthcoming). The resident assistants could not name any but handrails and grab bars. When we asked about the inverse, namely barriers to independence, they could come up only with toilets that are so low that residents require an aide to help them to a standing position.

What was the problem with this seemingly simple category? The answer is that this one category contains the root of all the others. Well-planned exit control, walking paths, personal places, social spaces, healing gardens, residential features, and a comprehensible sensory environment all contribute to residents' independence and autonomy. The better the design, the greater the independence residents have and the greater the self-determination that caregivers grant to residents. And the greater the impact of such environmental elements, the greater influence the environment has on residents' personhood, the richness of their lives, the suitability of staff care, and the responsiveness of family to residents.

The real independence and autonomy of residents, and the link between independence and the way caregivers and family treat residents, is central to providing residents with high quality of life despite their dementia.

Sensory Comprehensibility

In an Alzheimer's residence, sensory comprehensibility means that the environment's physical attributes, sounds, smells, and sights are understood by residents. Simplicity, clarity, and straightforwardness of residential design are major contributors to comprehensibility. The goal of these design elements is to enhance residents' abilities to negotiate the setting as well as to use their knowledge to feel in control of their own lives. These element contribute, therefore, directly to each resident's personhood. There are also beneficial side effects of this on staff and family. Staff who see residents managing on their own—going into the garden, for example, and tending a crop of tomatoes—treat residents more as whole people. Family members who are welcomed by residents in their own apartments and who see their relatives moving around with an independence they have not recently had also begin to think of their relatives as whole people and, as important, to think of themselves as separate individuals caring for someone else with dignity.

Hearthstone Alzheimer Care Treatment Residences: A Case Study

The principles discussed above have been put into practice at Hearthstone Alzheimer Care, a company that develops and manages assisted-living treatment residences for people in the middle and late stages of dementia. Hearthstone currently operates five Alzheimer's assisted-living residences in the Boston and New York City areas. Each includes a 24-hour residential program, a respite program for families that need to have a family member cared for only occasionally for a week or two, and a day program for residents who are cared for by family members at night.

A Care Continuum

Each residence is a wing of a larger assisted-living complex, providing seniors with a continuum-of-living arrangement, from relatively independent assisted living to assistance with problems of frailty and dementia. This cooperative arrangement enables seniors to take advantage of an even fuller range of options. A resident can live full-time at Hearthstone; or a couple may live in an assisted-living apartment with the member of the couple who has dementia participating in the day program. And some couples live sep-

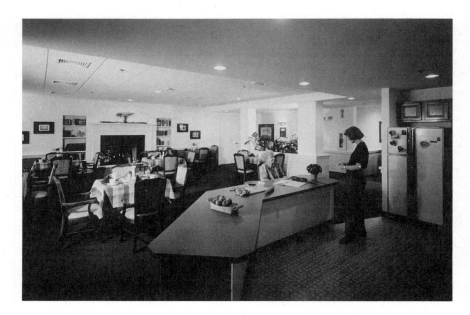

FIGURE 7.2. The hearth kitchen at Hearthstone Alzheimer Care

arately, with the person who has dementia living in the Hearthstone program while the spouse lives in an independent apartment. The particular arrangement is planned to maximize the quality of life of both members of the couple.

The Life-Quality Program

A typical Hearthstone day starts with each resident getting up when they wake up and not on a regulated schedule. The morning includes a shower, grooming, dressing, and a breakfast served individually in the hearth kitchen, the central design feature of each treatment residence (see figure 7.2). After breakfast, the staff engages residents in activities such as cooking, laundry, bingo, seated aerobics, and gardening, which help residents maintain a sense of self while developing a sense of the group as a whole. Lunch is another group activity, after which many residents rest in their rooms. The afternoon is full again, with several activities for small groups of about seven residents each. Residents move to another activity when they lose interest or their attention wanders. After dinner, residents generally gather around the player piano to sing and dance before getting ready for bed. If a resident wakes in the middle of the night, aides will engage her in conversation or play a game until she is tired again and goes back to bed.

Family members come to the residence often either to make informal visits during evening and weekends or for organized occasions such as birthday parties or holiday celebrations. Support groups, in which family members can share their experiences and joys and troubles, are run by program directors once a month. Family members are also regularly involved with resident's medical needs—making decisions regarding medications and taking residents to doctors' appointments.

The Environment

Each residence responds to the particular context created by the larger assisted-living context. One is located on three floors of a wing of a convert-

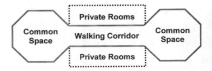

FIGURE 7.3. *Dumbbell, or dog bone, design scheme*

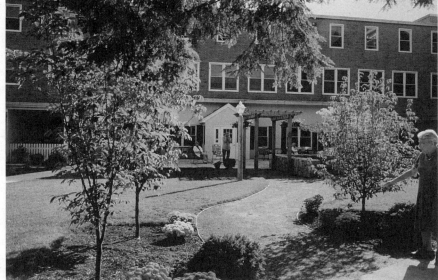

FIGURE 7.4. *Healing garden at Hearthsone Alzheimer Care*

ed school; another on the seventh floor of a New York residential hotel; a third on the ground floor of a newly constructed building. Each, however, follows a basic program that reflects the design principles described earlier in this chapter.

A basic design concept that connects each design is the dog bone, or dumbbell, scheme (see figure 7.3). Rather than putting social spaces in the center or having circular wandering paths, Hearthstone residences have straight walking paths with large social spaces at both ends. Social spaces generally include the hearth kitchen, a living room, a therapeutic laundry area, and a garden (see figure 7.4). The staff has a small office; there are private offices for the program director, the nurse, and the life-quality activity coordinator. Private suites include singles and rooms for two residents separated by a full wall or high piece of furniture. The walls along the walking path are decorated with photographs chosen by residents. Outside each private room is a shadow box—a framed-in glass box—which residents' families decorate with photographs and mementos of achievements.

Future Directions

The future of Alzheimer care and assisted living holds many exciting challenges in theory, design, research, and practice. Theory in this area reflects new approaches to Alzheimer's disease and treatment. Professionals in medicine, social work, design, and other areas are only beginning to answer the critical question, Can the remaining cognitive strengths of people with dementia serve as the basis for providing a high quality of life? The theoretical questions to be answered include:

—What is quality of life? How can it be more clearly defined? Does it include happiness and satisfaction? Does it have spiritual dimensions? How can it be assessed and measured?

—How do the needs of people with dementia correspond to our understanding of the psychological and social well-being of those who are not cognitively impaired? Are the theoretical concepts of the social and psychological sciences transferable to this population?

—How essential are cognitive capacities to life and satisfaction? Can the emotional intelligence that remains in many people with Alzheimer's make up for their loss of cognitive function?

—Do environment-behavior concepts such as territoriality, wayfinding, and privacy need to be redefined for this group, or do entirely new concepts need to be developed to understand their reality?

—In studying people with Alzheimer's disease, is a new model of life and its quality on the horizon, not only for the cognitively impaired but also for the population at large? Can we redefine our understanding of this unique and ubiquitous disease?

Design questions raised by trying to serve people with dementia in assisted living are also many. The most general of these is whether environment is really a treatment for disease. Can design really contribute to people's health and healing? More specifically:

—Is the commonly rejected thesis that design can directly and predictably influence people's feelings and behaviors—environmental determinism—actually false? Are there environments (other than prisons) that control behavior? And do they control in positive as well as negative ways? What are the attributes of such settings?

—If we are to explore the relation between environment and health, do we not need to include all environmental stimuli such as smell, sounds, and texture as well as built form?

—Once these principles have been understood, what role will the designer and design play in realizing such environments? Or will this task always fall to other professionals, such as programmers, health professionals, and gerontologists?

—What will determine high-quality design when the health impacts of design are understood? What will be the role of esthetics? of function?

Are research issues, including methodological and study design, also affected by questions of design and treatment for people with dementia?

—How can researchers test the effects of design without scientific models, much like that used to bring medications and drugs to market? Does society have the resources to carry out such rigorous tests?

—Does research into the health impacts of design not have to merge with research into other health strategies? Does the measure of the impact of assisted living on people with dementia have to measured in the same terms—delay in nursing home placement—as drugs to treat the disease?

—What special methods need to be developed for studying this population, which is essentially unable to express itself on intellectual matters? Are existing social science and environment-behavior methods applicable? Do we underestimate the capacities of those with dementia as subjects?

Practice will yield perhaps the richest information for the future of this area. Applications in development, design, caregiving, medicine, neuropsychology, and the social and psychological sciences all will have to stand the test of the market and of time—harsh judges of the effectiveness of health interventions.

—Are people ready and willing to accept an approach to dementia health care that eschews technological medical approaches for nonpharmacological design and communication therapies?

—Are developers and financial institutions going to be willing to invest in the construction and business necessary to support this approach? Are new building types going to emerge that will change the landscape of hospitals, clinics, and nursing homes?

—Will new diagnostic and evaluation techniques emerge that enable health practitioners to apply these concepts to practice? Will continuing education courses be developed that enable professionals to retrain themselves in new ways of working?

The future will tell if the approaches being developed at the end of the twentieth century in environmental design and caregiving for people with Alzheimer's disease and other dementias take hold in the twenty-first century or are discarded as short-lived fads.

References

Jarvik, L., and C. Winograd. 1988. *Treatments for the Alzheimer Patient*. New York: Springer.

Maslow, A. 1954. *Motivation and Personality*. New York: Harper and Row.

———. 1968. *Toward a Psychology of Being*. New York: Van Nostrand Reinhold.

Zeisel, J., and P. Baldwin. Forthcoming. *Residential Options for People with Dementia*. Ottawa: Canada Mortgage and Housing Corporation.

Zeisel, J., J. Hyde, and S. Levkoff. 1994. Best practices: An environment-behavior (E-B) model of physical design for special care units. *Journal of Alzheimer's Disease* 9:4–21.

Zeisel, J., J. Hyde, N. Silverstein, and S. Levkoff. Forthcoming. *Environmental Design Influences on Patient Outcomes in Special Care Units*. Washington, D.C.: National Institutes of Health.

Zeisel, J., and P. Raia. Draft ms. Alzheimer's: A treatable disease rather than a hopeless condition.

CHAPTER 8

Models for Environmental Assessment

MARGARET P. CALKINS
GERALD D. WEISMAN

The past two decades have seen a radical increase in alternative residential and care options for older adults. Although there are numerous options, ranging from continuing care retirement communities (commonly referred to as CCRCs) to congregate housing to home-sharing programs, the most rapid growth has been in what is increasingly being referred to as assisted living. Assisted living can be broadly defined to include services that range from light personal care to 24-hour nursing care. What services facilities offer vary significantly from state to state and even within a state. Indeed, a recent policy study by the U.S. Department of Health and Human Services cites seven definitions "that vary widely in specificity" (Regnier, Hamilton, and Yatabe, 1995, 2). Although there is no consensus on what assisted living is, there is consensus on what it is not; it is not a nursing home (Kane and Wilson, 1993).

With the proliferation of assisted-living facilities, there is increased interest, from both regulators and clients, in being able to assess the quality of these settings. The challenge is finding appropriate assessment tools for this task. As nursing homes began as subacute or chronic care medical centers, many of the strategies used to assess the setting and outcomes of the setting are medically oriented. Assisted-living facilities, on the other hand, do not define themselves primarily in terms of the medical services they may (or may not) provide. Therefore, assessment protocols designed to assess and evaluate nursing homes are likely not appropriate for assisted-living facilities. Thus, there is a need to examine and define an appropriate framework for assessing assisted-living facilities. This chapter seeks to provide such a framework. Because the basis of assisted living is fundamentally different from that of nursing homes, this chapter begins by exploring several environmental models for the aging, which provide the foundation for evaluating potentially useful assessment strategies.

Defining Assisted Living as a Setting

Before exploring the environmental models, it is useful to explore assisted-living facilities as a setting, or place type. It can be argued that much of what differentiates assisted living from traditional skilled nursing care is its foundation on a different set of therapeutic goals. While traditional nursing homes operate within a medical model, in which the emphasis is on the quality of care, assisted-living facilities place a more fundamental emphasis on quality of life (Regnier, Hamilton, and Yatabe, 1995). Several recent books on this topic differentiate assisted living (a positive and supportive setting) from nursing homes (taken to be institutions) by arguing that the physical, social, and organizational environments of assisted-living facilities are more supportive of personal control and autonomy, continuity with past routines and patterns of behavior, and independence (Calkins, 1995).

Much of the more innovative work in this area has been in the arena of dementia care. This is true in terms of both the evolution of the care setting and the assessment instruments. This is perhaps not surprising, given the increasing percentages of people with dementia residing in all types of residential care settings. Research suggests that as many as 60 percent of nursing home residents may have dementia or cognitive impairment (Office of Technology Assessment, 1992) and that 75 percent of residential care facilities (of which assisted living is one form) house residents with dementia (Hawes, Mor, and Wildfire, 1995). However, several studies suggest that the similarities between people with dementia and people without dementia residing in care settings (nursing homes and residential care settings) are not very significant (Rovner et al., 1990; Office of Technology Assessment, 1992). Thus, although some of the work referenced relates specifically to people with dementia, the principles are equally applicable to non-dementia-specific settings.

The Need for Models

Despite the proliferation and diversity of residential care settings for elderly persons that have developed over the past decade, there has been little attempt to develop a framework for understanding these settings and how they operate. Myriad references are available on the importance of staff training, on strategies to improve the physical environment, and on programming activities, particularly for people with dementia. However, there are surprisingly few attempts to integrate these aspects of the care setting into a comprehensive, holistic conceptualization of the setting. Thus, it is useful to return briefly to some early conceptual models of environment and aging relations.

The earliest conceptual model that recognized the relationship between the individual and the environment was by Lewin (1951), who formulated the ecological equation

$$B = f(P, E).$$

That is, behavior is a function of both the individual and the environment. This was quite revolutionary, as it suggested that behavior not only comes from within the individual but also is a consequence of the environment. Unfortunately, Lewin's model had limited direct impact on the field, in large measure because the term *environment* was overly broad and undifferentiated. Real advances in the field began to emerge after some of the landmark work of Lawton (1980), who suggested a modification to Lewin's equation. The new equation,

$$B = f[P, E, (P \times E)],$$

suggests that it is necessary to include more than E, or the objective environment; that an individual's perception of the environment (person $\times$ environment) is a necessary component to understanding behavior and refers to the experience of being in a setting or a place.

Lawton also began to explore in greater detail what was meant by the terms *person* and, more important, *environment.* His early work proposed a five-part conceptualization of the environment. The *personal environment* consists of the significant other people in the life of the individual. The *group environment* is the set of presses attributable to the behaviors of individuals acting together as a group. The *suprapersonal environment* includes the characteristics of the aggregate of people around the individual, regardless of whether the individual has actual contact with these people. The *social environment* is the role of larger social phenomena, such as social movements, political movements, economic cycles, and cultural values. Finally, the *physical environment* includes the natural and the built environment, reducible to objective and measurable terms. The combination of specific definitions and the role of place experience represented a significant epistemological, conceptual, and practical advancement for the field of environment and aging.

In the following years, numerous authors built on the foundations of Lawton's work, further defining the components of place and place experience. Despite their representing such diverse fields as psychology, sociology, and architecture, there is remarkable congruence among these models, although many were not as inclusive as Lawton's model. The work of Kahana on person-environment fit, for instance, deals almost exclusively with the $(P \times E)$ component: the needs, perceptions, and desires of residents and staff are priorities. Congruence between person and environment is defined in terms of segregate, congregate, institutional control, structure, stimulation engagement, affect, and impulse control.

Moos and Lemke present a somewhat different approach to conceptualizing the environment in their work on the multiphasic environmental assessment procedure (MEAP) (Lemke and Moos, 1989; Moos et al., 1979). Their work, which focuses specifically on sheltered care settings for elderly persons, is primarily concerned with the factors that influence the social environment of these facilities. The MEAP is composed of distinct rating scales for four domains of factors: the type of facility or level of care provided, the physical and architectural features, the policies and programs of the organization, and the aggregate characteristics of the residents and staff (similar to Lawton's suprapersonal environment). The development of the MEAP was heralded as a significant advance in the field, as it provided the means for not only conceptualizing sheltered care settings but also assessing them. Unfortunately, the MEAP does not appear to have lived up to its potential: it is used relatively infrequently in research on the environment and aging. In exploring the reasons, two explanations appear plausible. First, the authors were trying to develop a single assessment protocol that would be suitable for a broad range of setting types, from independent living (federally assisted apartment houses) to residential care facilities to nursing homes. It may be that these settings are different enough that what is suitable for one setting is not suitable for another. Second, and perhaps more important, the primary focus of their conceptual model is the social climate of these settings, which is defined in terms of cohesion, conflict, independence, self-exploration, organization, resident influence, and physical comfort. Unlike Lawton's model, this model deals with residents not as individuals but as aggregate parts of a larger organizational system.

Weisman (1981) developed a tripartite model of place by grouping the type of facility and policies and programs under the rubric of organizational factors. By explicitly incorporating Lawton's (P × E) factor, he suggests that the environment can be conceptualized in terms of properties (objective and measurable characteristics) and attributes (experiential or relational characteristics). He drew on the work of Windley and Scheidt (1980) in defining the relevant attributes: sensory stimulation, legibility, comfort, privacy, adaptability, control/territoriality, sociality, accessibility, density, meaning, and quality/esthetics. This model suggests that people, organizational factors, and the physical environment interact to create the environment as experienced.

A Proposed Model

In the model proposed here, the (P × E) component is represented as the environment as experienced by people with dementia (see figure 8.1). The integrative model of place (IMP) posits that a setting is composed of a complex system of relationships among four distinct dimensions: individuals, social context, organizational context, and physical setting.

The IMP follows Lawton's work by distinguishing among the characteristics, needs, abilities, and behaviors of an individual in a setting and the various characteristics and actions of groups of people associated with that setting. However, the IMP differs from Lawton's model by combining all aspects of groups of people into one category. The model concurs with

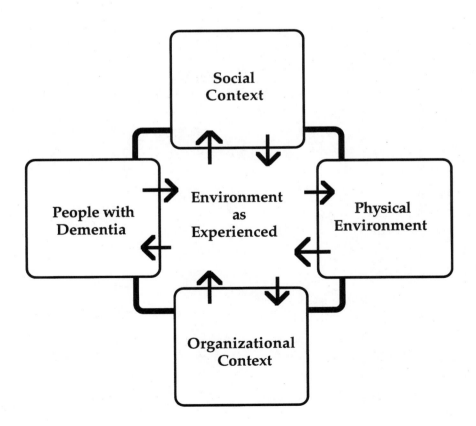

FIGURE 8.1. The integrative model of place

Table 8.1. Comparison of therapeutic goals for environments for the elderly

Physical and Architectural Features (Moos and Lemke, 1980)	Evaluative Criteria (Lawton, Fulcomer, and Kleban, 1984)	Environment-Behavior Issues (Calkins, 1988)	Therapeutic Goals (Cohen and Weisman, 1991)	Domains (Sloane et al., 1993)	Environment-Behavior Principles (Regnier and Pynoos, 1992)	Environmental Characteristics (Zeisel, Hyde, and Levkoff, 1994)	Desired Attributes of Place Experience (PEAP) (Weisman et al., 1993)
Orientation aids	Enhance memory and orientation	Wayfinding/orientation	Awareness and orientation	Presence of cues	Wayfinding and orientation	Noise comprehension	Awareness and orientation
Social recreational aids and activities	Increase social interaction	Socialization	Opportunities for socialization	Seating, staff-resident interaction	Social interaction	Common space structure	Social interaction
Expectations for functional ADL assistance	Increased autonomy in activities of daily living	Competence in daily activities	Support functional abilities through meaningful activities		Accessibility and functioning	Wandering paths	Support functional abilities
Physical amenities	Enhance sense of self	Personalization	Ties to the healthy and familiar	Home-like furniture, personalization	Personalization and familiarity	Residential character	Continuity of self
Provision of privacy		Privacy	Privacy	Privacy in bedrooms	Privacy	Individual away places	Privacy
Prosthetic aids and safety features		Safety and security	Safety and security	Handrails and grab bars	Safety and security	Exit control	Safety and security
Resident control			Autonomy		Control and choice	Autonomy support	Personal control
Architectural choice			Flexibility				
Access to community				Access to courtyard, views to outside		Outdoor freedom	
Staff facilities							
Tolerance for deviance	Increased meaningful use of time			Resident involvement in activities			
				Maintenance	Aesthetics and appearance		

Note: This table is organized so that similar constructs are aligned across the rows. Empty cells indicate that this construct or dimension was not included in the work.

Moos and Lemke regarding the importance of organizational factors related to a setting, although here again the multiple categories (type of facility, level of care, and policies and programs) are consolidated into one category, as in Weisman's model. And like the other models, the IMP recognizes the important role of the physical environment. One important difference between the IMP and the other models described above is that it is fundamentally interested not in the determinants of behavior but in the experience of place. Thus, Lawton's equation could be rewritten

$$P = f(I, E_{sop} (I \times E_{sop}),$$

where P = place experience, I = individual, E = environment, s = social environment, o = organizational environment, and p = physical environment.

The Attributes of Place Experience

The quadripartite conceptualization of the IMP allows for a detailed examination of the components of place and place experience. However, even with this level of specificity, it is necessary to further define the critical variables or components of a setting or setting type. After all, what is important in an auto mechanic's shop is likely to be different from what is of value in an assisted-living setting. Thus, the next step in this process of understanding these places is to explore which aspects of this setting are most important; in other words, what are the salient attributes of place experience of an assisted-living facility. There have been several attempts to define the salient characteristics of residential and care settings for elderly persons, often referred to as therapeutic goals (see table 8.1).

Most lists of goals are specific to population (people with dementia) (Lawton, Fulcomer, and Kleban, 1984; Calkins, 1988; Cohen and Weisman, 1991; Sloane et al., 1993; Zeisel, Hyde, and Levkoff, 1994), while others are specific to setting. The environment-behavior principles by Regnier and Pynoos (1991) were developed specifically for assisted-living facilities. Despite being developed over a span of fifteen years, for different settings and populations, and by different methods (rational and empirical), there is a high degree of congruence among these conceptualizations. Almost all address the issue of environmental stimulation, either in terms of amount (regulating it so it is not overwhelming) or in terms of quality (minimizing negative or noxious stimuli). Recognition that the environment can be structured to help compensate for both physical and cognitive changes that impair an individual's ability to continue to be independent is another common element. Maximizing awareness and orientation (both temporally and spatially) reflects concern over the increasing disorientation common to dementia. Providing a safe environment addresses the increasingly impaired judgment of people with dementia, preventing them from using an environment in a conventional and safe manner. Also included are attributes that relate to opportunities for both privacy and social interaction. This congruence suggests that these therapeutic goals are likely to be relatively robust across settings and for people with differing abilities. These refer to characteristics these experts think a setting should have, however, and do not necessarily reflect what, in reality, it does have.

The therapeutic goals listed in table 8.1 are similar to the environmental attributes defined by Windley and Scheidt (1980) and used by Weisman (1981) in his model of place. The high degree of congruence suggests that, despite the emphasis placed on the special needs of older adults, their underlying needs may be more similar to those of the general population than is sometimes thought.

Environmental Assessment Protocols

A major aim of this chapter is to explore strategies for assessing assisted-living environments. Before examining specific assessment protocols, it is useful to introduce the difference between global and discrete conceptualizations of environment, as this has an impact on how assessment protocols are structured.

In any systematic exploration of a setting, there are fundamentally different ways of conceptualizing that setting, which directly impact how an evaluation is conducted (Weisman, Calkins, and Sloane, 1994). Global, or macro, conceptualizations view the setting as a single treatment and tend to examine the impact of the whole setting on the individual being studied. An example is a study of the impact on residents of relocating to a new care setting (Lawton, Fulcomer, and Kleban, 1984). Discrete, or micro, conceptualizations treat environment as a set of discrete, and usually independent, variables. Typically, studies that reflect a discrete approach focus on one or a few characteristics, such as lines on the floor at exit doors to limit egress, disregarding (or controlling for) the myriad other aspects of the setting (Hussian and Brown, 1987).

One of the earliest, but also most complete, assessments is the MEAP, developed by Moos and Lemke (1980) to assess the social environment of residential homes for elderly persons (nursing homes, veterans homes, residential apartments). This work was conducted before assisted-living facilities, as such, were developed. The MEAP includes separate scales for policy and program information, resident and staff information, physical and architectural features, social climate, and a generalized rating scale. The physical and architectural features (PAF) checklist is most relevant to this discussion; it addresses community accessibility, physical amenities, social and recreational aids, space availability, safety features, staff facilities, orientational aids, and prosthetic aids. However, there are significant limitations to the MEAP, in addition to the issues discussed above. Many of the MEAP's questions require a relatively high degree of subjective interpretation and do not reflect the most recent research in aging-environment relationships (see Weisman, Calkins, and Sloane, 1994, for a discussion).

Lawton, Fulcomer, and Kleban's set of attributes (see table 8.1) was developed as evaluation criteria to conduct a postoccupancy evaluation of the newly constructed Weiss Institute at the Philadelphia Geriatric Institute. The Weiss Institute was the first care setting specifically designed for people with Alzheimer's and related dementias. A number of hypotheses about the supportiveness of the environment were incorporated into the design; the goal of the evaluation was to assess the impact of these features. While the results of the research were compelling regarding the extent to which a supportive environment can maintain functioning despite continuing decline in basic cognitive abilities, the authors expressed frustration with their inability to understand the interplay of a broad array of environmental features. The independent variable in the study was the new care unit, a global variable that obviously incorporated myriad distinct but related components. When this study was conducted in the late 1970s, almost no assessment instruments were available that could disentangle these components.

Advances have been made since the early 1980s; several instruments have been designed to specifically assess special care units as a setting. The therapeutic environment screening scale (TESS) has evolved from a twelve-item to a thirty-seven-item descriptive assessment instrument (Sloane et al., 1993). Domains covered in the expanded version, TESS2+, include general design, maintenance, space and seating, lighting, noise, resident rooms, privacy and personalization, and programming orientation. While conceptually related to these domains, the individual items in the TESS2+ are concrete, objective characteristics of the physical environment. Being primarily a descriptive instrument developed to differentiate the environments of special care units from traditional care settings, there is almost no attempt to identify one response category as better than another (the exception being maintenance and lighting). Thus, the TESS2+ is particularly useful for describing similarities and differences between the physical environments of a large number of special care units.

Zeisel, Hyde, and Levkoff (1994) developed their E-B model concepts from a combination of literature review and an expert consensus process. Each of the eight E-B (environment-behavior) concepts (see table 8.1) can be defined in terms of two dimensions, which together form a matrix for evaluating a special care unit. For example, when considering the E-B concept of common space structure, the related dimensions are quantity and variability of spaces. A unit would be rated on the extent to which multiple spaces were available (many or few) and the extent to which these spaces were distinctive (high or low variability). These two ratings (which are fundamentally descriptive) are then combined into an evaluative rating: units with many distinctive shared social spaces are better than units with a single, undifferentiated social space. Thus, this instrument includes both descriptive and evaluative assessment of the special care unit. It also combines aspects of both the global and discrete perspectives. Each environment-behavior concept can be seen as combining two discrete variables into a more global variable. Most of the dimensions, however, relate only to the physical environment and are rated on a dichotomous scale.

A somewhat similar format can be found in the professional environmental assessment protocol (PEAP). Like the E-B model concepts assessment, the PEAP is directly based on the attributes of place experience: maximize awareness and orientation, maximize safety and security, provide privacy, support functional abilities, regulate quality and quantity of stimulation, provide opportunities for personal control, enhance continuity of self, and facilitate social contact. It goes beyond the E-B model concepts assessment, however, in that it includes many indicators to evaluate the extent to which a setting meets each goal (as opposed to only two). It also deals with more than the physical environment and specifically includes components of the social and organizational environment as well. Each of the nine dimensions is rated on a five-point scale, plus optional intermediate points as

Table 8.2. Sample Ratings for Awareness and Orientation

Rating	Description
5	Exceptionally high support: Such a setting is highly supportive of awareness and orientation in all of the ways described above: structural characteristics (small unit size and/or use of loop or cluster plan rather than traditional long corridors); easy visibility of key activity areas; clear differentiation of spaces in terms of both program and architecture (furniture, finishes, variation in size and character of individual spaces); and the use of multiple forms of environmental information (color, signs, pictograms, personal memorabilia).
4	High support of awareness and orientation: Such facilities (through initial design or renovation) most typically provide clear differentiation of areas through furnishings and finishes (if not overall architectural character), and an effective way-finding system. Corridors may be somewhat longer and visual access somewhat more limited than optimal. Programmatically, there should be a clear and unambiguous location for each activity.
3	Moderate level of support: Use of multiple cues for orientation, efforts to provide a degree of differentiation in what may have been a traditional institutional setting, clear and unambiguous activity program with clear locus for each activity.
2	Low support of awareness and orientation: Few orientation cues in a traditional, visually undifferentiated unit with long corridors. Diverse activities are held in a limited number of spaces.
1	Unusually limited support for awareness and orientation: Little or no differentiation of environment at any level, with long corridors, few views into activity areas or to exterior, multiple (conflicting) activities within the same space(s), irregular schedule.

plus or minus (Norris-Baker et al., 1995; Weisman et al., 1993). The ratings for awareness and orientation are provided in table 8.2.

Although it is relatively new, the PEAP appears to be a promising tool. When the PEAP was pilot tested in twenty nursing homes in Kansas, reliability (kappa) for individual dimensions ranged from .69 to .85. Additional data collected from both nursing homes and assisted-living facilities highlights some notable differences (see figure 8.2).

Despite wide variations among assisted-living facilities, they are fundamentally different and distinct from nursing homes. The literature suggests that issues such as privacy, autonomy, and continuity of self are typically given higher priority in the design and operation of assisted-living facilities than they are in nursing homes, which tend to focus on the physical needs of the residents. What the field needs, however, is a framework for articulating these differences. The examination and analysis of the eight sets of therapeutic goals, developed over a number of years and derived through several methodological approaches, suggest that these may be an appropriate framework for differentiating assisted-living facilities from more traditional nursing homes. Despite minor differences in the various conceptualizations, the commonalities suggest a robustness of the underlying constructs. Thus, one might expect that an assessment protocol based on these therapeutic goals, such as the PEAP, would generally rate assisted-living facilities higher than nursing homes.

The data support this hypothesis. On every dimension, assisted-living dementia care units rate higher—that is, more supportive—than special

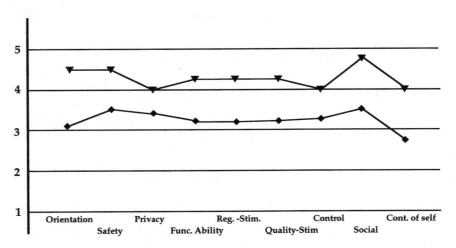

FIGURE 8.2. *Mean scores from PEAP in nursing homes and assisted-living facilities*

◆ SCUs in Nursing Homes
▼ Assisted Living Facilities

care units in nursing homes. Overall, these differences averaged 1.04 (on a 5-point scale), suggesting a moderately substantial difference. The three dimensions with the most significant difference between assisted-living facilities and special care units in nursing homes are awareness and orientation, social contact, and continuity of self (with differences of 1.37, 1.25, and 1.25, respectively). The magnitude of these differences is not surprising for awareness and orientation and social contact, given how highly these are rated for assisted-living facilities. However, the difference between the scores of nursing homes and the scores of assisted-living facilities on the continuity-of-self dimension is particularly interesting, given that the score of 4.0 for assisted-living facilities is the lowest rating given (also given to privacy and control). It appears that special care units in nursing homes (or at least in the nursing homes included in this analysis) do a particularly poor job of providing for continuity of self. While the sample of facilities assessed by the PEAP is still too small to generalize to assisted-living facilities as a whole, these results suggest that assisted-living units for people with dementia may address the issues incorporated in the therapeutic goals embodied in the PEAP better than do special care units in nursing homes. Although the PEAP is still under development, it appears that it reflects the IMP model by combining multiple dimensions of the environment (social, organizational, and physical) and by specifically dealing with the experience of place.

References

Calkins, M. 1988. *Design for Dementia: Planning Environments for the Elderly and the Confused.* Owings Mills, Md.: National Health Publishing.

——. 1995. From aging in place to aging in institutions: Exploring advances in environments for aging. *Gerontologist* 35:567–71.

Cohen, U., and G. Weisman. 1991. *Holding on to Home: Designing Environments for People with Dementia.* Baltimore: Johns Hopkins University Press.

Hawes, C., V. Mor, J. Wildfire, et al. 1995. *Analysis of the Effect of Regulation on the Quality of Care in Board and Care Homes: Executive Summary.* Research Triangle Park, N.C.: Research Triangle Institute and Brown University.

Hussian, R., and D. Brown. 1987. Use of two-dimensional grid patterns to limit hazardous ambulation in demented patients. *Journal of Gerontology* 42:558–60.

Kahana, E. 1975. A congruence model of person-environment interaction. In P. Windley, T. Byerts, and F. Ernst, eds., *Theory Development in Environment and Aging.* Washington, D.C.: Gerontological Society of America.

Kane, R., and K. Wilson. 1993. *Assisted Living in the United States: A New Paradigm for Residential Care for Frail Older Persons?* Washington, D.C.: American Association of Retired Persons.

Lawton, M. 1980. *Environment and Aging.* Monterey, Calif.: Brooks-Cole.

Lawton, M., M. Fulcomer, and M. Kleban. 1984. Architecture for the mentally impaired elderly. *Environment and Behavior* 16:730–57.

Lemke, S., and R. Moos. 1989. Personal and environmental determinants of activity involvement among elderly residents of congregate facilities. *Journal of Gerontology* 44:S139–48.

Lewin, K. 1951. *Field Theory in Social Science.* New York: Harper & Row.

Moos, R., and S. Lemke. 1980. Assessing the physical and architectural features of sheltered care settings. *Gerontologist* 3:571–83.

Moos, R., M. Gauvin, S. Lemke, W. Max, and B. Mehren. 1979. Assessing the social environments of sheltered care settings. *Gerontologist* 19:74–82.

Norris-Baker, L., G. Weisman, M. Lawton, P. Sloane, and M. Calkins. 1995. Assessing special care units for dementia: The professional environmental assessment protocol. In S. Danforth and E. Steinfeld, eds., *Measuring Enabling Environments.* New York: Plenum.

Office of Technology Assessment. 1992. *Special Care Units for People with Alzheimer's and Other Dementias: Consumer Education, Research, Regulatory, and Reimbursement Issues.* Washington, D.C.: Government Printing Office.

Regnier, V., and J. Pynoos. 1992. Environmental interventions for cognitively impaired older persons. In J. Birren, B. Sloane, and G. Cohen, eds., *Handbook of Mental Health and Aging.* New York: Academic.

Regnier, V., J. Hamilton, and S. Yatabe. 1995. *Assisted Living for the Frail and Aged: Innovations in Design, Management, and Financing.* New York: Columbia University Press.

Rovner, B., P. German, J. Broadhead, et al. 1990. The prevalence and management of dementia and other psychiatric disorders in nursing homes. *International Psychogeriatrics* 2:13–24.

Sloane, P., G. Weisman, M. Calkins, J. Teresi, and M. Ramirez. 1993. Therapeutic environment screening scale, 2+. Unpublished assessment protocol.

Weisman, G. 1981. Modeling environment-behavior systems: A brief note. *Journal of Man-Environment Relations* 1:32–41.

Weisman, G., M. Calkins, and P. Sloane. 1994. The environmental context of special care. *Alzheimer's Disease and Associated Disorders* 8 (supp. 1): S308–20.

Weisman, G., M. Lawton, M. Calkins, and P. Sloane. 1993. PEAP: Professional environmental assessment protocol. Unpublished manuscript.

Windley, P., and R. Scheidt. 1980. Person-environmental dialectics: Implications for competent functioning in old age. In I. Poon, ed., *Aging in the 1980s: Psychological Issues.* Washington, D.C.: American Psychological Association.

Zeisel, J., J. Hyde, and S. Levkoff. 1994. Best practices: An environment-behavior model for Alzheimer special care units. *American Journal of Alzheimer's Care and Related Disorders and Research* 9:4–21.

PART III THE PROVISION AND
CONSUMPTION OF CARE

CHAPTER 9

Dementia Care in Assisted Living
A Case Study of Copper Ridge

CAROL L. KERSHNER
CARMEL ROQUES
CYNTHIA D. STEELE

Assisted living is a popular term used today to describe many alternatives in living arrangements that offer an array of services for older persons who require some assistance with activities of daily living. The American Association of Homes and Services for the Aging defines assisted living as a program that provides or arranges for the provision of daily meals, personal and other supportive services, health care, and 24-hour oversight to persons residing in a group residential facility who need assistance with activities of daily living and instrumental activities of daily living. It is characterized by a philosophy of service provision that is consumer driven, flexible, and individualized and that maximizes consumer independence, choice, privacy, and dignity. It is helpful to agree upon this definition as the basis of the description of a specific assisted-living program, Copper Ridge, which has been developed to respond to the special needs of the person with dementia (Gulyas, 1995).

Copper Ridge is a 126-bed facility dedicated to caring for those affected by memory impairment illness (see figures 9.1 and 9.2). Opened in July 1994, the facility serves 60 residents in private assisted-living rooms, 66 residents in skilled nursing care and more than 350 patients who are followed in an outpatient assessment clinic. Faculty from the Neuropsychiatry and Memory Group of Johns Hopkins University School of Medicine provide psychiatric services. FMS, a medical group practice operating on-site provides primary care physicians, dental care, and rehabilitation services. Copper Ridge is as an example of a successful synthesis of innovative building and a program designed to create an exceptionally accommodating environment for persons with dementia. The dynamic relationship between the design features and a social model of a daily life program provides an opportunity to test the effectiveness at all levels of a nonmedical setting for persons with dementia. The experience of four years of planning and three years of operation are reflected in this chapter.

Assisted-living facilities have historically provided a low-cost alternative for the frail elderly person who requires assistance with daily life functions or who is at risk for needing health care. These settings, typically, appeal not only because they are economical but also because they emphasize independence and choice. The combination of the noninstitutional environment of these settings with their informal care system has proven to be effective for people with dementia. The physically frail or the cognitively intact older person is provided with care on an individual basis. Each person is assessed with respect to the degree and kind of assistance he or she requires.

This model of care, which is consumer driven, breaks down when applied

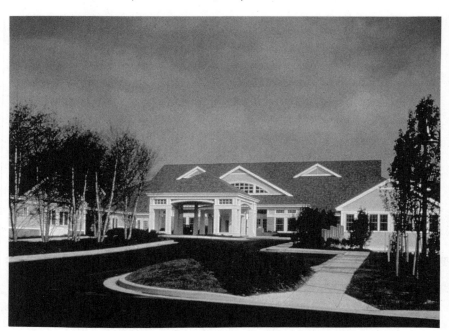

FIGURE 9.1. *Copper Ridge, Sykesville, Maryland, front elevation*

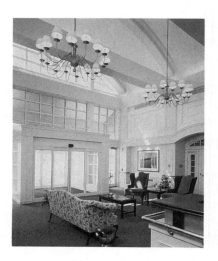

FIGURE 9.2. *Entry lobby at Copper Ridge*

to the cognitively impaired person for whom physical frailties are usually secondary to issues of judgment and memory. At every stage of decision and care, differences between traditional assisted-living and dementia-specific units emerge. The initial point of entry for dementia care is likely to be sought by concerned family members, not by the resident consumer. Issues leading to the decision for placement typically involve incontinence, deficits in ability for self-care, failure to recognize familiar surroundings, aggressive behavior, and the general inability of the family to maintain the person safely in the home environment (Pfeiffer, 1995).

The setting and services required for the safety and security of the memory-impaired person with these deficits are significantly different in kind and scope from other assisted-living arrangements. Facilities for people with dementia require greater emphasis on health care, supervision, and monitoring. These differences mitigate the economic incentives usually associated with assisted living, particularly if there is a commitment to aging in place. Providing dementia care in noninstitutional environments is philosophically consistent with the value we place on the older person. It is ethically important however, to dedicate the necessary attention and resources to provide care in a responsible way. Assisted living is not a low-cost alternative for dementia care; the option exists only for those with minimal cognitive impairment. Unfortunately, advancing illness is predictable in most cases.

The discussion about dementia care in assisted living, then, centers on the mix of services typical of traditional assisted care and those more often associated with the higher-cost health care model. Aspects of assisted-living settings that are important in caring for residents with a dementia-related illness include the aesthetics of a noninstitutional environment and an emphasis on normal daily life routines. Opportunities for choice and the ability to exercise independent judgment must be planned so that manageable levels of risk are involved. For example, it is acceptable to choose to go

Table 9.1. Attributes of Assisted-Living Facilities, Nursing Homes, and Assisted-Living Facilities for Persons with Dementia

Attribute	Assisted Living	Nursing Home	Assisted Living for Persons with Dementia
Philosophy of care	Residential	Medical model; protectionist	Philosophy of residential care with focus on supporting residual function
Admission decision	By resident	Medically driven	Admission decision made by family or caregivers
Formality of program	Minimal	Very structured program	Program well defined though based on flexibility
Independence	Supported; limited supervision	Dependence based on physical frailty; 24-hour supervision	Independence limited by issues of judgment but emphasized programmatically; 24-hour supervision
Freedom of choice	Supported	Limited; institutionally defined choices	Choices modified to manage risk; opportunities for participation provided
Freedom of movement	Supported	Limited mobility, controlled access	Mobility managed; security for safe wandering provided
Administration of medications	Self-administered	Intensive nursing care; administration of medications by staff	Nursing care as necessary; administration of medications by staff
Assistance with activities of daily living	Some assistance for minimal dependence	Assistance for total care, as required	Moderate assistance on bathing, dressing, and management of continence
Coordination of medical information	Minimal	Intensive medical care; coordination of medical information	High degree of medical management for physical and psychiatric health-related needs
Staff training	Minimal	Staff education and training focused on health-related needs	Staff education and training focused on dementia care
Regulations	Minimal	Highly regulated	Variable regulation

outdoors in an enclosed and secured environment, even though the risk for falling while unsupervised in that outdoor space exists.

Supports for the memory-impaired person must be planned through all aspects of the facility and reinforced by the program structure. Attention must be given to both the medical and the psychiatric care needs of the resident. Considerations include everything from building features to staff training. The formal planning that is required resembles more closely the health care model than the common assisted-living arrangement, since the very fine details of resident needs must be addressed. The final product of the planning must appear to be effortless and informal, since the outcomes depend greatly upon the extent to which the setting is comfortable and non-institutional. It is this apparent discrepancy, along with the higher costs, that create the greatest challenges in providing assisted living for dementia care. Assisted living for dementia care bridges assisted living and nursing home care (see table 9.1). Differences among these settings highlight the importance of careful and structured attention to individual resident needs. The attributes of the melded model balance the two settings, although they do not precisely fit either the nursing home or the traditional assisted-living setting.

Program Philosophy

Meeting the needs of the person with dementia is the single most important reason to adopt the assisted-living philosophy. Without a commitment to the basic dignity and humanity of the person with dementia, there is no compelling reason to address the difficulties inherent in going the extra mile to provide care in this way. Nursing home care for people with dementia assumes that the provider will play a protective role and have superior knowledge. This model is based on the need for medically related care. Post (1995) describes people with dementia in early stages as dependent on structures of meaning to make sense of their condition, to make sense of their loss. If it is important to support the struggle to retain dignity, then assisting persons with dementia to remain in noninstitutional settings and in control of their environment has value.

The philosophy of the program at Copper Ridge is explicit: "The philosophy of care for all programs is to emphasize and support the dignity distinctive to all persons through approaches that maximize each person's functional abilities." Building on this foundation, the facility program begins to address and to support functional abilities through all aspects of daily care.

Marketing and Admissions

The consideration of who will be served is more than a market issue. The continuum of care comes into focus as providers describe the criteria for who may come and who must be discharged to more supportive environments. Regulatory and reimbursement issues will necessarily drive decisions in many states. Public funds are limited for assisted-living settings, and most families are concerned about how long private resources will last, given the extended length of dementia-related illnesses.

Family members commonly become the decision makers for the persons with dementia and often choose the care setting for their loved ones. Most families do not seek care until there are significant problems within the home setting; therefore, the assisted-living facility must deal with multiple and complex care issues. Typically, families are unfamiliar with the costs associated with 24-hour care when they seek placement. Comparisons between assisted-living facilities that provide dementia care and assisted living for the frail elderly is likely to be unfavorable to the former. Services for the cognitively intact can be priced on a fee-for-service basis, based on cogent decisions by the resident, whereas dementia care must assume a level of need based on the inability of the resident to make informed choices. For these reasons, facilities that provide special care for dementia struggle to price care at affordable levels to provide sufficient income to cover building costs and staffing expenses. When providers choose to tackle this challenge, it is an affirmation of their philosophical commitment. However, it is imperative that families become informed consumers in order to distinguish between facilities that merely advertise dementia care and those in which the setting and the program actually address the special needs of this population.

Program Focus

The focus of assisted living for persons with dementia must be on provision of a continuum of services that address complex care needs while maintaining a residential lifestyle. The setting must be able to address cognitive impairment, behavioral and psychiatric symptoms, physical frailty, and illness.

Such programming is directed toward supporting and enhancing residents' remaining areas of health and ability in the least restrictive environment. It draws upon residents' preserved areas of cognitive functioning, including highly learned material and remote memory. By consciously organizing the day around normal activities of daily life, medical care and psychiatric issues become the basis of support but do not assume the central organizational role in residents' life. The daily life of residents reflects natural cycles of eating, sleeping, waking, and activity. Thus, a residential quality of life is enhanced through schedules and routines based upon residents' preferences and needs rather than upon staff convenience.

This principle has been addressed at Copper Ridge through a programmatic approach called the daily life program. The key elements of this program are discussed below.

Recognizing the Dignity and Uniqueness of Each Person: To recognize the uniqueness of an individual, it is essential to focus the program on the individual, not on the collective unit. Residents with dementia do not readily engage in programs for a large number of participants. To be meaningfully engaged, it is usually necessary for the group size to be small and the activity of short duration. This type of programming is labor-intensive and requires that all staff members who come in contact with residents understand challenging behaviors and are able to support each resident with dignity.

Supporting Normative Activities of Daily Life: The resident with dementia in assisted living requires varying degrees of support, cueing, and hands-on assistance to engage in the normal activities of daily life. Ensuring resident involvement and success in these activities requires a supportive building design, a staff trained to work with the residents, and a commitment to the underlying assumption that self-care behavior leads to an increased sense of well-being. At Copper Ridge, residents are involved in the daily life of the unit by helping to set up for meals, folding napkins, making their beds, and dusting the common areas, just as they would do in their own homes (see figures 9.3 and 9.4). Participating in his or her own personal care and household chores is part of the structured daily life plan for each resident.

Providing the Least Restrictive Environment: The program should provide structure without increasing regimentation. The daily life plan serves as a guideline for the resident and the staff, not as a rigid schedule to be adhered to for staff convenience. Creating a plan for the day that is predictable but that offers choices greatly increases residents' sense of control and decreases excess disability.

Caring for the Resident and the Family: The family of the person with dementia, the consumer, is an integral part of the care team. The resident cannot be well served unless the needs of the family are addressed. At Copper Ridge, this is done systematically through regularly scheduled care plan conferences, family council meetings, family support groups, and the individual sharing of information about the resident with the family. The as-

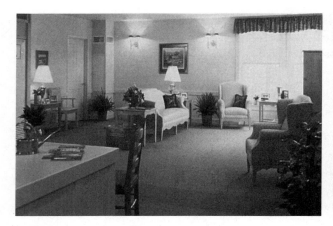

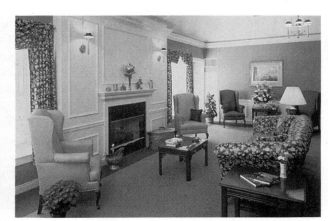

FIGURE 9.3. *Resident lounge staff work area at Copper Ridge*

FIGURE 9.4. *Fireplace room at Copper Ridge*

sumption is that each family circumstance is unique and requires an individual plan of care, just as the resident does.

Universal Staff Participation in Activity Programming: Engaging all employees in the provision of social and recreational opportunities for the resident is a successful mechanism for implementing the daily life plan. Universal staff participation in activity programming helps personnel to relate to residents outside the context of their specific job spheres. This keeps every staff person focused on the resident as a unique individual and creates a dementia-sensitive culture.

As part of employee orientation at Copper Ridge, staff persons are asked to identify hobbies, interests, and skills that they would enjoy sharing with others. Following orientation, employees are guided in designing an activity that meets the needs of the residents, based on individual employees' talents. This approach provides a mix of residents and staff involved in normal daily pursuits. Staff and residents together enjoy baking, singing, walking, reading the Bible, playing cards, looking through fashion magazines, nail manicuring, working on a simple craft project, or weeding the garden. The value and dignity of each person is supported by this approach and allows the staff to spend time enjoying the company of residents.

Residential Spaces

The role of the architectural environment as a therapeutic intervention has recently gained greater recognition. Studies carried out in many settings indicate a positive relationship between homelike settings and the ability of the cognitively impaired person to function within the space. While architectural design alone does not provide a therapeutic milieu, the least restrictive environment results from creatively combining building design features with flexible and creative programming (Cohen and Weisman, 1991).

Copper Ridge is consciously planned for this synergy. Private rooms, many small, decentralized activity spaces, staff work stations placed in the midst of residential lounges, a variety of bathing systems, and security systems at exterior doors serve to increase personal choice and reduce reasons for confrontation. Good building planning supports both resident and staff functioning (see chapter 14).

Building features include residential finishes and furnishings and unobtrusive props such as way-finding mechanisms to help residents feel secure and at home. Props also include Dutch doors, identity boards, and interior finishes distinctive to each housing cluster. The Dutch doors function effectively to help residents identify their own room and to reduce wandering and rummaging behavior. The identity board at each resident's door, with a photograph or a memento, further cues the residents. These features have the secondary effect of helping to create a sense of community. Identity boards also help residents find their neighbors; the Dutch doors allow for casual conversation similar to those held over the garden fence.

The issue of providing for privacy while promoting community has been addressed through the use of cluster design and small sitting areas scattered throughout the building. Each of the three "houses" is divided into smaller clusters of ten residents, with decentralized utility and bathing areas. The seating areas function as a destination for residents who wander. Soft music is played, and games or other objects are left out on the tables. Staff members direct residents to these areas for one-on-one socialization or for time out from the more active areas in the unit. Families use these areas for socialization with their loved ones and other residents.

The use of substations has resulted in greater staff and resident interaction and has enhanced the ability of resident assistants to unobtrusively monitor residents. However, the substations' effectiveness in meeting these program objectives has greatly reduced their usefulness as staff work areas. Residents naturally gravitate to these areas, seeking attention from the staff and handling or moving paperwork left unattended.

Security for Outdoor Wandering

The ability of residents to move about in the greater world diminishes greatly once the need for care is being met outside a home setting. While this is also an issue for the physically frail, access to spaces that are interesting and normal can be provided for residents with dementia only if careful thought is given in the planning and building stages. Security against egress must include both indoor and outdoor spaces. The ideal is to provide residents with access to outdoor spaces at will—gardens where the staff can visually observe them. Philosophical questions to be addressed include whether residents should wear identification, whether an alarm system should be triggered by residents, or whether an electronic locking system should be used to secure the facility against egress. Fire protection systems that require all doors to unlock in the event of fire, while necessary, present a special challenge for a dementia care facility. The experience at Copper Ridge indicates that outdoor spaces also need to have elements of interest to attract residents to the outside. Gardens that include observable events appear to be more used than serene areas where nothing is happening.

Dining Services

Food-related responsibilities and mealtime activities form a significant portion of time and attention for able and independent adults. Retention of some ability for independent food preparation is a major focus for traditional assisted-living facilities, since it is important to the resident. Typically, there is, at a minimum, a communal kitchen available for preparation of snacks, like toast and tea. Residential-style dining service is important for the cognitively impaired for several reasons. In addition to the daily pleasure of socializing in the kitchen around food-related tasks, the cueing of mealtimes and the stimulation of appetite from the aromas of food preparation combine to create a positive experience (Calkins, 1988).

The meal program at Copper Ridge builds on concepts from the daily life program, and normal mealtime patterns are reinforced. Primary meal preparation occurs in a centralized, off-unit commercial kitchen and are completed in the kitchens of the unit in which the meal is served. Choices are made at mealtime rather than selected in advance. Breakfast, though served at a specific time, is available to residents when they waken in their natural cycle and can be earlier or later than the scheduled meal. Snacks are provided in refrigerators that are accessible to residents at all times. To preserve safety in the kitchen when the staff are unavailable, stoves and appliances such as coffee pots and toasters are wired to one locked on/off switch.

Many social activities are planned around food. Baking cakes or preparing Jell-O involves residents, who may either sit and watch or engage in the preparation. Just as in the common home environment, the kitchen becomes a center for other activities. It is furnished with rocking chairs and window seats, which enhance the homelike environment (see chapter 14).

Medical Care

Medical care is often very limited in assisted-living settings. Although some models seek to substitute for nursing care, the typical arrangement coordinates provision of medical care by community-based physicians outside the facility. Due to the complex care needs of the population at Copper Ridge and the importance of addressing underlying medical problems promptly, physician services are easily accessible, readily available, and comprehensive. It is a hardship on residents and care providers to schedule routine medical appointments outside of the facility. Thus, the most practical and effective medical care provision is regularly scheduled physician visits in the facility. These services are provided at Cooper Ridge by the on-site medical group practice, which allows the physician to assess residents in their natural setting. The primary care nurse assumes an important role as resident informant and coordinator of medical and psychiatric care. While most settings may not have access to this level of medical service, it is recommended that dementia care assisted-living settings make arrangements for medical providers to come to the facility. This practice is less disruptive for residents and more valuable to caregivers and family members.

Neuropsychiatric Services

In traditional assisted-living environments, physical frailty and chronic physical ailments related to aging are the primary focus. Dementia-related illnesses, such as Alzheimer's disease, involve the brain. Obviously, mood, memory, and behavior may be affected by such illnesses. A holistic approach to resident treatment includes psychiatric and mental health services as an essential component of care—for a variety of reasons. Despite the prevalence of dementia in aging populations, many primary care physicians are not familiar with symptoms and treatment options for these illnesses.

Psychiatric disorders other than Alzheimer's, such as depression and behavior disturbances, are common among residents with dementia and may result in combativeness or wandering. In fact, these problems are strong risk factors for seeking 24-hour care settings and so should be expected to be common even in assisted-living facilities. These psychiatric and behavioral complications often pose the most significant challenges to staff members who provide daily care, and they are the most frequent cause for discharge from assisted living to more physical-health-related levels of care. Thus, the characterization and monitoring of behavioral and psychiatric symptoms are essential to the success of such a program. These illness can be managed effectively, and the consequences of dementia are often reversible or stabilized with a good treatment plan (Lyketsos and Steele, 1995).

The basic components of neuropsychiatric care are a comprehensive assessment, the monitoring of a resident's condition over time, and the development of specific interventions. Information is ideally collected before admission through an interview and a direct examination of the resident and an interview with an informant who knows the resident well, since the person with dementia cannot be an accurate informant. The assessment can be completed by other members of the staff trained to work in conjunction with the psychiatrist and the physician.

Personal and Social History: The personal and social history provides the basis for developing a care plan that fundamentally respects the individuality of the resident. The history includes demographic information, a summary of daily life experiences, education, work history, marital status and the quality of the marital relationship, religious faith, previous and current activities and interests, and current social supports. Before placement, the primary care provider, typically a spouse or an adult child, has been the "expert" on the resident. Honoring this relationship is essential and establishes the foundation for developing a successful partnership in care. Engaging the family in this aspect of the assessment process provides an individualized picture of the resident and a natural beginning for the important relationship between the family and the facility's staff.

Medical and Psychiatric History: Each resident's medical and psychiatric history is also important in building a baseline assessment. There is increasing understanding of the fragile and intimate relationship between the medical health and the mental status of an elderly resident with dementia. Even small medical problems, such as bladder infections and dehydration, can produce broad and abrupt changes in mental state and behavior. Psychiatric history is important, since individuals with a previous history of psychiatric illness are more likely to exhibit similar symptoms in the context of a dementia-related illness.

Mental Status: Mental status is evaluated in a standardized way, using any of the rating scales for cognition. One example is the Folstein Mini-Mental State Exam (Folstein, Folstein, and McHugh, 1975). In addition to cognition (memory, language, comprehension, and attention), an assessment includes an evaluation of the person's mood state (from depressed to manic). The person is also directly questioned about the presence of hallucinations (seeing visions, hearing voices) and delusional beliefs (such as fixed suspicions). The presence or absence of additional psychiatric symptoms, such as a depressed state or a delusion, will greatly impact on the resident's ability to cooperate with care and to benefit from an assisted-living environment.

Function in Activities of Daily Living: Data about the ability to function in activities of daily living are gathered from an informant and from direct observation of the person by the staff. As is the case with cognition, there are many excellent rating scales for functional ability.

Behavioral Problems: An assessment of behavioral problems is critical to developing a plan of care that adequately addresses issues of quality of life and safety for both residents and staff. Clear, descriptive data on behaviors may be gathered through a variety of instruments, such as the Behavioral Pathology in Alzheimer's Disease Rating Scale and Psychogeriatric Dependency Rating Scale. Behavior is then rated in terms of consequences to the resident and the care provider. It is important for the staff to understand the origin of behavioral problems in order to develop appropriate interventions. Careful evaluation is particularly important to rule out treatable underlying causes. Failure to adequately assess behavioral problems and address them proactively may have serious consequences for the resident and the facility.

Diagnosis of the Dementia Syndrome: The last element of an assessment is establishing a diagnosis for the dementia syndrome. There are many conditions that cause dementia in the elderly, and different underlying diseases, such as Alzheimer's disease and vascular dementia, have different symptom profiles and prognoses. The diagnosis is relevant to treatment planning and requires evaluation by a physician or psychiatrist.

Integrating Neuropsychiatric Services into the Overall Program

While dementia care assisted-living environments are planned to support those with cognitive impairment, each resident will unavoidably respond differently in the setting. Thus, individuals must have their impairments and strengths carefully measured and monitored. For example, two people who have had Alzheimer's disease for five years may be very different in their ability to function and in their psychiatric symptoms and behavioral disturbances.

Most conditions causing dementia are progressive and result in deterioration over time. As this happens, care needs also to change. Thus, ongoing monitoring of each resident is important to anticipate difficulties and to respond to changes promptly. An important example of this occurs when residents become delirious from an infection or medication toxicity. In this instance, it is essential that the change would not be attributed to "just more dementia"; rather, the underlying physical cause must be identified and treated.

Interventions are diverse, innovative, and creative and rely on all of the facility's staff members to effect. With residents who have even moderate degrees of cognitive impairment, traditional talking therapy is usually not appropriate. Such residents are not able to have insight into their difficulties. Certainly, empathy on the part of professionals and others who deal with residents is very important. Thus, when residents are upset, they should be treated with empathy—an appreciation of their distress and an affirmation of their feelings without agreement or argument.

Disruptive behavior is seldom attributable to a single cause. A holistic approach to these psychiatric and behavioral problems is necessary to pinpoint the aspects of the environment, the resident's physical health and underlying cognitive impairment, and the caregiver's approaches that may have contributed to producing a particular disturbance. After surveying all factors, a plan of care establishes interventions, which may include a change in approach to care, a change in the environment (such as moderating the noise or activity level), and the prescription of a psychotropic medication. The goals of treatment here are quite different from those of traditional care. The focus is on residual capabilities, meaningful activity, and helping the resident achieve maximal function.

It is not usual for an assisted-living facility to arrange for on-site psychiatry services. Dementia care assisted-living facilities can significantly improve their ability to manage and care for residents if they have such a partnership, and neuropsychiatry services provided within the facility are most effective. It is rarely possible for professionals in an outpatient office to understand a problem in isolation from the environment in which the problem is occurring. Additionally, the caregiving team, in communication with psychiatric practitioners, will allow the most consistent care. In this approach, neuropsychiatry care is both anticipatory and crisis oriented. It is anticipatory in recognizing and preventing problems wherever possible, and it is crisis oriented at managing problems and behaviors. Neuropsychiatric care must also be integrated with medical care.

While it is expected that most circumstances can be managed and treated within the assisted-living setting, with appropriate support, there are circumstances when more intense intervention is required. Occasional psychiatric inpatient stays to stabilize residents when a symptom or behavior disorder becomes unmanageable in an assisted-living setting can often result in the resident being able to remain in the setting rather than requiring discharge to a higher level of care. It is ideal if the team in the facility is associated with a team in an inpatient setting that also is experienced in caring for the elderly person with dementia and who shares the optimism that residents can, indeed, be helped. This approach to management of short-term, acute episodes has been very successful at Copper Ridge.

As with other aspects of care, family intervention is an important element in providing psychiatric and medical care to the resident. This consists of educating families about the resident's decline in function over time and offering them emotional support throughout the years of care. Occasionally, family members will need their own psychiatric therapy and this can also be provided.

Another effective intervention in use at Copper Ridge is a neuropsychiatry round, a regularly scheduled meeting that includes medical and psychiatric staff, managers, and caregivers. Such meetings provide a setting for group problem solving, education, and support to the staff. Information from these meetings can also help families understand the care needs of their family members.

Training and Education Issues

Studies on special care units in nursing facilities highlight staff education as a necessary component of a dementia-specific program. In this area, dementia care assisted living mirrors the health care field rather than traditional assisted-living facilities, which often rely on the universal worker approach. While the staff may be cross-trained in dementia care assisted-living programs, all members of the staff who come in contact with residents require basic training on care and management skills necessary to understanding resident behaviors.

At Copper Ridge, staff education begins with orientation and continues throughout employment. Staff members often have many concerns about working with residents with dementia. These are dealt with through sensitive, concerned education and through opportunities for discussion. Teaching methods must match the employees' style of learning. It is most effective to provide a variety of experiences, including films and role-playing. Staff members must learn creative ways to assist a person who may deny the need for help or who may actually resist attempts at assistance.

Most behavioral outbursts of residents occur during personal care; teaching staff members how to gain the cooperation of residents is essential. Not all combativeness can be prevented; therefore, training staff members in techniques for minimizing the consequences of outbursts, such as escaping a hair pulling, can avoid injury to staff members and residents. At Copper Ridge, experience has shown that well-trained staff are calmer and more confident of their ability to keep themselves and residents safe from injury. Such self-defense techniques are also essential in the transfer of agitated and combative residents to acute care hospital settings.

Caregivers are typically nonprofessionals, even in dementia care assisted-living settings. Ongoing training is essential to develop an increasing base of knowledge. This training is also accomplished through hands-on demonstrations and discussions in the context of caregiving (clinical rounds). Information shared in rounds is relevant to the working world of the staff, who can discuss resident problems they face during caregiving. This forum also provides a means to support the staff, who may interpret residents' noncooperativeness as willful. Understanding resident behaviors can be reinforced as the staff reviews these occurrences, which result from a multitude of factors rather than deliberate intention. The staff must understand that residents have a variety of vulnerabilities and are easily stressed. This understanding will enable the staff to respond to residents with empathy, even as they deal with difficult behaviors.

Conclusion

Assisted-living environments for the person with dementia are more complicated and more costly than typical assisted-living settings for frail elderly persons who are cognitively intact. While most assisted-living facilities also deal with many residents who have symptoms of memory-impairing illnesses, there is probably inadequate attention to many of the factors described in this chapter. The result is frequently the precipitous discharge of residents when events overtake the ability of the facility to manage particular circumstances or particular behaviors.

With proper planning, careful thought to admission and discharge criteria, appropriate assessment prior to admission, and a programmatic structure to support residual functional abilities, residents with significant dementia can successfully reside in assisted-living settings. The need to account for the difference between physical frailty and loss of memory and judgment is the distinguishing factor.

Residents with significant memory loss have traditionally been placed in nursing homes because there were no alternative settings. Assisted-living settings that include appropriate modifications for dementia care provide a very positive alternative. While they are more costly than typical assisted-living settings, these facilities are likely to be less costly than a traditional medical setting. The emphasis on dignity, individual strengths, and home-like settings are all favorably compared to the institutional environments of nursing home care. Assisted-living settings that responsibly provide care for dementia through careful planning and appropriate programs can maintain the resident into very late stages of the illness, when health-related needs assume priority. While there is no cure for these illnesses at this time, there are positive ways to provide care for residents and their families.

References

Calkins, M. 1988. *Design for Dementia: Planning Environments for the Elderly and the Confused.* Owings Mills, Md.: National Health Publishing.

Cohen, U., and G. Weisman. 1991. *Holding on to Home: Designing Environments for People with Dementia.* Baltimore: Johns Hopkins University Press.

Folstein M., S. Folstein, and P. McHugh. 1975. Mini-Mental State: A practical method for grading the cognitive state of patients for the clinician. *Journal of Psychiatric Research* 12:189–98

Gulyas, R. 1995. *AAHSA's Position on Assisted Living.* Washington, D.C.: American Association of Homes and Services for the Aging.

Lyketsos, C., and C. Steele. 1995. The care of patients with dementia. *Reviews in Clinical Gerontology* 5:179–97.

Pfeiffer, E. 1995. Institutional placement for patients with Alzheimer's disease. *Postgraduate Medicine* 97:125–26.

Post, S. 1995. *The Moral Challenge of Alzheimer Disease.* Baltimore: Johns Hopkins University Press.

CHAPTER 10

Primary Care in Assisted Living
A Geriatrician's Perspective

PAMELA Z. CACCHIONE
JOHN E. MORLEY

Primary care providers in geriatrics are consistently challenged to identify the appropriate level of care for their patients. Assisted-living units have added a very exciting level of care. Assisted living fills a void between independent living and nursing homes that has been long felt. Many individuals who are in assisted living today would have gone to a nursing home five to ten years ago. The long-term care continuum depends heavily on the individuals' ability to care for themselves or to receive assistance from others. As an individual's functional status declines or the support system becomes overburdened, frequently a more supportive environment is required (see figure 10.1).

Older adults who flourish in an assisted-living setting are those requiring both assistance in managing their medications and meals and emotional or cognitive support. These people may have a psychiatric illness that requires consistent medication management, or they may have a cognitive deficit that inhibits them from taking medications properly. The frail elderly often require the emotional support and socialization provided in an assisted-living setting. Often, the ultimate benefactors of assisted-living settings are the families, who have been struggling to provide a sheltered environment for their aging family members. This chapter describes the experience of the Division of Geriatric Medicine at St. Louis University in caring for patients at Lake St. Charles, an assisted-living setting.

Lake St. Charles is a twenty-six-bed unit. The Geriatric Medicine Division follows at least twenty of the twenty-six residents at any given time. The average age of the residents is 83. They are primarily female (84.6%; see table 10.1). Their cognitive function is fair, but they are frequently depressed. The telltale signs for their need for assisted living come from an evaluation of their activities of daily living (ADLs) and instrumental activities of daily living (IADLs). The average ADL score is 5 of 6, but the average IADL score is 2 of 8 (see table 10.2). The need for assistance with IADLs mandates assisted living. Once ADL scores of the residents in assisted living start dropping, a more supportive environment such as a nursing home becomes necessary.

Lake St. Charles was developed in response to a need for a more supportive environment for some residents of an independent-living apartment complex. The administrators of the senior apartment complex identified a group of elderly residents whose quality of life was suffering due to lack of support and structure in their independent apartments. The administrators were attempting to provide a continuum of care for their elderly residents. However, the administrators were frustrated by having to refer seniors, whose functional status had declined due to a medical, cognitive, or emo-

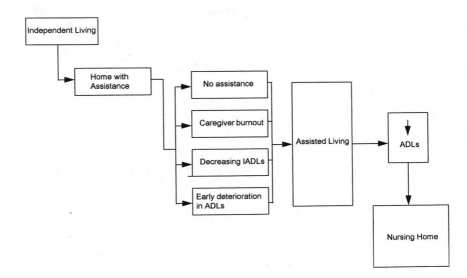

FIGURE 10.1. *The long-term care continuum*

tional deterioration, to other assisted-living facilities. Functional decline, with limited supports, creates an unsafe environment for frail older adults, a situation that precipitates a move to a more sheltered environment. The continuum of care before the development of Lake St. Charles included only a nursing home, which was a block away from the independent apartments.

A plan was developed to carefully remodel apartments and storage areas on the ground floor of the apartment complex into twenty-six assisted-living apartments, each with a bedroom and bath. The number of apartments was chosen based on how many would be necessary to make an assisted-living setting fiscally viable. There are two common living rooms, a common dining room, and an activity room. The corridor between the assisted-living facility and the restaurant for the independent apartments houses a beauty shop, a common kitchen, an exercise room, and a chapel. The unit was designed to provide the greatest quality of life for the assisted-living residents as well as the independent-living residents.

Lake St. Charles has been extremely successful. There has been a long waiting list for rooms, and the facility now accepts applications only from seniors who live in the independent setting. Therefore, future plans include building an additional thirty assisted-living apartments at the same site to meet the needs of the residents who are now in independent living and those from the community who are now excluded due to the long waiting list. This assisted-living unit is considered a residential care facility II, defined by the State of Missouri as any premises other than a residential care facility I, an

Table 10.1. Number, Age, and Medication Status of Assisted-Living Residents

Item	Number/Age
Number of residents	26
Male	4
Female	22
Average age (years)	83
Male	82
Female	83
Average number of medications	
Routine medications	6
As-needed medications	3

Table 10.2. Average Scores on Functional and Cognitive Screens

Measure	Mean	Range
Katz's activities of daily living	5/6	4/5–6/6
Lawton's instrumental activities of daily living	2/8	0/8–4/8
Folstein's Mini Mental Status Exam	21/30	11/30–30/30
Yesavage Geriatric Depression Scale	7/30	2/30–15/30

intermediate care facility, or a skilled nursing facility that is used by its owner, operator, or manager to provide 24-hour accommodation, board, and care to three or more residents who are not related within the fourth degree of consanguinity or affinity to the owner, operator, or manager of the facility and who need or are provided with supervision of diet, assistance in personal care, storage and distribution or administration of medications, supervision of health care under the direction of a licensed physician, and protective oversight, including care during short-term illness or recuperation (Division of Aging, 1995).

The criteria for becoming and remaining a resident of Lake St. Charles include the following:

— Residents must be able to mentally and physically negotiate a path to safety unassisted. They may use assistive devices. They must be able to open the exit door with an understanding that the door does go to the outside of the building.
— They must have a mental understanding of "fire" and "emergency."
— They must understand the boundaries of the complex and must be able to remember to tell the staff when they are leaving the complex. The doors are not equipped with alarms; therefore, they must know where they live.
— If they use a wheelchair or an electric cart, they must be able to transfer from that wheelchair or electric cart to a bed or a chair unassisted.
— They must be mentally able to respond to a bowel and a bladder training program if they are having difficulty with continence.
— They must be free from infection or infectious diseases.
— They must not be in need of intermediate or skilled care.
— They must be mentally stable and not a danger to self or others.
(Reprinted with permission from National HealthCare, 1996).

These criteria are provided to potential residents, their families, and their physicians before admission.

Primary Care Models

There are two models for the provision of primary care for residents of assisted living. One is the standard primary care office practice, which depends on the ability of the resident to travel to the primary care provider's office. A major barrier to this model of primary care is the absence or high cost of appropriate transportation to the primary care provider's office. This model is convenient for the physician but requires close communication with the staff of the assisted-living unit. Patient problems are managed over the phone, by additional office visits, or through emergency room visits. Unfortunately, this model is often very taxing for the patient and the family.

The other model brings the primary care team to the assisted-living setting on a regular basis, to provide home visits for the patients in the facility. This model is obviously most cost-effective if there is a large group of residents to be followed in a facility. This model has multiple benefits to the primary care provider as well as the patient: the provider can see several patients in a facility at one time; the provider can observe the patient's functional status in the home environment; communication between facility staff and provider is enhanced; and rapport between the facility's nursing staff and the provider is developed, which cuts down on the number of visits required and improves their quality. Almost everything that can be done in an office practice can be done in the home setting with the proper equipment and contracting laboratories and mobile imaging companies. The Division of Geriatric Medicine has had great success getting x-rays, electrocardiograms, ultrasounds, and echocardiograms performed in the assisted-living setting. Eliminating the need for residents and their families to travel to their primary care provider's office is a major advantage and a positive marketing tool for any practice. Few assisted-living facilities provide transportation to medical appointments, due to the frailty of the residents.

The Lake St. Charles experience has shown that an arrangement for providing primary care in assisted living works best if the primary care practice has admitting privileges at a nearby hospital. This facilitates continuity of care and prevents the loss of revenue to a practice when a resident goes into the hospital. If admitting privileges are not available at a local hospital, the next best thing is to develop a close working relationship with a geriatrician in the community who is willing to follow the assisted-living residents when they are hospitalized. There are mutual benefits to such an arrangement: the community physician has a higher hospital volume, improving his or her revenue, and the assisted-living residents are well taken care of by a colleague of choice in the community hospital.

Assisted-living facilities provide opportunities for providers' education. The Lake St. Charles practice includes the medical director, a gerontological nurse practitioner, and a rotating geriatric fellow. Frequently, medical students, nurse practitioner and clinical nurse specialist students, physician assistant students, and dental fellows evaluate patients as part of their geriatric education. It is essential that primary care providers in the field of gerontology have a good understanding of this growing level of care. A nurse practitioner can be instrumental in providing primary care visits to residents in the assisted-living setting. Nurse practitioners (NPs) are, as of 1991, master's-degree-level registered nurses educated to perform advanced physical assessment, to order and interpret laboratory tests, to provide health promotion and disease prevention, and to manage and monitor acute simple health problems and chronic health problems. Nurse practitioners function under their own licensure and certification and enter into collaborative practice agreements with physicians. The physician then provides the patient care that is beyond the NP's scope of practice and serves as a resource person to the NP (Mezey and McGivern, 1993). Physician's assistants (PAs) can provide similar services in an assisted-living primary care practice when the physician is present. Physician's assistants have multiple levels of entrance into practice, from associate's degree to master's level preparation. Their functions include performing diagnostic, therapeutic, preventive, and health maintenance services in any setting in which a physician is rendering care (Jones and Cawley, 1994).

Primary care in geriatrics is a multidisciplinary effort. Assisted-living units are no different; there is the obvious collaboration between nursing and medicine in most levels of care. When residents are in need of psychological support, it can be facilitated through collaboration with psychologists, psychiatrists, social workers, and psychiatric clinical nurse specialists.

Lake St. Charles has a working relationship with a group of licensed social workers, who provide psychotherapy in the resident's assisted-living apartment. This has been extremely helpful for residents with depression and anxiety. The social workers are reimbursed for their services through Medicare and bill the patient or secondary insurance for the Medicare co-payment.

Rehabilitation services are also essential for the frail geriatric population and can often mean the difference between assisted living and a nursing home. Being able to transfer independently is an essential criterion for entering and remaining in most assisted-living settings. Developing a close working relationship with a home care agency that provides physical therapy, occupational therapy, and speech therapy is very beneficial for the residents in an assisted-living facility. The assisted-living setting under discussion has a working relationship with the rehabilitation services at the nursing home. Therapists from the nursing home come to see residents in their assisted-living apartments.

The Division of Geriatric Medicine has a philosophy of aging that focuses on preserving function for as long as possible; it emphasizes physical, emotional, social, and cognitive functional status. The comprehensive multidisciplinary approach to care of residents in assisted living is an essential part of the division's philosophy. Included in this comprehensive approach is the reality of the end of life; death as a part of life is probably most widely accepted in the practice of gerontology. However, the concept of dying with dignity requires communication and advance planning on the part of the elderly, their families, and their primary care providers. The Division of Geriatric Medicine recommends the use of a durable power of attorney for health care, which designates a surrogate decision maker should residents become unable to make decisions for themselves. This works best when the surrogate decision maker is a family member or close friend who has had end-of-life discussions with the resident. Residents who are unable to communicate their end-of-life decisions due to depression, psychiatric illness, cognitive decline, and so forth, a prior value history is helpful in guiding the decision making.

Due to the limited amount of nursing care provided in assisted living, it is unusual for residents to actually die in the assisted-living setting. If death does occur there, it is usually sudden. Frequently, residents must be transferred to an acute-care setting or a nursing home to receive the care they have requested. Depending on the resident's decision, this care may be aggressive intervention to preserve life to the very end or supportive, palliative care requiring extensive nursing care. Hospice care is frequently instituted in an assisted-living setting and continued in a nursing home or an inpatient hospice once the resident's functional status has declined to the point of requiring too much nursing care for assisted living to provide.

Common Medical Conditions

Cardiovascular disease, including hypertension and coronary artery disease, is the most common medical diagnosis (81%) of residents in assisted living (see figure 10.2). This diagnosis is followed by recovery from fractures (65%), dementia (58%), sensory impairment (50%), arthritis (42%), depression (27%), cerebral vascular accident (27%), malnutrition (23%),

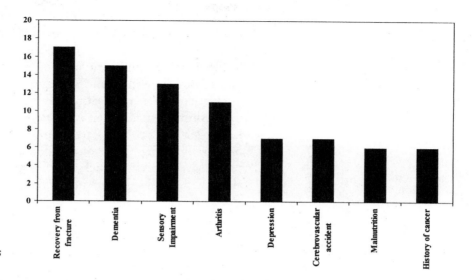

FIGURE 10.2. *Common medical diagnoses of patients in assisted living (N = 26)*

and history of cancer (23%). Laboratory screening is done for all residents with a diagnosis of dementia upon admission to the assisted-living units to determine if there are any reversible causes for the resident's cognitive impairment. Screening includes a chemistry panel, a complete blood count, thyroid function tests, and tests for vitamin B_{12} and folate levels. If the resident is on digoxin, a digoxin level is checked, particularly when weight loss is a concern. Along with the physical exam, the Folstein Mini-Mental State Exam (Folstein, Folstein, and McHugh, 1975), the Yesavage Geriatric Depression Scale (Yesavage and Brink, 1983), Katz's activities of daily living (Katz et al., 1963), and Lawton's instrumental activities of daily living (Lawton and Brody, 1969) are completed at the initial evaluation.

Weight loss is a common problem in geriatrics and often precipitates admission to an assisted-living setting. Three meals a day are provided and supervised by the staff of the assisted-living facility. Even with the provision of three daily meals, however, some residents lose weight. When this occurs, an acronym can guide the evaluation: MEALS ON WHEELS is used to focus an investigation into the cause of the weight loss (Morley, 1991).

—*M*edications (e.g., digoxin, psychotropic drugs)
—*E*motional (depression)
—*A*norexia (nervosa or tardive) or alcoholism
—*L*ate-life paranoia
—*S*wallowing disorders

—*O*ral factors (e.g., loss of teeth)
—*N*o money (absolute or relative poverty)

—*W*andering (dementia)
—*H*yperthyroidism or hyperparathyroidism
—*E*ntry problems (malabsorption)
—*E*ating problems
—*L*ow-salt or low-cholesterol diet
—*S*hopping and food preparation problems

Two of the causes of weight loss identified in the acronym should be automatically eliminated by the move into an assisted-living facility: no money, and shopping and food preparation problems. The meals are included in residents' monthly rent, and the food is prepared and served for them. The most frequently identified causes for weight loss found in assisted living are depression, medications, thyroid disorder, and dental problems. The most common medication culprits are digoxin and diuretic therapy. Medication-caused problems are addressed by decreasing or eliminating the medication. Weight loss due to depression usually requires a more comprehensive approach, including antidepressant therapy, psychotherapy, along with meal supplements such as ice cream, milk shakes, or frequent snacks.

The Division of Geriatric Medicine discourages the use of low-salt or low-cholesterol diets for frail older adults, who are already at great risk of developing orthostatic hypotension and malnutrition without the addition of a restrictive diet. Falls due to orthostatic hypotension are extremely common in elderly persons. Many factors contribute to the problem of orthostasis, some of which are poor autonomic function due to multiple disease states, multiple medications (antihypertensives, antidepressants, diuretics, etc.), venous insufficiency, malnutrition, and dehydration. Orthostatic hypotension can often be treated by liberalizing the resident's salt intake, providing compression stockings, and teaching the resident to change positions slowly. Changes in medications may also be required. Falls are a major concern in the assisted-living setting and often precipitate hospitalization, loss of function, nursing home placement, or even death. The evaluation of falls begins with a review of the resident's diagnoses and medications, followed by a history of how the fall occurred and a physical exam. The physical exam includes orthostatic blood pressure, gross visual exam with visual fields, muscle strength, the Tinnetti Gait and Balance Test (Tinnetti, 1986), and a general physical exam to evaluate for any acute illness. An environmental assessment of where the fall occurred is also done to evaluate the safety of the patient's environment, especially when the fall was in the patient's room or bathroom. The room is assessed for extension cords, furniture height, throw rugs, footstools, and lighting. The bathroom is assessed for handrails around the commode and safety rails and shower chair in the shower or tub.

The most frequent cause of falls at Lake St. Charles is gait and balance disorders due to generalized weakness and arthritis. The most common intervention for residents who frequently fall is gait and balance training by physical therapists and an evaluation for an appropriate assistive device. Walkers with seats and baskets adapted for oxygen tanks are prescribed for residents who fatigue easily or who require continuous oxygen. On rare occasions, personal alarms are used to alert the staff when someone who is suffering from weakness and imbalance is attempting to get up without assistance. This is usually done as a last-ditch effort to avoid nursing home placement. Residents who require assistance with all their transfers are no longer appropriate for assisted living. It is essential that the residents be able to independently transfer and move about safely to stay in this assisted-living facility.

It is also essential that residents be able to maintain continence. As residents with dementia progress through the stages of dementia, incontinence often becomes a problem. Frequently, the primary care provider is asked to treat residents' incontinence so they can remain in the assisted-living setting. Residents moving into assisted living must be continent. Therefore, cases of urinary incontinence in assisted living are all acute onset. The most common causes of acute incontinence are summarized using the mnemonic DRIP (Kane, Ouslander, and Abrass, 1994):

— *D*elirium, depression
— *R*etention, restricted mobility, restraints
— *I*nfection, inflammation, impaction
— *P*harmaceuticals, polyuria

The most common causes of acute-onset urinary incontinence in assisted lving are delirium, urinary tract infection, and diuretic therapy. Urinary tract infection and diuretic therapy can often be easily treated in the assisted-living setting. Antibiotic therapy and encouraging the drinking fluids often is sufficient in treating a urinary tract infection. When the diuretic cannot be reduced or eliminated, frequent toileting following the taking of the diuretic will often suffice. In some cases, it may be necessary to do further evaluation, including a daily voiding diary, a postvoid residual check, or even bedside urodynamics. If the primary care provider is unfamiliar with these techniques, nurse consultants may visit facility to perform bedside urodynamics.

Delirium is a geriatric syndrome frequently encountered in the assisted-living setting. The hallmark of delirium is the sudden worsening of confusion, inattention, and disorganized thinking and an alteration in sleep patterns. Delirium is frequently caused by medication reactions, infections, electrolyte imbalances, and dehydration. An astute nursing staff, who know the residents and identify signs of delirium early, can seek out intervention quickly and frequently can prevent a transfer of a resident to the hospital. The most common episodes of delirium encountered at Lake St. Charles are caused by simple infections, medication reactions, and electrolyte imbalances. With early recognition by the nursing staff, timely evaluation through blood work and x-rays, and rapid institution of treatment, hospitalization can often be avoided without undue burden on the assisted-living staff.

Many of the residents in assisted-living settings have had previous psychiatric illness and behavior management issues. Other residents may have progressive dementias or agitated depressions that exhibit problem behaviors. A motivated nursing staff can frequently individualize care to help manage behaviors. For residents who want to call their families constantly, a behavior-modification program of tapering calls to once a day works well. For residents who are agitated and wandering, individualized attention with milk and cookies or other dessert has worked wonders. There is no replacement for excellent nursing care.

Occasionally, of course, individualized attention, distraction, or other techniques are not sufficient to manage behavior and keep the residents safe. Medications are then required. Major tranquilizers are a last resort, when residents exhibit such psychotic behavior as hallucinations and delusions.

The Division of Geriatric Medicine frequently uses low-dose trazodone (Desyrel) for residents with agitated depression or agitation associated with dementia. Buspirone hydrochloride (BuSpar) is another choice for long-term management of anxiety and agitation. Some of the new selective serotonin reuptake inhibitors (SSRIs) have also been found to be helpful in managing troublesome behaviors. In an acute episode, or outburst, a midrange-acting benzodiazepine, such as Ativan (Lorazepam) may be useful when used in low doses of 0.5 mg. If the resident is paranoid or delusional, 0.5 mg. of haloperidol or 0.25 mg. of resperidone may be needed for the short term. These medications should be reviewed at least monthly.

The Role of the Medical Director

Assisted-living residents who become a danger to themselves or others because of, for example, aggressive behavior or wandering, are no longer considered appropriate for assisted living. Residents may also be found inappropriate for assisted living if they become too dependent in the activities of daily living or if their incontinence cannot be managed by frequent toileting. The medical director may be called on to help facilitate the transfer from assisted living to a nursing home, especially when there is a lack of recognition by the family, the resident, or even the resident's private physician that the resident is no longer safe in the assisted-living setting.

The medical director is also responsible for facilitating proper care of residents by their primary care providers. Each resident must have a primary care provider, who must respond when needed by the nursing staff. The primary care provider must see the resident at least yearly for the resident's annual physical exam. There are no assisted-living unit guidelines requiring the primary care provider to see the resident more then once a year. Another responsibility of the medical director is to oversee employees' health, including the management of infectious diseases, particularly, tuberculosis. The medical director must assist the staff in determining when someone requires treatment for tuberculosis. The medical director, in conjunction with the state's local health department, also participates in the ongoing management and evaluation of employees who require tuberculosis treatment. The medical director is also often called on to meet with families at family forums and to be a resource person for all residents and their families.

Conclusion

The assisted-living setting is a very exciting area to have a primary care practice. It is essential that primary care providers be aware of the capabilities and limitations of each particular setting. Assisted living is a supportive environment, but it does not provide the level of care a nursing home provides. Patients are often inappropriately transferred back to assisted living following hospitalization, although they require more nursing care than is available there. Following hospitalization, residents frequently require short-term rehabilitation in a skilled nursing facility before returning to assisted living. The responsibility for determining the appropriate setting following hospitalization falls on both the nursing director of the assisted-living unit and the patient's primary care provider.

For many older adults, assisted living is often an appropriate and positive alternative to nursing home placement. It is essential that primary care providers be aware of the continuum of long-term care settings available in their communities.

References

Division of Aging. 1995. *Long-Term Care Facility Regulations and Licensure Law for Residential Care Facilities I & II, Intermediate Care Facilities, Skilled Nursing Facilities.* Jefferson City: State of Missouri Department of Social Services.

Folstein, M., S. Folstein, and P. McHugh. 1975. Mini-Mental State: A practical method for grading the cognitive state of patients for the clinician. *Journal of Psychiatric Research* 12:189–98.

Jones, E., and J. Cawley. 1994. Physician assistants and health system reform: Clinical capabilities, practice activities, and potential roles. *Journal of the American Medical Association* 271:1266–77.

Kane, R., J. Ouslander, and I. Abrass. 1989. *Essentials of Clinical Geriatrics.* New York: McGraw-Hill.

Katz, S., A. Ford, R. Moskowitz, B. Jackson, and M. Jaffee. 1963. Studies of illness in the aged: The index of ADL, a standardized measure of biological and psychosocial function. *Journal of the American Medical Association* 185:914–19.

Lawton, M., and E. Brody. 1969. Assessment of older people: Self-maintaining and instrumental activities of daily living. *Gerontologist* 9:179–86

Mezey, M., and D. McGivern. 1993. *Nurses, Nurse Practitioners: Evolution to Advanced Practice.* New York: Springer.

Morley, J. 1991. Why do physicians fail to recognize and treat malnutrition in older persons? *Journal of the American Geriatrics Society* 39:1139–40.

National Healthcare. 1996. Criteria for Assisted Living. Internal Document. Murphysboro, Tenn.: National HealthCare, L.P.

Tinetti, M. 1986. Performance-oriented assessment of mobility problems in elderly patients. *Journal of the American Geriatrics Society* 34:119–26.

Yesavage, J., and T. Brink. 1983. Development and validation of a geriatric depression screening scale: A preliminary report. *Journal of Psychiatric Research* 17:37–49.

CHAPTER 11

"I Live Here, but It's Not My Home"

Residents' Experiences in Assisted Living

JACQUELYN FRANK

Few words in the English language embody emotional power of *home*. For people of all ages, the word carries meanings of shelter, security, and protection (Rybczynski, 1986; Lawrence, 1987). At the same time, home is also an intensely personal idea. Experiences conveyed by the notion of home span one's entire lifetime. During childhood, individuals become familiar with the idea of home not only as a place they live but also where they find comfort and refuge. As one grows older, the concept of home stays with us, yet its meaning expands to encompass more intangible qualities: cultural norms, social values, and personal memories (Fogel, 1992). Ultimately, with the passing of time, the meaning of the word is enhanced: the older a person becomes, the more enriched the notion becomes. By the time people reach their elderly years, their concept of home is often independent of place and has been integrated into their personal identities (Howell, 1985; Saile, 1985; Csikszentmihalyi and Rochberg-Halton, 1989).

Although the meaning of home can be separated from a physical place, home is still considered to be "where the heart is." This may be especially true for older adults who no longer live in their own dwellings and often associate home with somewhere they used to live. Elderly persons who move into life care facilities do not automatically feel at home in their new living arrangement. Frequently, the cause for this discomfort is the physical environment: it is too institutional and too unlike their former homes.

The concept of assisted living was born from a collaborative effort by architects, providers, and scholars in an attempt to remove the stigma attached to housing for seniors. Assisted living is a promising housing alternative for elderly persons who are no longer able to live independently in their own homes but who do not require 24-hour nursing care. The foundation of assisted living is a philosophy of care that emphasizes choice, control, independence, and autonomy in a homelike environment (Regnier, 1991; Kane and Wilson, 1993; Kalymun, 1990). One of the distinguishing characteristics of assisted living is its material design. The diverse architecture and the design of the physical environment brings a residential setting to an institutionalized population. The physical environment is emphasized because it is the context in which the philosophy of care can be put into practice both during and after an individual facility is planned and constructed.

Because so much attention is placed on the design of assisted living, the majority of research and literature on the subject focuses solely on the physical environment. Indeed, my own research originally focused exclusively on residents' perceptions of the architecture of their assisted-living facility. Although the importance of design should not be downplayed, we place too much emphasis on the architecture of assisted-living settings. Providers and scholars have been grappling with ways to improve the environment for residents, and they have succeeded. Paradoxically, however, residents perceive architecture as the only major difference between assisted living and a nursing home. The aim of assisted-living proponents is not simply to change the appearance of housing for seniors; their true goal reaches beyond physical environment to philosophy of care: the purpose of assisted living is to create a supportive social setting that elderly residents can really call home. Thus far, however, regardless of the alterations that have been made to the physical design of assisted living, by far the majority of residents in my study were unable to make it their home. The critical question is, Why?

Using findings from eighteen months of fieldwork, this chapter attempts to address this question as it relates to residents at two assisted-living sites in Chicago, Illinois. Both providers' and residents' voices are interwoven throughout the discussion in order to flesh out the gap between providers' goals in assisted living and residents' experiences.

Dealing with Loss and Transition

Providers of assisted living sometimes have difficulty understanding residents' reality because they see only what their facility offers residents: the potential gains they might make in health, social life, and well-being. What providers often forget is how much older adults have to give up when they move into assisted living. Residents at Kramer and at Wood Glen, the two assisted-living facilities I studied, constantly told me that outsiders could not possibly understand how it feels to leave one's home after many years and move to a strange place with unfamiliar people.

Entering assisted living means giving up one's home and, often, the outside world. The process of leaving one's dwelling is referred to as "breaking up the home" (Shield, 1988, 1990), during which the elderly person must decide what items to take along and what items to dispose of. "Breaking up a home means losing ties with many people, objects, and places. Most recall the loss of loved ones—a spouse, children, a friend—with whom they once made a home. Their histories store memories of birthdays, weddings, and other times when someone now gone, was somehow linked to them. . . . Breaking ties with objects blurs a set of sentiments as does breaking ties with people. . . . The familiar trivia of everyday life are often the hallmark of solid ties" (Shield, 1988:132). Loss of one's home encompasses every other loss the elderly person experiences. Perhaps that is why remaining in their homes is so important to older adults.

The transition to assisted living is often difficult. The activities, meal choices, and services that providers offer do not replace the freedom and independence residents experienced in their own homes. Residents at both Kramer and Wood Glen share this opinion. Eighty-nine-year-old Kramer resident Katie Jacobs, who has been in group living for more than ten years, claims, "I've been in these places [group living] long enough to know that no place is better than your own home." One reason residents do not think of assisted living as home is because home is a place where they have complete control. Residents at Kramer and Wood Glen claim they do not have a sense of control over their lives. Instead, they feel a sense of loss.

What happens after these elderly people move into assisted living and try to settle in? Many residents of Kramer and Wood Glen never complete the transition from their home to their assisted-living facility. They reside in a limbo of sorts. An explanation of how and why this occurs can be found in the anthropological literature on rites of passage. In cultures throughout the world, rites of passage occur to mark the transition from one stage of life to another. According to Van Gennup (1960), rites of passage have three components: *separation* from the old status, *transition* (or liminality) between old and new roles, and *reincorporation* into the new life role. During rites of passage, initiates must learn about the new position they are about to acquire. Rituals that take place during such rites help to make the transition less stressful for the initiates. The liminal, or transition, phase is considered the most precarious of the three stages because the person has no defined role. Turner (1967) further developed the idea of liminality, applying it to any situation in which people are defined as belonging to neither one category nor another. Turner also stresses the idea of *communitas*, or the bonding that initiates usually experience when they undergo a rite of passage together. Shield (1988) applied these concepts to elderly residents in one particular nursing home and argues that elderly residents undergo an incomplete rite of passage when they enter a nursing home because, although they leave their role as community-dwelling adults, they have no new role to assume in the nursing home. According to her, residents experience no *communitas*; they do not bond with others when they move into the nursing home, and they do not assume new roles once they settle in.

My own research at Kramer and Wood Glen reveals much the same process happens in assisted living. A number of residents told me they feel useless and that they have no role to undertake in assisted living. They feel suspended: they have no clearly defined role in the facility and do not know how long they will stay there. In their own homes, residents knew what role to assume and how they fit in. At Kramer and Wood Glen, residents frequently seem lost. For example, Wood Glen resident Sara Vernon contrasts her current liminality with her former roles and relationships in life. "I lived in a two-flat originally until I was married. Then I had my own two-flat and home after that. . . . I loved that two-flat best of all. Those were the ten best years of my life because my mother and father lived upstairs. I did not see them that much, but I knew they were there. And my husband traveled, so at night at least, I knew they were close by. My family was very close." Another example comes from Kramer resident Zelda Arnold. During this interview she demonstrates her pride in her past roles as wife and mother. "After I got married I lived in a twelve-room house in Portish Park. I had three children, three sons. I lived in this house for seventeen years, and my children grew up there. I stayed home and kept house and raised my children. My husband supplied everything. I had everything on God's green earth that any woman would ever want." These two women have a clear sense of their past roles in life but express frustration regarding their present position.

Providers can inadvertently enhance residents' sense of liminality. Although providers try to create and maintain the safest, healthiest, and most supportive assisted-living environments they can for residents, and although it is clear from my interviews that providers care a great deal for their residents and that they want them to feel at home, facility policies are often unclear to residents and this adds to their confusion and sense of uncertainty. At all ten assisted-living sites in my study, discharge policies are especially vague. Removing a resident from assisted living is a delicate issue, and most providers try to handle such situations on an individual basis. Nancy Simpson, social work liaison at Kramer, says that asking a resident to leave is "always a case-by-case decision. We have so many meetings before we come to that final decision. We really try everything possible here at Kramer. We usually talk to the family about our concerns, maybe Mom or Dad needs more help, maybe they need a companion. What we base that final decision on is their cognitive ability—if they are no longer oriented to person, place, or time. Or, if they are disruptive to the group. Also, if they can't meet their needs at Kramer, if we cannot provide a safe environment."

Many administrators stress safety as a key issue in deciding when a resident should leave. Bartholomew Home administrator Barbara Carns explains how she knows when it is time for a resident to leave assisted living: "Usually it is a safety issue. Often it will be repeated falls. . . . If there is . . . a problem that sends them to the hospital and when they return they are at a different level [of care.] Persistent incontinence—they will often try to hide that but then you begin to notice a very bad odor in their room. Sometimes confusion will get to the point where they are squirreling away food and they've got ants and cockroaches."

Even the philosophy of care can unintentionally reinforce liminality for residents. Fostering independence is a central component in the assisted-living philosophy of care. However, independence is often defined solely on physical capabilities. For instance, the number of activities of daily living (ADLs) that residents at Kramer and Wood Glen are capable of performing without assistance is often the only criterion providers use to label residents independent. Asking providers how they define independence for their residents elicits some valuable insights. Dr. Richard Arsk, physician at Wood Glen, defines independence for assisted-living residents as follows: "Able to do everything for themselves, such as dress, groom, take medicines, eat, socialize . . . be independent in their activities of daily living . . . independent in their day-to-day living." At Kramer, social work liaison Nancy Simpson describes independence in this way: "For Kramer, I think if a person is able to meet their basic needs, meaning able to feed themselves, clothe themselves, feed themselves. I don't think you need to define it as somebody who goes out on all the trips or who is very sociable."

It is curious that providers emphasize the ability to perform four or five activities of daily living as the sole criterion for staying in assisted living. The reasons for this observation are twofold: (1) if these older adults are able to accomplish most or all of their ADLs without any assistance, why would they have moved into assisted living? and (2) the main purpose of assisted living is to *assist* residents with their ADLs. Instead, the need for assistance often becomes the measuring stick providers use to remove residents from assisted living. Clearly, activities of daily living play a critical role in providers' definitions of independence.

Providers want to be flexible with policies but not turn their assisted-living site into what one Wood Glen administrator calls "a lessened nursing home." Again, the philosophy of assisted living is to promote independence while assisting increasingly frail residents via a unique physical environment. The foundation for assisted living rests on environments that can be flexible and supportive for residents as they require more help with ADLs.

This means an environment that adjusts to the residents, not vice versa. Why would providers want architects to design environments if residents are not going to use them? This point illustrates the fact that innovations in the physical milieu of assisted living do not always translate into a better social environment for residents. Often, providers seem to be saying, "If the resident cannot support the environment, then he or she will have to leave." This is never the case in a person's own home. Further, this statement contradicts both the design goals and philosophy of care inherent in assisted living. Such contradictions reinforce resident liminality. Among residents at Kramer and Wood Glen, this suspended state leads to perceptions of uselessness.

Feelings of uselessness can stem from many sources. Physical limitations, boredom, health problems, and age stereotypes combine to affect how residents perceive themselves. Elderly people want to feel that they can still contribute to society. Most of the residents at Kramer and Wood Glen are convinced they no longer serve a purpose in other peoples' lives. Their candid disclosures are illustrated in passing comments, such as, "I feel useless here." Looking over my transcriptions and field notes, I realized this was a serious underlying problem for residents. These statements also illustrate the strong contrast between their present feelings of uselessness and feelings of empowerment in the roles they previously held.

Finding a New Role

Before moving to Kramer, resident George Simon lived in a small group home for several years. When contrasting the two residences, George reveals considerable insight. He expresses his feelings toward his first group living site as follows: "There was a family atmosphere. There were only twelve people living there, and everyone was responsible for something—like setting the table or washing dishes. It made you feel useful." Wood Glen resident Wendy James says, "I like to try and keep busy and feel as though I am doing something useful. I don't want to sit around twiddling my thumbs." For many residents, feeling useful relates to daily chores. For example, eighty-nine-year-old Kramer resident Zelda Arnold is frustrated because at Kramer there is nothing for her to accomplish that she sees as purposeful. She has no new role to assume in her assisted-living setting. Her thoughts reveal liminality combined with uselessness.

> Since I am here I just got down in the dumps—*I don't do a thing!* I used to knit and crochet and do—my hands were always doing something, baking or something. Here, I haven't done a thing, so I am just thinking I better get myself doing something or else *I will go out of my mind!*
>
> I don't know. I just didn't have any project that I was working on and . . . you have to have something to do. This is no good just sitting around with nothing to do. When you have a house you always have something to do. It is either cleaning or cooking or baking. There is always something in a house and here there is really nothing.
>
> Well, that's the way I feel about it, everybody doesn't feel that way. Some people like to just sit and do nothing. Even in their younger years, you have people like that. I was always active and did something. . . . There is always something to do in your own house and here you go stark crazy!

Zelda believes that the activities and responsibility surrounding the maintenance of her home made her feel useful. Now she has no house to maintain and is bored. At Kramer she cannot cook or bake because the kitchens have no ovens. She cannot entertain because she has no private space except her bedroom. Zelda has not found a new role to undertake at Kramer, so she feels trapped in her liminal state.

Kramer resident Gail Young maintains a more general view of her predicament. "The useful, productive part of our lives is over. Now I can best be productive by trying to keep myself healthy." Gail has reduced her former active life to a struggle for mere survival and existence. Her reference to productivity reaches a deeper level than just activities of daily living; Gail is alluding to instrumental activities of daily living (IADLs). Included in this category are activities such as shopping, cleaning, cooking, and driving, which are considered instrumental to the independence of older adults. Assisted-living residents at Wood Glen and Kramer regard these tasks as pivotal to their sense of self-worth. These tasks go beyond merely existing or "trying to stay healthy." Residents claim that instrumental activities of daily living, such as shopping or paying bills, give them active rather than passive lives. Cooking and cleaning are activities that assisted-living residents (mostly women) performed in their former homes, that were part of their daily routines during the "useful" and "productive" part of their lives.

Providers at Kramer and Wood Glen often underestimate the critical importance of IADLs in residents' self-perceptions and are frequently oblivious to residents' desires to perform these tasks. Instead, providers are often proud of the fact that the facility essentially takes responsibility for residents' IADLs like cooking and cleaning so that residents can "feel free to relax and enjoy themselves." Residents counter that the only thing they "feel free" to do is sit and be idle. Providers often view IADLs as burdens, while residents view them as blessings.

Through the comments providers and residents at Wood Glen and Kramer offer, two "equations" emerge. The first is the *independence equation: ADLs minus assistance equals independence.* The more activities of daily living that residents are able perform without assistance the more likely they will be labeled independent. The second equation is created by residents and is applied to themselves and other residents (providers do not seem to be aware that the equation exists). It is the *usefulness equation: IADLs equal usefulness.* Older adults residing at Kramer and Wood Glen perceive themselves as useful only in relation to their ability to accomplish tasks such as cleaning, shopping, and driving. The lack of opportunity to carry out such tasks in assisted living leads many of them to feel useless. Zelda Arnold, George Simon, and Wendy James concur. Their statements above translate to the notion that if they cannot do something, then they must not be serving a purpose.

The most disturbing part of many residents' accounts is their hopelessness and resignation about their present purpose in life. Ninety-year-old Wood Glen resident Gertrude Farmer explains, "I can't say that I like anything here best. It is just that I have a roof over my head and I feel like my cares are taken care of. I am just biding my time and waiting for the day . . . that's all." Gertrude sees herself as suspended in time and waiting to die. Comparing their current situation to that of their former lives is a constant source of anguish for residents. Memories of their younger years serve as catalysts for their present feelings of uselessness, loss, and liminality.

One day, Kramer resident Gail Young turned to me and remarked, "You know, something we keep doing around here—in case you haven't noticed—we compare our lives now to how they were then. We don't have much to do now, so that's what we do." Another Kramer resident, Fannie Isaacs, a feisty and extremely independent ninety-six-year-old, remarks:

> All the people here are in the same shoes. We had houses, *we had lives*— they [other residents] made a living, and now they are sitting. Everyone I talk to, the same thing comes up. *Emptiness.* You eat, you drink, you sleep, *that's life? That's not life.*
>
> You cannot do this [feel useful] here. You are here. This place is a trash can for mothers and fathers—*it is the trash can of the world.* You bring your mother and your father here. *You* feel better that she's in a surrounding that if something happened [to her] somebody is here. *It is for you not for me!*

The comments of these residents illustrate the fact that many Kramer and Wood Glen occupants do not believe they possess the sense of purpose and fulfillment that they so desperately need. They want to *live* their lives not just *be* alive. Moving into assisted living and discerning no useful roles for themselves amplifies their sense of loss of control over their lives. Yet, residents do not blame their families or society: they blame themselves and they blame the clock.

One afternoon at Kramer, I overheard a conversation among five residents. They were discussing aging. One woman began, "I never expected to get this old." As the conversation continued, the residents discussed what it means to be old now compared to a generation ago. One resident interjected, "60 used to be old, and then 70 was old, and now . . . ." As she trailed off, the rest of the group sat in silence, perhaps contemplating what they thought it means to "be old." Then another resident suggested that perhaps humans today live too long and that maybe 90, 91, or 92 is simply *too old.* As the conversation among these five women continued, one bravely asked, "What purpose do you serve when you're that old?"

This outlook parallels the opinion of many assisted-living residents at Wood Glen and Kramer. My field notes are filled with entries regarding the frequency of comments such as, "Oh, I am old and have served my purpose," or "Oh, I am old and useless now." Residents almost exclusively link the words *old* and *useless.* When these people feel old, they feel useless, and when they feel useless, they feel old. It is a vicious cycle. Age is the key that connects all of the emotions involved in loss of independence, control, and freedom. Resident Yvonne Diamond claims, "You or anyone else who is not going through it cannot possibly understand what it is like to feel a loss of control because of your age." Fannie Isaacs adds the following: "If you come [here] from living forty years by yourself [as I have done] you have confidence. You come here and you look for something to hold on to. Sometimes you find it, and sometimes you don't. But we are old. You know it is very hard to be old, *very hard.* It is no Golden Age. Everything is gray."

Many processes contribute to an older adult's sense of uselessness. Both

Kramer and Wood Glen residents are often at a loss to pinpoint exactly what might give them some purpose in life. One thing on which residents agree is that they do not want to entertain themselves with facility activities. Most of these projects do not alleviate their boredom or build their self-esteem. Feeling useful in one's life and in the lives of others is a very individual matter. Residents have differing opinions about how they might feel useful again. Several residents simply do not know what could be done to make them feel like contributing members of society. Most residents at Wood Glen and Kramer agree that assisted living serves as a catalyst for their feelings of uselessness and of being "old." Zelda Arnold says, "There was always something to do in your own home, cook or clean—here, there's nothing." Yetta Davis agrees: "In your own apartment you kept busy, there were a lot of things to do." Residents believe that the chores they performed in their homes gave them some purpose. Now, according to one resident, they "sit all day" because they have no responsibilities beyond making their beds and keeping themselves alive. Ultimately, what I learn from these residents is that feeling useless is intricately intertwined with feelings of not only loss and liminality but also loneliness.

Friendships and Social Life

Isolation and loneliness pervade many of the conversations I had with residents. Although assisted-living residents are surrounded by other people, they often feel alone. A large part of what makes people comfortable in their environment is the people around them. In their own homes, these older adults knew their roles and could choose whom they lived with. This is not the case in communal settings such as assisted living. It seems logical that residents would be pleased to have companions. In a place in which residents are surrounded by other people of similar age, why is it that they are not more social? The answer is complicated and involves a variety of factors, the first of which is their perceptions of other residents.

I asked residents individually whether they find the other residents stimulating or interesting to talk with. The array of responses are mostly negative. Sara Vernon says,

> No [residents are not stimulating]. I don't know [why]. They are just somehow removed from my kind of thinking, and I look at some of them and I just know there is no point in even pursuing this. And then I have gone to many of the groups [activities], because there you can hear what they have to say. And there are very few [residents] that even read the newspaper! . . . I am just grateful that I have this friend here. If I did not have her I don't know if I'd be too comfortable. Because we can share some things. . . . You see so many people are not that observant and they weren't exposed to a lot of the things that she and I were.

Many residents want friends but seem to have difficulty finding them in assisted living. As a matter of fact, Wood Glen resident Tillie Von Deurst finds many of her fellow residents too annoying to befriend. "I find it irritating just sitting at a table with five old ladies. It is very catty, very petty, very backbiting. Somehow, I used to think that the older you got the more spiritual you got—but I don't find it that way. See? . . . I have difficulty loving these people." Surprisingly, residents at Kramer and Wood Glen have little to say about each other unless it is negative. Most of the respondents simply do not find their cohabitants very interesting. Part of the reason older adults enter assisted living is for friendship and companionship, but they do not always find it there. Kramer resident Yvonne Diamond believes she has little in common with other residents and, therefore, has not made many friends. "Well, you come in contact with a lot of different people here, and you have very little in common with them. You come from different—everything is different about your previous life—and it's not like they're your friends, you know. You come in and everybody has different ideas, and that's why it's not always easy to make friends. You can have—you can *know* everybody—but you're lucky if you get close with a couple of people."

Making friends is difficult not only because of the group living situation but also because of time constraints. Even if occupants do make new friends, they tend to be reluctant to spend a great deal of time with them. Kramer resident Gail Young explains it this way: "Even when you like someone here, you don't get too close because you know it won't be a long-term thing. It is really too hard to get close now." The fear of further loss with the death of a newfound friend keeps many residents at a distance. Residents like Gail want companionship but on their own terms. Gail adds, "Being in group living is hard. You come for the companionship, but you only seem to get it when other people want it. You don't seem to have a choice of when you get to be social."

Perhaps the reason that residents do not get close is that, in Gail's words, "Nothing here is permanent." The residents know that their health as well as the health of those around them will decline and realize that sooner or later, one way or another, people will leave assisted living. They see assisted living as a temporary stop and may not feel strong enough to take the emotional risk of making new friends. Assisted living seems to offer an opportunity to avoid being alone, *not to escape loneliness*. A consequence is that residents sometimes isolate themselves from others and spend a great deal of time alone, emerging from their rooms only for meals. Helen Finks says she believes that living at Kramer creates an "every man for himself type of attitude" and that "residents don't help each other out as much as they could." Many at Wood Glen and Kramer share this opinion. Unfortunately, such feelings lead to more detachment and time spent apart from other residents. Everyone shares the same dilemma, and yet they are all protecting themselves from being hurt or used. According to Gail Young, "You can't have feelings or be compassionate here or you'll never survive. People will take advantage of you. In this type of environment, you have to be looking out for yourself. You need to be selfish."

Such viewpoints, though totally counterproductive to obtaining companionship and social ties, are the reality for most of the residents I interviewed. Finding no solace in their common situation, they instead retreat even further. The outcome of this detachment is that no sense of community forms. Instead of gaining a sense of belonging to a group that offers emotional support and commonality of experience, residents remain suspended and isolated. They are detached from their old community and way of life, yet they have no real connection to their new setting. Residents are not given a new status, and therefore they never complete the rite of passage. Perhaps Fannie Isaacs best sums up the sentiments of her fellow assisted-living dwellers when she says "My children did not want me to live alone in South Carolina. So, now they move me up here [to Chicago and to assisted living], and I am still alone."

Residents need companionship for more than security reasons. To be sure, residents like to know that they are not alone if something should happen to them or if they become frightened, but true friendship transcends security. Many residents at Wood Glen and Kramer desperately want to connect with each other but feel too threatened or scared to do so. Residents also openly express resentment about being forced to live with people who are not to their liking. Inhabitants verbalize animosity toward cohabitants whom they perceive as being too opinionated, too cognitively impaired, or too dependent. I was regularly informed by residents that they "have nothing in common with *these* people," so they deprive themselves of the most beneficial aspect of life: interpersonal relationships. Residents speak about their past lives and relationships as the standard by which they judge their present and their future.

Residents also measure themselves against each other. This fact is most evident in the domain of physical health. They do not like to see those around them declining. Most of them informed me that assisted living should be reserved for "able-bodied" older adults and contend that many residents at Kramer and Wood Glen are too frail to be there. Sara Vernon is one resident who holds the view that assisted living must not degenerate into a nursing home. Sara, paralyzed on her right side from a stroke, is partially dependent on a wheelchair. She can, however, transfer independently and can walk short distances with a handrail. In terms of daily routine, Sara is almost completely self-sufficient. Sara holds very high standards of independence for all assisted-living residents at Wood Glen and vehemently explains her view of the first-floor assisted-living wing at Wood Glen. "I think this first floor is a *mockery!* Because, originally, they had said this was going to be independent. When I say independent, I thought they meant independent except for a little assisted help at times. I need to have my bed made and I need to have help with a shower, but other than that I need no . . . And the others . . . they have a *diapered person* on this floor! And now we have someone who is . . . she is ailing all the time."

Such a response leads to a closer examination of the term *independence*. I tried to clarify Sara's definition of independence by telling her that I was interpreting her definition of independence to mean trying to do things for oneself, to attempt to do as much as possible. This is her reply: "Wouldn't you *want to do it*? If you had to depend upon someone to get a towel or toilet paper? . . . I'll go get it! If I don't know where it is, then I go find someone who will go and bring it to me. I can't see being waited on!" Sara maintains a fiercely autonomous view of how functional assisted-living residents should be at Wood Glen. There is little doubt that her passion is influenced by her own physical constraints as a result of her stroke. Sara wants to fight for independence, and she cannot understand why someone more mobile than herself would not want to do the same. Other Wood Glen residents agree. While I was interviewing Wendy James, she lowered her voice, leaned toward me, and said: "They've got some people here that shouldn't be on the assisted-living floor. This woman next door to me . . . it has upset us to a certain extent. I think the first floor should be as independent as possible. Like, I make my bed, I change my linens. I do everything myself except vacuum and clean the bathroom." I asked Wendy if she likes performing these tasks for herself. She replied, "Yes, I want to feel independent. That way I am my own boss, you know?"

Residents at Kramer and Wood Glen should not be viewed as totally uncaring. On the contrary, they care a great deal about their fellow residents and voice genuine compassion about the failing health of those around them. Kramer resident George Simon declares, "it kind of breaks my heart when I see people here with walkers and canes. But, we all have some sort of health problem, that's why we're here." Yvonne Diamond's concern is clear. "This woman here, this woman who can't see, who can't get around, who can't . . . she's got Alzheimer's. I pray every day that she does not get hurt on the stairs. Yesterday she got mixed up even on the elevator. Now it's time for her to leave, and they [the staff] know this. I'm sure that they are working on something for her. They want to do the best for her, which is good. . . . But see, this woman, well, she's senile and [virtually] blind, she goes in and out of it. It is going to kill her when they tell her she has to leave."

Aging in Place

Residents told me that before moving into Kramer they were led to believe that no "sick" elderly persons would be present at their assisted-living site. Then, after moving in, they compared themselves to those around them and wondered why deteriorating residents were being allowed to stay. Healthy residents want sick residents removed. An explanation for this behavior is that healthy residents really do not want to admit the obvious: that populations at Kramer and Wood Glen are not static. People who are 85 and 90 years old will very likely decline over time. Residents do not want to face this reality for three major reasons. First, it is very painful to befriend someone and then watch them slip away. Second, the scenario of infirm residents in assisted living is contrary to what they thought they were promised when they moved in. Third, residents are fearful. They are not being cruel when they say "there are people who really do not belong here." Rather, they are scared for themselves.

The inner conflict that residents face with the sickness and decline of those around them speaks to a larger issue: whether or not residents should be allowed to age in place. The aging-in-place/continuum-of-care debate underlies all the issues discussed thus far.

The continuum-of-care model is medically oriented and emphasizes the health care environment and nursing services. Under this model, assisted living is seen as a bridge between residing independently in the community and living in a nursing home. The proponents of this model believe that assisted living serves a very useful role as part of a progression of increasingly medicalized environments. Supporters of the continuum-of-care model do not believe it is appropriate to allow older adults to remain in assisted living if their health declines significantly. The continuum-of-care model is currently the standard in the United States. The alternative model of assisted living is the aging-in-place model. Proponents of this model believe that elderly persons should be allowed to remain in assisted living until they die. Supporters believe not only that the residents' quality of life will be enhanced by staying in a more residential environment but also that residents will not constantly worry about when they will have to leave. Losses, liminality, and loneliness are all influenced by the friction between these two models of care. It is useful to address these two models as they are negotiated in the everyday lives of Kramer and Wood Glen residents. The dilemmas these two models present for residents combine to make assisted living less than an ideal home for them. The discord between the models becomes most evident when residents ask the question, How long can I stay?

Residents at both Kramer and Wood Glen have strong but mixed feelings on the subject of aging in place. Although the presence of very frail and dependent residents upsets them, still they themselves want to be able to age in place, to know they will not be cast out when they become more impaired. Residents voice compassion and concern for their cohabitants who are in failing health. "It could be me" and "There but for the grace of God go I" are common sentiments. Still, long-time assisted-living residents also express distress at the increasing numbers of frail and cognitively impaired elderly who are living at Kramer and Wood Glen. If regulations do remove assisted living from the continuum of care, allowing residents to remain until they die, healthier residents are likely to become even more depressed than they already are. Kramer and Wood Glen residents definitely do not want to see their fellow residents ailing. In many ways, residents would rather cling to their liminality than face the issues of impairment and death. Yet, some residents are annoyed that Kramer and Wood Glen accept "unsuitable candidates." Retaining the continuum-of-care model might mean that these facilities could maintain a more noninstitutional ambiance. Many residents draw a direct link between increasing frailty among fellow residents and their inability to call their assisted-living facility home. Perhaps tenants such as those I interviewed might feel more comfortable in assisted living if impaired residents continue to move into advanced-care facilities. Paradoxically, they will never think of assisted living as home unless they can remain there indefinitely.

The aging-in-place model of assisted living supports residents' capacity to age in place, to stay where they are until they die. Proponents of this model assert that assisted living would then target a much broader range of potential residents because providers would not have to worry about inappropriate placement. Another asset would be the general move away from nursing home placement and all of the institutional trappings that accompany it. As Kane and Wilson (1993) say, "Assisted living can be seen as a promising way to change the paradigm for delivering care to persons with substantial disabilities" (xviii). Providers could spare themselves the agonizing decision about when a resident should be asked to leave.

As noted earlier, assisted-living providers in the Chicago area find that discharge criteria is one of their most difficult policy-making areas. Many share the dilemma between allowing and preventing aging in place. Providers want to allow residents to remain in the homelike setting that assisted living offers, but because of policies, resident pressure, and state regulations, they cannot or will not always do so. For the short term, most of these providers are willing to reshape the rules so that a resident may remain in assisted living longer than might have been previously considered appropriate. However, providers do not interpret aging in place to mean

177

that occupants can remain in assisted living until they die; most interpret aging in place as prolonged residence, which means that residents can stay in assisted living until some undetermined point in time when they need assistance with most or all of their activities of daily living. Then their prolonged residence is terminated, and they are moved to a higher level of care. Is this what proponents of assisted living are striving for? Prolonged residence does not do justice to the aging-in-place model. It also brings into question the necessity of design innovations and environmental alterations. Why make the environment more accessible and more homelike if residents cannot remain there to use it?

In their daily life, residents do not want to witness others' medical decline. They want to maintain the facade of good health as long as possible. Residents at Kramer and Wood Glen cling to the notion that out of sight is out of mind. In effect, they do not have to face the problem if it is not there. A pivotal finding from my fieldwork is that many residents would rather undermine their own long-term residential security by supporting a policy that asks residents to leave than have to be constantly confronted with the issues of declining health and death that are presented by ailing residents. The essential choice residents are making is to prioritize their present desire to dwell among "healthier" residents over their future security of aging in place. At present, the healthier, more cognitively intact residents at Kramer and Wood Glen prefer to have those who are languishing to be out of their sight and to ignore the possibility of their own failing health and potential eviction. Residents choose to hold on to the ideal that they may not decline to the point of eviction rather than accept sicker residents living with them. Most residents do not perceive that their liminality will diminish over time in assisted living. Rather, they see themselves as remaining in the same indeterminate state whether or not they are allowed to stay in assisted living until they die. The major result of this uncertainty among residents is a tendency toward the continuum-of-care model of assisted living.

The conflict for residents is great. They do not want to be cruel to other residents, yet they do not want to be forced to live among the more impaired elderly. They seem to have a literal interpretation of aging in place, considering it to mean remaining where they are until they die (not prolonged residence). In addition, prolonged residence makes residents noticeably nervous. A troubling question in their minds is, How long can I stay? Providers cannot reasonably answer this question. How could they? Every case is different. But residents comprehend the issue in a much harsher light: they want to know that they can either stay in assisted living or, when a designated ailment occurs, they must leave. How can they call a place home if they do not know how long they can stay? If assisted living is, as one provider says, "a way station," why would anyone *want* to try and settle in? The liminality of prolonged residence frightens them.

It is enlightening to find that assisted-living residents' reactions are more in line with the continuum-of-care model than with the aging-in-place model. Despite their desire to settle in and feel at home, most residents at Kramer and Wood Glen would rather sacrifice their future for their present. They would rather risk eviction than watch fellow residents deteriorate.

The Notion of Home

This discussion leads back to the issue of a homelike environment in assisted living. Maybe the circular argument about the homeyness of assisted living within and without the continuum-of-care model is actually moot. After all, as many Kramer and Wood Glen residents say, assisted living will never be home. This fact has little to do with the physical environment. In fact, the residents at Kramer and Wood Glen are least concerned with the architectural design. Although residents consistently voiced positive opinions about the design and decor of their assisted-living settings, they do not prioritize the physical environment.

When I began my exploration of assisted living, the literature pointed to design as the key to residents' happiness. During the interviews, I asked residents many questions regarding the physical setting: Do you like the decoration? Do you like the neighborhood setting? What do think of the building? What features do you like best? Very few of the residents interviewed or surveyed complained about the physical environment, except about the lack of cooking facilities (see note). Residents say quite plainly that assisted living is not home, but they are content with the physical environment. In effect, the physical environment is a priority for scholars, not for residents.

This finding actually translates to high praise for designers. Architectural forethought and attention to planning help to make assisted living much more homelike than a nursing home could ever be, and the residents themselves agree. Unfortunately, residents are still unhappy. Why? Because they use a different measure than providers do. Providers compare assisted living to nursing homes, while residents compare assisted living to *their own homes*. Therein lies the paradox of assisted living. The points of reference for providers and residents are completely different. Residents' homes represent their past identities, roles, and relationships. Now, when they think about assisted living, they think about their losses, their liminality, and their loneliness. Providers compare assisted living to a nursing home environment and see the benefits of the assisted-living setting as it compares to the institutional surroundings of a nursing home. Providers examine the architecture and design and say, "This is fantastic. It is *not a nursing home*." Residents examine the architecture and design and say, "This is *not my home*."

The gap in perspective points to the emotional connection between elderly people, their homes, and their past. Assisted living lacks the emotional bond that their own homes symbolize. Throughout this chapter, residents from Kramer and Wood Glen illustrate the fact that assisted living exemplifies their disconnection from life. When they look back on their former homes and what they represent, they see a time when their lives were full of relationships, responsibilities, and purpose. Sara Vernon describes her notion of home this way: "It is where the heart is, to be cliché-ish. But it is where your children are and where there is . . . where you are loved and where you love. Where people care about each other and share their lives, whether it is painful or not. You share, and that is all that matters."

Kramer resident Wendy James eloquently expresses her notions of home in this manner: "Home? *That's where the heart is* (chuckles). Home is one or two people that are congenial and like [the same things] . . . but not always . . . you don't always have to like everything that the other party does. It is nice to have a companion, but if you don't then you have yourself and you have something that means something to you [material things] . . . whether

179

it's expensive or not, it's up to you. *And you've got it around you and it's like a coat.* I don't know what else to say."

These definitions reveal that for many people, *home* is a very emotional term. What these descriptions have in common is that they are personal, abstract, and lifelong. Residents hold notions of home based on their past experiences. Memories of former homes are often idealized, because they symbolize a time when these older adults were young and independent. Realizing this fact, Kramer and Wood Glen residents try to avoid living entirely in the past. They comprehend the distinction between the ideal of the past and the reality of the present. The question remains, What is their current perspective on assisted living?

For Sara Vernon, assisted living does not feel like home because she is living with people she hardly knows. "You see, home is where you are with your own people and I am . . . these are all strangers to me, and they will forever be strangers." Zelda Arnold highlights the relationship between instrumental activities of daily living and her inability to call assisted living home. "A home is where you have your family together. You have your kitchen and you can do everything you want. We don't have that here." Fannie Isaacs synthesizes the perspective of most of the assisted-living residents at Kramer and Wood Glen: "Home is everything. It is *in* you. Every place could be a home. When I used to come home [before moving here], I was sitting in *my* home, not a *borrowed* home. And . . . people are very nice here, but I have no connection."

How do these emotion-laden descriptions of home help us draw some conclusions about assisted living? Creators of assisted living strive to establish a home*like* environment for residents. *Homelike* is a word that combines both the ideal and the reality of residing in a communal setting such as assisted living. Ideally, the setting will be *like a home* in that it will be comfortable, cozy, and familiar. At the same time, the term *homelike* acknowledges the fact that assisted living is not the resident's true home. It may contain characteristics that make it similar, but it will not truly be a home for reasons such as those expressed by Fannie Isaacs: lack of connection, lack of history, and lack of an active role. Most residents say, "I live here, but it's not my home." Past life experiences inform the way they view their current residence; they compare assisted living to their *own homes,* a point of reference entirely different from that of providers. The discontinuity is evident. Further, residents do not think this gap in viewpoint can be bridged by providers, expressing their firm belief that providers are unable to "stand in their shoes." These residents repeatedly told me that until people face the aging process themselves, they cannot comprehend the loss, the liminality, or the loneliness that they experience daily.

Residents agree that assisted living is home*like.* The architecture and interior design do make the environment less institutional. The residents of Kramer and Wood Glen clearly see the distinction between the physical environment of assisted living and that of a nursing home. Creators of assisted living have indeed succeeded in creating a more livable environment for older adults. This leads back to the troubling yet still unanswered question: Is the architecture the *only real difference* between assisted living and nursing homes? The answer is complex.

After speaking to many assisted-living providers and spending several years investigating the subject, I claim that there are differences between assisted living and nursing homes that transcend design. The philosophy of care is enmeshed within the physical structure. Assisted-living providers do encourage independence, autonomy, and choice among their residents. Administrators at Kramer and Wood Glen *want* their residents to create a real home in assisted living. However, providers' ideals and residents' realities continue to conflict. Providers plan based on ideals but residents live in the reality that emerges from those ideals. Assisted living's multilayered philosophy embraces architecture, design, health care, sociology, and policy. Yet, residents at Kramer and Wood Glen often experience only one layer: the physical setting. The major difference residents notice between assisted living and a nursing home is the design. Because they cannot reconcile the principles, philosophies, and goals of assisted living with their losses, liminality, and loneliness, they cannot call assisted living home. The philosophy of assisted living is like a foreign language for residents: they cannot decipher it. Providers and residents are not speaking the same language.

Can assisted living proponents develop ways to translate the philosophy of assisted living into a reality for residents? Is this an impossible task? This chapter clearly illustrates the enormous losses, frustration, uncertainties, and health problems residents face. Are these problems insurmountable? Researchers and developers need to bridge the gap by helping residents translate assisted-living ideals into realities. In accomplishing this task, there is much to be gained for both providers and residents. By accepting the fact that a homelike environment is not necessarily home, providers will gain insight into the social and emotional needs of residents. Attention could then shift to the social and interpersonal environments so critical to residents in assisted living. Refocusing on the social environment could help increase residents' sense of competence, community, and empowerment despite the losses and liminality they experience.

Note

This research took place from 1991 to 1993. It consisted of formal, tape-recorded interviews with residents and staff, informal conversations, surveys, and participation in daily activities at two assisted-living sites. Kramer, in suburban Chicago, is a freestanding assisted-living site housing twenty-nine residents. Wood Glen, in the city of Chicago near a busy commercial district, is a nursing home with one floor, with a capacity for eighteen persons designated for assisted living. With the exception of several well-known scholars in the field of assisted living, all names of persons and places are pseudonyms.

I conducted formal interviews with people involved in all areas of assisted living. These interviews can be loosely placed in three categories: experts in the field of elderly housing; assisted-living providers (people whose professional lives involve daily contact with an assisted-living site); and assisted-living residents. I interviewed a total of forty-one people, some more than once, and conducted a total of fifty-two formal, tape-recorded interviews.

Four of my interviews were conducted with housing experts in California, Massachusetts, Florida, and Washington, D.C. Twenty-seven of the interviews were with twenty-two assisted-living providers. I formally interviewed eight administrative personnel at Wood Glen, several of them more than once. At Kramer, I interviewed all five administrative personnel, some more than once. Tape-recorded interviews were conducted with fifteen residents, for a total of twenty-one interviews (eight of the twenty-five Kramer residents; seven of the twelve Wood Glen assisted-living residents). I would have liked to interview a greater number of residents at both sites. However, many residents I approached declined an interview or refused to be tape recorded.

Besides Wood Glen and Kramer, I toured eight other assisted-living sites. In general, the people I interviewed at the eight sites were friendly and forthcoming. At several locations, I was given a sales pitch for the facility. At a few sites, more than one person spoke with me about the facility, which offered me multiple perspectives on that location and showed me that providers were committed to the development of assisted living.

The only major complaints about the physical environment at Kramer and Wood Glen were with the kitchens—or lack thereof. At Wood Glen there are no kitchens and at Kramer, although there are shared kitchens (three people to a kitchen), there are no working ovens (which were considered unnecessary by planners). Residents, however, want fully functioning kitchens, where they can cook and bake. They also want refrigerators and access to more individualized food storage space.

References

Csikszentmihalyi, M., and E. Rochberg-Halton. 1989. *The Meaning of Things: Domestic Symbols and the Self.* Cambridge: Cambridge University Press.

Fogel, B. 1992. Psychological aspects of staying at home. *Generations: Journal of the American Society on Aging* 16:27–35.

Howell, S. 1985. Home: A source of meaning in elders' lives. *Generations: Journal of the American Society on Aging* (Spring): 58–61.

Kalymun, M. 1990. Toward a definition of assisted living. *Journal of Housing for the Elderly* 7:97–131.

Kane, R., and K. Wilson. 1993. *Assisted Living in the United States: A New Paradigm for Residential Care for Frail Older Persons?* Washington, D.C.: American Association of Retired Persons.

Lawrence, R. 1987. What makes a house a home? *Environment and Behavior* 19:154–68.

Regnier, V. 1991. Assisted living: An evolving industry. *Seniors Housing News* (Spring): 1–3.

Rybczynski, W. 1986. *Home: A Short History of an Idea.* Harrisburg: Donnelley and Sons.

Saile, D. 1985. Experience and use of the dwelling. In I. Altman and C. M. Werner, eds., *Home Environments.* New York: Plenum.

Shield, R. 1988. *Uneasy Endings: Daily Life in an American Nursing Home.* Ithaca: Cornell University Press.

———. 1990. Liminality in an American nursing home: The endless transition. In J. Sokolovsky, ed., *The Cultural Context of Aging: Worldwide Perspectives.* New York: Bergin and Garvey.

Turner, V. 1967. *The Forest of Symbols: Aspects of Ndembu Ritual.* Ithaca: Cornell University Press.

Van Gennup, A. 1960. *The Rites of Passage.* Chicago: University of Chicago Press.

PART IV   **DESIGN: WHO CARES?**

CHAPTER 12

Assisted Living
An Evolving Place Type

BENYAMIN SCHWARZ

In its broadest definition, assisted living is a reconceptualization of long-term care services for special-needs populations such as the frail elderly, the physically disabled, and the cognitively impaired. Assisted living is both a residential model, which combines housing and supportive services in a noninstitutional setting, and a vehicle to meet confined demands for supportive services, personal care, and skilled nursing services in elderly housing (Mollica and Snow, 1996). As one of the fastest-growing options for long-term care in the United States, assisted living has appealed to investors, consumers, care providers, and advocates for the elderly as an alternative to the nursing home.

Those who have studied nursing homes are all too familiar with the negative attitudes that these institutional settings provoke. Despite a myriad of improvements that this building type has undergone since its inception, it still stirs up thoughts of "the dreaded nursing home" in the minds of most elders and their families. Nursing homes are regarded as frightening, depressing places in which residents experience deterioration in their health and quality of life stemming from a diminished sense of control. The American nursing home in its current form is viewed as a costly building type that is profoundly influenced by the medical model. With its emphasis on regimented routines, safety, and efficiency, the medical model exerts a subtle and pervasive influence on the design and ambiance of the nursing home environment.

In contrast, the new housing and care model of assisted living is an attempt to achieve a different set of objectives. Through a different philosophy of care and a different configuration of the setting, it strives to maximize tenant dignity, autonomy, privacy, and independence. Wilson (1996), who designed, developed, and managed Oregon's first assisted-living facility, articulates the philosophy of this model as follows:

Assisted-living's philosophy is to provide physically and cognitively impaired older persons the personal and health-related services that they require to age in place in a homelike environment that maximizes their dignity, privacy, independence, and autonomy. Assisted-living maximizes dignity, privacy, and independence by providing a range of personal and health-related services (including supervision and assistance with scheduled and unscheduled needs on a 24-hour basis) designed to accommodate and support the needs and preferences of individual tenants in private residential units. To meet the goal of tenant autonomy, assisted living emphasizes individuals' rights to make decisions about their own care and to take responsibility for certain risks that may result from those decisions, consistent with the individual's capacity to make decisions and the provider's exercise of prudent risk management through negotiated risk agreements. Autonomy is reflected in opportunities for self-governance, protection of individual rights, the exercise of autonomy within the context of bounded choice, and negotiated levels of risk agreed to by the individual (or his/her designated representative) and management. (10)

This chapter explores assisted living as a *place type* for the provision of long-term care. It investigates this blend of shelter and personal care with special attention to the association between the complex concept of home and the homelike model of care. The aim of the chapter is to dispel some of the ambiguity of assisted living and to discuss the reciprocal relationships between people and their total environment with reference to this model. Clearly, these relationships cannot be taken for granted. Studies over the past several decades demonstrate that "the architectural setting is more than a background variable" and that it "may exert significant influence on the behavior and quality of life of both individuals and groups" (Cohen and Weisman, 1991:4). Conceivably, the most important factor that designers can influence in housing arrangements for frail elders is the degree of autonomy and individual choice given to the residents. The architectural framework can provide or inhibit opportunities for privacy, independence, control, and choice. Thus, it is important to study those environmental attributes of assisted living that attempt to translate program philosophy and therapeutic goals into a place type that supports the personal autonomy of its tenants.

Ultimately, our interest in buildings begins with a focus on the people who occupy them. While a building needs to serve a social purpose, it is an instrumental good and not an end in itself. Architecture has always been about the values held by the people who had it built—their attitudes about life and their assumptions (sometimes conscious, sometimes not) about what is real and what is important (Gowans, 1992). Therefore, the thing we wish to know about the assisted-living place type is the same thing we wish to know about anything else people make: How does it serve the most important purpose, that of fulfilling the task that is unique to people? Namely, how does it perfect their nature and allow them to pursue the pleasures that are uniquely available to people as people?

I begin with a discussion of the major differences between the medical model and the residential model, then review the various entities of assisted living to distinguish among the building types that encompass assisted living. A substantial portion of the chapter is devoted to the concept of building types and the manner in which we experience them as they convey the latent and manifest purposes of designed places and the philosophies or ideologies behind their construction and occupation. Two studies are presented, focusing on the identification of environmental attributes in assisted-living arrangements. The conclusion discusses aspects of integrative and innovative research regarding the nature of the settings of assisted living and raises the basic questions that must be answered in order to achieve this goal.

Models of Therapeutic Environments for Frail Elders

Implicit in the development of purpose-built therapeutic environments for frail elders has been the assumption that physical as well as interpersonal aspects of the environment affect outcomes (Carp, 1987). This assumption originates, inevitably, in a kind of environmental determinism. It implies that the relationship between environment and behavior is based on a cause-and-effect linkage and that the environment is a major determinant of human behavior. Accordingly, given a physical setting, it is clear that some choices are more probable than others and that what people are able to do in this environment is consistent with, and limited by, the environmental or spatial opportunities available to them. Essentially, in creating built environments, designers necessarily put limitations on people's behavioral opportunities by establishing the general context for those opportunities (Tiesdel and Oc, 1993).

Therapeutic environments for frail elders have different meanings. In some cases, therapeutic environment means simply a location in which healing and care take place. In other cases, therapeutic environment means that the environment itself is therapeutic (Canter and Canter, 1979). Be that as it may, there appears to be a great deal of confusion as to the nature and value of environments designed for therapy. On one hand, we find statements such as, "Let us first dismiss the idea that we can ever design an environment which will be in any significant way 'therapeutic,' nor should we claim that the users of design are 'happier,' 'get along better' or 'are better adjusted,' *because of design*. There is nothing we can say about someone's internal state of satisfaction or health which can be causally related to his interaction with the physical environment" (Charles W. Rusch, cited in Moore, 1970:280).

On the contrary, scholars such as Jones (1962), Cummings and Cummings (1964), Cohen and Weisman (1991), Ulrich (1995), Malkin (1994), Kane (1995a), Regnier (1994), Davidson (1995), Brawley (1997), and others (including several contributors to this volume) suggest that the environment has a significant, perhaps central, role and that it contributes to or enhances therapeutic processes directly. The proponents of this view recognize that no one aspect of the provision of therapeutic facilities, be it care providers, policies, or environmental attributes, can on its own produce a therapeutic environment. They acknowledge that environment does not control behavior—a hard architectural determinism—but rather that environment influences, limits, or affords opportunities.

Those who support this view argue that the therapeutic process is facilitated by the environment and is influenced by the practical and symbolic messages conveyed by aspects of form and use of the physical surroundings. Therefore, each and every design process of a therapeutic setting needs to clearly specify the "therapeutic aims which enable the setting to be considered as a direct facilitator of those aims" (Canter and Canter, 1979:8). Failure in the creation of environment for therapy can be traced frequently to an inadequate definition of these goals. However, given the complexity of the organizations involved in provision of care and the ambiguous forms in which the goals of therapeutic settings are established, it is likely that only the central themes that underlay the central assumptions about the facility will be communicated. Consequently, "the only real message on which agreement is achieved can be characterized as a central stereotype or model of the nature of the therapeutic situation" (12). The idea of a model may be helpful in identifying the nature of an organization's approach to a particular therapeutic setting.

Various housing arrangements for elders have also been affected by the *prosthetic* model. In its essence, this model attempts to make up for deficits of behavior or individual disabilities by providing compensation for certain lost or diminished skills (Kushlick, 1975). Prostheses may take forms of environmental attributes, such as handrails and specially designed furniture, or of social support, such as home health care, in which another person, and not mechanical devices, provides the frail individual with a substitute for lost skills. The prosthetic approach recognizes the increasingly diminishing competence vis-à-vis biological, social, or economic factors—those accompanying the aging process—and seeks environmental supports that can help maintain acceptable levels of personal and social functioning (Lipman and Slater, 1979). Designers of housing for older people frequently exploit the potentialities of selected physical elements and spatial arrangements in order to maintain resident independence and autonomy. Since individuals' ability to function in a setting is determined by matching their competence with their environment, the provision of social and physical prostheses for a long period of time and at increasingly excessive levels may have negative consequences. Mismatches that create undersupport can result in diminished levels of functioning and increased levels of stress, whereas those that create oversupport tend to lead to dependency (Lawton and Nahemow, 1973).

Another model at issue is the *medical* model. "Largely because of the migration of the medical model into the nursing home, the emphasis is on medical or nursing care even though there seems to be little such care actually given" (Agich, 1993:66). Grounded in the medical model, the nursing home came to look and function much more like a miniature hospital than a home. Two forces shaped the standard setting of the American nursing home: time pressures and concerns about possible catastrophes.

> Faced with the task of creating standards quickly for a modality of care that was largely unfamiliar, federal and state bureaucracies turned to models that were available. One of these was the small hospital. A federal program to support the construction of rural hospitals had created blueprints and standards for construction and staffing. Hence, there was a great temptation to envision these nursing homes as miniature hospitals, a view not at variance with that of the program's framers. At the same time, there was a great fear of headline-grabbing catastrophes, especially fires. Thus, the regulations placed strong emphasis on issues of life safety (wide corridors, fire doors, sprinkler systems). These were elements already incorporated into the hospital plans used as templates. (Kane, 1994:25)

In many ways, the nursing home is as much the victim as the perpetrator of the problem. However, with its emphasis on curing illness in patients that rarely can benefit from this endeavor, the medical model has misguided the design of the nursing home since its inception. There is little doubt that the medical approach has achieved dramatic successes in the area of general medicine. However, in the case of the nursing home, the medical model has had influences that are clearly counteractive to therapeutic philosophy. Nursing homes and hospitals are absolutely different entities in the character of their residents, the kinds of services they are expected to provide, and the way they are controlled and governed. A double-loaded corridor, for example, with a nurses' station strategically located to allow good observation of patients' rooms, makes considerable sense in an acute-care setting, in which people are temporarily subjected to medical treatment. It is much less desirable, however, in a place in which people live for an extended period of time and expect to maintain their quality of life. Similarly, the concept of semiprivate rooms is more suited to an efficiency-oriented hospital environment than to a setting that is supposed to encourage privacy and autonomy among residents who often age in the same place for the remainder of their lives.

Kane (1990) identifies four Rs—*routine, regulation, restricted capacity*, and *resource constraints*—as enemies of personal autonomy. All are prevalent in the nursing home environment. The four Rs interact. Routines established for administrative convenience have a dampening effect on resident autonomy. Regulations are peculiarly intensive in the nursing home sphere; unfortunately, the same regulations designed to protect residents often restrict them in minute and intimate ways. And resource constraints militate against creating the environment and the staffing ratios that might permit autonomy to flourish. Thus, restricted by their individual impairments, residents of nursing homes are incarcerated by the routines and regulations of the institution and by the relatively fixed entity of their physical environment.

The long-term care system in the United States has a strong bias toward the use of nursing homes, and reimbursement policies remain institutionally biased despite the preference of elders to remain in their own homes or to be cared for in noninstitutional environments: "Despite the growth of home and community-based care, Medicaid spending reflects a bias toward institutional care. Of the program's $40.3 billion expenditures on long-term care in 1995, $36.2 billion was for institutional care, while $4.1 billion was spent on home and community-based care. Nationally, over 70% of all long-term care expenditures in 1995 were for nursing home care, though less than 20% of all people receiving paid services are institutionalized" (National Academy on Aging, 1997).

There are signs, however, that the nursing home in its current form has reached a limit—or at least a turning point. Older Americans are not entering nursing homes at the same rate they did in previous years. The growth in the home care industry is significantly attributable to the fact that many older persons are no longer going into nursing homes to receive care that they can get in their own homes. Despite a significant increase in the population of persons aged 65 years and older, there has been a decline in the number of nursing home residents in the same cohort as well as a continuing decline in the ratio between the number of nursing home beds and the number of residents aged 65 and older (Strahan, 1997).

Despite its short life, the nursing home as an entity for the provision of long-term care for elderly persons is a building type from another era and has outlived its time. The shift has developed against the background of demographic projections, government expenditures, and the growing recognition that continued reliance on nursing home care as the primary service option for frail elders is neither economically wise nor socially desirable. The nursing home is beginning to lose favor in the eyes of government policy makers, who now speak of its limited usefulness for the majority of older people. There is a growing realization that the nursing home as we know it—an institution that could never be mistaken for a home—is appropriate only as a last resort. It "should be reserved for people who cannot interact with their environment, who are so medically unstable that they need hospital-like medical attention, and who perhaps need intensive rehabilitation on an inpatient basis" (Kane, 1995b:182).

A new set of priorities is beginning to gain favor as advocates and policy makers struggle to develop new models of care. Some of the new trends are funding and creating nonmedicalized residential alternatives for frail elders, limiting the use of nursing homes through changes in Medicaid eligibility criteria, and creating managed care programs for older adults that prevent or postpone institutionalization. These reorganizations are driven by the government's fiscal motivation to save public dollars, limit spending, and restrict Medicaid access.

As one of the preferred modalities of care, assisted living focuses on two desirable objectives. One objective is provision of comprehensive, flexible care and service options that meet the changing needs of individuals with increasing levels of disability. Crucial to this objective is the ability of residents and their families to choose and evaluate the services periodically and the ability of staff to maintain residents' dignity and autonomy. The second objective centers on developing the least restrictive therapeutic setting that promotes privacy, comfort, independence, and social interaction like that experienced at home.

The Many Forms of Assisted Living

The term *assisted living* raises a fundamental question because it stands for major classes of entities. Assisted living represents an entire range of buildings and programs that serve older, functionally impaired people who, on a continuing basis, need personal care to compensate for limitations in the activities of daily living (Kane and Wilson, 1993). Settings that meet these requirements include residential care facilities, personal care homes, catered living facilities, retirement homes, homes for adults, community residences, residential care in continuing care retirement communities, parts of independent-living arrangements, and special residential sections of nursing homes. These entities differ in the way they are used (level of care, the people they serve, their cost), in their physical properties (a wing of a nursing home, a freestanding residential-appearing structure, a midrise apartment complex), in the way in which they are regulated and ruled (as a residential care facility, as a special care unit for dementia, as a medically modeled health care center), and in the way they are understood by diverse interpreters (a stage between independent living and nursing home, a residential setting that maximizes a resident's ability to age in place).

Clearly, the term *assisted living* is ambiguous, confusing, and controversial. While a common standard definition of assisted living is unlikely, there seems to be an agreement about its residential, rather than institutional, character. Mollica and Snow (1996), who studied assisted living and board-and-care policies in all fifty states, argue that "while many observers equate institutional with medical, the distinction between medical and social lies less with the services delivered than the setting itself" (i). The researchers discuss three models of assisted living that reflect the various state approaches to licensure, unit requirements, and service level. The first model may be found in institutional settings or board-and-care facilities characterized by shared bedrooms without attached baths. They restrict admittance to eligible residents or limit the provision of nursing services. The second model pertains to housing and services. These facilities are usually apartment settings and restrict admittance and care to eligible tenants. Their philosophy stresses resident autonomy and independence and their regulations for the physical environment and services are more flexible than those of the first model. The third model focuses on the service provider, whether it is the facility itself or an outside agency. This model simplifies the regulatory environment by concentrating on the services delivered to the tenants rather than on the physical setting.

As for architectural design, assisted living differs from conventional housing for elderly persons chiefly by the way in which many of these arrangements attend to the concrete experiences of the settings and the manners in which they shelter their users: "Buildings designed and built as assisted living tend to have higher lighting levels in common spaces, more common spaces for activities and socialization, different flooring, small refrigerators raised above floor level, handicapped-accessible bathrooms in every unit, roll-in showers, wider corridors with handrails, two-way voice communication, and other features. Conventional elderly housing generally may not have been renovated to accommodate the decreasing independence of residents needing care" (Mollica and Snow, 1996:12).

Moore (1996) distinguishes among three fundamental market models of assisted living. The first is the integrated model with independent-living housing arrangements, which allows communities of independent living to provide their residents with extended care without forcing them to move directly to extended-care facilities. The second is the integrated model with extended-care arrangements in hospitals or nursing homes. This market model assists sponsors of these facilities in attracting a wide range of patients and residents while improving their economies of scale. The third is the stand-alone facility, the housing model of the 1990s. Freestanding assisted living reflects the market's preference for a social and residential model rather than the medical model. Ideally developed assisted living, however, is far more than just shelter and quality food and services. It "must have a strong—but largely invisible—medical basis as the solid foundation for its operating philosophy and market position strategy" (14).

Experiences with assisted living suggest that it is possible to repackage nursing home services for many current users into alternative housing arrangements that offer a better quality of life at no substantial risk to quality of care. Designers of assisted living consistently attempt to interpret therapeutic goals, such as dignity, autonomy, privacy, and independence, and to express them via architectural elements. Furthermore, architects and interior designers aim at redefining the role of the physical environment in these settings by rendering a new therapeutic building type, which has its typological roots in residential housing (Regnier, Hamilton, and Yatabe, 1995; Kane and Wilson, 1993). Freestanding assisted-living communities are typically small and are characterized by their residential appearance (Kane and Wilson, 1993; Regnier, 1994; Regnier, Hamilton, and Yatabe, 1995; Roush and Grape, 1995). Normally, these facilities comprise a limited number of residential units with private bedrooms, bathing facilities, and adequate cooking areas. The common areas are usually composed of a dining room, a health clinic, and spaces for recreational and social activities. Services can include assistance with bathing, dressing, housekeeping, laundering, and monitoring medications. The facilities frequently offer self-contained apartments and supportive services, which may be purchased separately or included in the monthly fee.

Regnier, Hamilton, and Yatabe (1995) list several attributes that influence the form and organization of assisted-living dwellings. These include the size of the facility, its service autonomy, the scale of the building, its appearance, and whether it was originally designed as an assisted-living facility or was remodeled from another use. "However," they argue, "the major challenge in developing an attractive and viable facility is achieving a compelling *residential* character while satisfying the economies of scale necessary to deliver a range of personal-care services cost-effectively" (30–31). Moreover, the authors prescribe design directives for the setting of assisted living through broad environment-behavior principles that emphasize images of residential character in the building's interior and the surrounding areas.

A similar notion is echoed in the works of Cohen and Weisman (1991) and Cohen and Day (1993) regarding special care units for people with dementia. Design guidelines in both of these publications focus on the transactional relationship between residents, the physical environment, the social setting, and the facility's policies and management. Their emphasis on "holding on to home" suggests strong interrelationships between the therapeutic goals for people with dementia and the building type that accommodates their needs and that draws on residential characteristics.

Wilson (1995) also stresses the appearance of the setting and its environmental attributes as a significant aspect in the creation of assisted living. She argues that a residential model as assisted living requires the following: "(1) An architectural style that is commonly associated with places where people have lived and that they recognize thematically as being tenantial; (2) Community common space with recognized public functions; (3) Accommodation of cultural preferences for privacy and control of personal space; (4) Amenities in public and personal space in keeping with lifelong experiences; (5) A scale appropriate to support tenantial feeling; (6) Features to enhance the ability of the individual to age in place" (141).

One typical rule of the care philosophy in assisted living has been the concept of managed risk, which recognizes that allowing individuals to make choices about their level of perceived and enacted independence can have consequences concerning their physical safety or their psychological health. In its essence, this concept is a revisionist response to a dialectic that lies at the heart of person-environment relations in later life, namely, the tension between autonomy and security (Parmelee and Lawton, 1990). In assisted-living facilities with managed risk, tenants are allowed informed individual choice and responsibility within supervised care arrangements. This care philosophy reflects a shift in values of long-term care provision, which increasingly seeks to find the right balance between degree of security and personal autonomy for frail elders.

Aging in place is an additional goal commonly promoted in assisted living. Aging in place represents a transaction between an aging person and his or her dwelling that is characterized by changes in both the inhabitant and the residential setting (Lawton, 1990). Most American elders want to age in place. The American Association of Retired Persons has repeatedly conducted housing surveys with regard to aging in place. The results of their recent study indicate that 83 percent of the surveyed people agree with the statement, "What I'd really like to do is stay in my home and never move" (AARP, 1996); 70 percent believe they can accomplish this goal. However, when elderly people are faced with the circumstances that force them to move out of their homes, most of them want to avoid having to move again, and they do not want to face the nursing home as their only option.

Aging in place in the context of assisted living presents an enormous social management and operations challenge, because the objective is helping residents remain in their dwelling units as long as possible. In an ideal situation, it means helping tenants remain in their units until their death, avoiding institutionalization in a medical setting by providing ancillary services on-site. This goal challenges the long-standing assumption in the regulatory system of housing for older adults, which typically forces people to move into "service-rich" housing arrangements as they become more frail and their care needs increase. For fire safety and health reasons, several states prohibit the very frail or bedridden from staying in retirement homes, which are licensed to help tenants mostly with routine activities like grooming, taking medicine, and perhaps cooking. It is becoming increasingly apparent, however, that residential settings such as assisted living can provide all the care and services to persons who need assistance in activities of daily living or who require more intensive health care services (Pynoos and Liebig, 1995).

From the designer's perspective, the question is, What type of building can support these needs? Furthermore, what should be built for the provision of assistance in living? Or what attributes of which existing building types can be useful to create an adequate place for providing long-term care for frail elders?

Assisted Living and the Concept of Building Type

Like other evolving building types, assisted living has been applied to the particular circumstances of a given architectural problem and continues to adjust to that state of affairs. Building type is a fundamental concept in architecture and is often associated with general categories of use or construction. In this sense, *type* is understood as a term of functional or structural taxonomy. Professional journals, for example, routinely classify building types for the aged as "congregate housing," "shared housing," "board and care," "assisted living," "continuing care retirement communities," "nursing homes." The rationale behind this classification is that the purpose that each of these buildings is expected to serve actually defines the type of building it is. Type, in this context, means a building in principle, a design's essence, the building's nature, an ideal design. In other words, the building type of each category is a generalized idea of a building containing within it all the possible examples of actual buildings of that type that have been and can be built. Types are the generative means by which buildings receive their configurations. The idea or essence of each type develops differently in each society according to the specific circumstances generated by patterns such as a country's climate, the mores and lifestyles of its inhabitants, and its institutions. It has been suggested, however, that the idea of a building type should not be treated as an answer or the assumed end point, because building types change over time, and their nature cannot be assumed to be fully understood.

Robinson (1994) notes that types are "idealized forms with generally agreed-upon names that stand for a set of concrete objects. Associated with each idealized form and name are concepts and physical elements that characterize the type" (180). She distinguishes between *basic type*, which is what lay people ordinarily use to create order among objects for functioning in daily life, and *classificatory type*, which is used by professionals to make distinctions between objects in order to delineate and to define boundary conditions. For example, a house and an apartment are basic types of dwellings, whereas a single-family house and multifamily housing are classificatory types. The design process necessitates the use of both of these kinds of type—the first as a means to understand the nature of the selected type; the second as a method to adjust, respond to, or match the ideal type and the particular situation.

Basic types are shared within a given cultural context and are useful for communication because they allow members of similar backgrounds to agree about a limited set of objects. Moreover, basic architectural types are used to delineate design context. Categories (schools, factories, hotels, hospitals, nursing homes) and labels (institutional, residential, commercial, industrial) follow particular cultural usages with regard to physical form. As Robinson (1994) observes: "Basic types represent simultaneously: (1) a set of architectural attributes that can be described; (2) a set of rules for construction and for organization of space; (3) a set of behaviors and defined roles that take place within it; and (4) a set of qualities it should exhibit" (183–84).

A case in point is the environment of the nursing home with long, double-loaded corridors, sparsely furnished residents' rooms, and pivotally located nursing stations, all of which constitute a set of distinct architectural attributes. The spatial organization of this setting is governed by a strict system of regulations, construction rules, and reimbursement controls. The behavior of nursing home residents is determined by inflexible routines, which compromise residents' privacy and autonomy in the name of cleanliness, efficiency, and safety. The social structure is formally defined by a regime of inequality, which stems from the great dependence of one group of users on the other group of users. A "plan of care" governs every waking and sleeping hour, every morsel of food consumed. Each phase of a person's daily ritual is rigidly fixed and is carried out in the company of others, who are all treated alike. The staff enforce the activities of daily living as part of an overall plan designed to fulfill the aims and the qualities of this institution (Schwarz, 1996a).

Buildings or architectural settings can be classified in four ways: (1) based on the way they are used, (2) based on their physical properties, (3) based on how they are made, and (4) based on how they are understood. Classified according to intended use, assisted living can be grouped by the people they serve, by the functions they perform, by the level of their services, or by cost. The same settings may be grouped according to their physical properties. This can be done based on taxonomic categories, such as construction method (e.g., wood frame, metal frame, concrete structure, masonry infill), floor plan, and space configuration (e.g., courtyard buildings, atrium buildings, clustered form buildings, linear buildings), scale or size (e.g., low-rise, high-rise, residential scale), and style (e.g., Victorian, Georgian, modern). Though style and type are understood by some scholars as unrelated, style is an object of judgment, while the constructive and utilitarian side of building type is an object of proof. In this context, type refers to the compositional pattern relative to function, while style refers, as Vilder (1977) puts it, to "clothing for an otherwise 'naked' object" and capable of being changed at will.

Rules and processes, which control the ways buildings are made, is another way to categorize assisted-living settings. The nursing home, for instance, is a category of housing responding to federal regulations that generally govern structure, process, and outcome developed to ensure basic, decent, and humane care for the frail elderly and people with disabilities. Nevertheless, these generative processes become a distinct set of rules that define the architectural form of a particular building type. Overlap between categories is often apparent. Functional intentions and expectations may be linked through floor plan configuration to the way environments are made, just as categories of scale are linked to materials, which frequently overlap with categories of form and style. Categories of regulations and codes may be generative and at the same time may respond to intended use. Similar overlap occurs vis-à-vis methods of financing and construction, as in the nursing home design process, which is controlled by regulation, financing, and reimbursement systems (Schwarz, 1996b). Thus, groupings are rarely used in their pure forms. Rather, the categories are used as tools for design and analysis in a combining and overlapping fashion.

The fourth taxonomic classification, how environments are understood, is perhaps the most complex because it is value loaded, subjective, and grounded in personal and cultural interpretation. Associational and symbolic, this category deals with a variety of meanings that evolve through human experience with form, function, and space. An enormous body of scholarly and critical work, involving iconography, art criticism, semiotics, and subfields of the behavioral sciences has been generated by the analysis of meaning. Grounded in two epistemologies, the visual arts and the behavioral sciences, buildings express values or meanings that are received and interpreted by their users. If the content of architectural expression refers to whatever is expressed or implied by a building and, likewise, if the content of architectural interpretation pertains to whatever an interpretation about a building implies, the question is whether these two contents coincide. Expression and interpretation in architecture often overlap, but they do not necessarily coincide, as Canter and Canter (1979) note: "The fact that other people may 'read' from the physical setting the potential interactions which may take place and, as a consequence, elaborate from those interpretations ideas about, say, isolation or aloofness, which were not originally intended, helps to illustrate how seemingly small details may nonetheless grow to have great implications for symbolic interpretations. Hence 'institutional' colour schemes or imposing entrances may have an impact beyond their immediate function" (1979:5).

While a building type suggests how certain purposes ought to be accommodated by a building, circumstances do not always allow it to be so. Thus, the importance of knowing circumstances and conventions, as well as types, becomes apparent the moment we notice the departure from the norm to accommodate an actual situation. This is particularly important in the case of the evolving building type of assisted living, in which, in addition to the physical attributes of the building aimed at communicating domesticity, the intentions are focused on provision of the attributes of home, such as comfort, involvement, caring, bonds among tenants and caregivers, and domestic services. Two additional questions regarding the meaning of places may be asked: Is the meaning implied by the building intentionally embodied in it by those responsible for it? Are the messages of this intentionality recognized and understood by the users of this setting?

Answering these questions is far from simple. We experience buildings through form, function, and space (Markus, 1994). Form refers to the geometry of a building's volume, its degree of enclosure, its texture, color, transparency, the way light and shade express surface properties, and the furnishings and ornamentations that are part of these environments. Experiencing form is immediate and direct and pertains mostly to what things look like in the building. We can experience a building's function by either participating as actors in the setting or by observing other actors in the setting. We can deduce what is done in a building and what each of the spaces is for from its location in the total structure and from its adjacencies to other spaces. In short, we understand the building's function. We describe each of the elements by function-related words such as "entrance," "corridor," "dining room," "bedroom," "bathroom." Within a given culture, each of these words carries a rich package of meanings. The terms *residential setting* and *institutional setting*, for instance, do not define simply a physical environment but a sequence of spaces in which particular activities take place and "a culture whose essence is a set of complex relationships between people, things, places, and ideas. Such words serve not only to *de*scribe what exists but to *pre*scribe what is to come into being" (Markus, 1993:16). Space is experienced through whatever is done in a building—because it is done in a space that is related to surrounding spaces and to outside space. The adjacencies of these spaces can reflect the social relationships among the users of the building. These topological relationships relate to encounters between people and mirror the way in which control and power are distributed in the setting (Hillier and Hanson, 1984; Robinson, 1993).

Through our experience with form, function, and space in a building, we can extract a variety of meanings. Form acts as metaphor, sign, or symbol, although it may be interpreted in various fashions. Function speaks directly of social relationships and reveals the status, role, and purpose of each user. Space, on the other hand, speaks indirectly of the same relationships. However, form, function, and space are intrinsically independent. In other words, there is no internal connection between the three elements. Services and activities in an assisted-living setting, by way of illustration, may be performed in any spatial structure or style. By the same token, a Victorian-looking building that serves frail elderly persons can rarely describe the function or the spatial structure of its interior. Although buildings reflect the institutions they house, there is no predictable relation between form and function. The setting conveys "a distinct meaning that, within a culture, signifies a known set of relations, and within a stable building tradition implies a limited and easy-to-recognize range of forms and spatial structures" (Markus, 1994:151).

Home: The Conceptual Foundation of Assisted Living

Searching for transferable residential attributes that symbolize the home environment has been at the heart of the design of and research about assisted-living settings. Designers and scholars of environment-behavior studies promote the concept of homelike, in spite of the ambiguous nature of the concept of home (Rapoport, 1995) and the pitfalls of its interpretation and realization in public domains. The concept of homelike contrasts with the concept of institutional "because home environments, unlike traditional institutions, encourage independent action and stimulate continuing growth on the part of the resident" (Robinson et al., 1984:5). Just as the literature seems to reflect a bias toward residential environments over institutional ones, the preference among residents' families is for residential care settings that maximize tenant autonomy and dignity. The preference among providers is also to change existing settings to reflect a more homelike ambiance for marketing purposes. Consequently, many facilities assert that they provide care in residential settings.

Recognizing that the physical environment inhabited by older persons is an integral part of a larger system of social and operational patterns of therapeutic care, designers are concerned with the design of dwellings as manifestations of space, structure, and order but have had difficulty in touching upon the more subtle, emotional, and diffuse aspects of home. In addition, while the majority of assisted-living facilities described in the literature reflect a preference for homelike settings, there is no agreement on what constitutes a residential, or homelike, setting. The ultimate question is, Which attributes of the home can be effectively transferred to create an environment that evokes the perception of home? While there are many claims that a given institutional environment is homelike, there is little in the way of objective measures that can be used to determine what these residential characteristics are and which of these characteristics, either individually or in combination, are necessary to create a residential environment in assisted living. Before laying out the attributes of homelike, we have to clarify the concept of home, since its multidimensional nature seems to stimulate the search for a homelike ambiance.

Much of the research about home suggests that the need for a home is a fundamental human imperative, providing a locus of order and control in a world of chaos. Home imparts a sense of identity, security, and belonging (Rowels, 1987). The phenomenon of home consists of a tangible relationship between people and the places in which they dwell. The common dimensions of home as identified by Hayward (1975) are as follows: "Home as physical structure," "as territory," "as locus in space," "as self and self-identity" and "as a social and cultural unit." This analysis suggests that affective qualities and human relations are as significant as physical dimensions. In this respect, it is noteworthy that the terms *house* and *home* seem to be used too often interchangeably in the literature. However, the two concepts have distinctly separate meanings. While a house is an object, a part of the environment, a home is best conceived of as a relationship between people and their environment. The term *home* refers to an experiential phenomenon rather than to the house, place, or building that may or may not represent its manifestation in built form. Thus, home is not an empirical variable whose meaning can be clearly defined, measured, or transferred like a marketable product. A home in its essence breaks away from the physical properties of house into the psychological territories of identity, memory, habits, and culturally conditioned reactions and values.

Evidently, then, home is not a building but, rather, a complex condition that fulfills a hierarchy of human needs. Home has a psychological and metaphysical significance over and above being a shelter in which to conduct everyday life. Home is a set of rituals, personal rhythms, and routines of everyday life that need their temporal stability and continuum to develop. The passage of time appears to be central in the process of developing attachment to a place, and consequently the home is a gradual product of the dweller's adaptation to the world. Pallasmaa (1995) raises the question of whether a home can be an architectural expression: "Home is an individualized dwelling, and the means of this subtle personalization seem to be outside of our concept of architecture. Dwelling, or the house, is the container, the shell for home. The substance of home is secreted, as it were, upon the framework of the dwelling by the dweller. Home is an expression of the dweller's personality and his unique patterns of life. Consequently, the essence of home is closer to life itself than an artefact" (132).

Clearly, the concept of home is complex, and the idea that one can simply extrapolate the concept of home to the concept of homelike perhaps is naive. Yet designers and developers of assisted living have undertaken just such a task because they believe that a home has also some recognizable physical characteristics. In his attempt to embrace the idea of home for assisted living, Brummett (1997) lists four potential contradictions of the concept of home embedded in the assisted-living residence: (1) resident dependence on staff for the provision of their needs, (2) compromises of privacy and territoriality resulting from living with other people in a group, (3) staff and caregiver needs, and (4) higher levels of safety standards and concerns with regard to the well-being of residents. This list may be extended to include the attitudes of administration and staff toward the implementation of programs, the size and number of residents in the setting, the characteristics and the mix of residents, and the modification options of the existing physical environment. While modification of a house for achieving a homelike setting may be relatively simple, it is "virtually impossible to eliminate a sufficient quantity of cues to make an institution's image change from institutional to homelike" (Robinson et al., 1984:10).

The homelike concept contains the promise of the home experience. The interpretation in assisted living has been characterized by the effort to create an environment that is the direct opposite of an institution. In this view, the institution has staff intent on performing instrumental tasks as routine; conversely, in a homelike setting, caregivers care for residents almost like children in a family caring for beloved parents. In an institution, the resident is a case; in a homelike setting, the person is seen as a parent, grandparent, or friend. The institutional facility allows little personal autonomy; in the homelike environment, individuals are encouraged to set their own schedules and to control their surroundings. Residents of an institution are isolated from the community; members of a homelike facility are encouraged to be involved in the community. The institutional environment is sterile and cold; the homelike setting is warm and cheerful. Homelike attributes offer a psychological and physical comfort steeped in remembrance of one's own home experiences: "Homelike is an ideal philosophy of care that explicitly aims to recreate a sense of *home* in a public place. The essence of this outlook is to preserve residents' prerogatives to exercise personal control while maintaining necessary levels of physical and social support. It is a complex of person and place in which all the various activities of daily life are undertaken as people not patients" (Pastalan et al., 1993:10).

One of the difficult tasks of this line of inquiry is the measurement of homelike attributes. This complication arises from the attempt to identify the tangible and intangible properties of home and to determine which of these many attributes could be successfully transferred to a public place, such as assisted-living housing. The assumption is that it is theoretically possible to transfer a sufficient type and number of attributes to approximate a residential situation. It is also theoretically possible to assess settings and to determine which of them is the most successful in providing for the presence of these attributes and, therefore, which is the most homelike. Researchers acknowledge, however, that for every home attribute that can be successfully transferred to create a homelike ambiance, there is a need for not only an appropriately designed environment but also a program and policy that supports domestic activities and a committed staff that tirelessly and continuously implements such intentions.

Two Studies of Environmental Attributes in Assisted Living

Pastalan and University of Michigan colleagues (1993) developed a 158-item instrument for the assessment of homelike attributes in special care units for people with dementia. They directed attention to the physical environment, the staff and caregiver characteristics, and the programs and policies that have an impact on a residential ambiance. There are sixty-eight physical attributes, which refer to issues such as appearance, scale, configuration of space, adjacency of spaces, use of spaces, lighting control, acoustic control, and finishes and furnishings. The program and policy section covers seventy-six issues, such as accommodation of deviance, family involvement, visitation schedule, group activities, mealtime ambiance, personalization of resident units, access to public spaces, accommodations for individual schedules and preferences, accommodations for privacy, and recognition of residents' accomplishments. The staff and caregiver section includes fourteen items, such as staff/resident ratio, caregiver and resident relationship, caregiver continuity, caregiver attire, staff facilities, and recognition of residents' pasts.

In translating abstract concepts of home attributes into particular questions and guidelines for observation, the items were objectified. Dealing with the concept of autonomy, for example, the translation needed to identify aspects of the physical environment that facilitate or constrain residents' expression of autonomy. For instance, is there evidence that residents use their own furniture to personalize their rooms? Are there mementos depicting histories of self and family? What are the window, wall, and floor treatments? Are there private phones, television sets, secured storage, and acoustic control in residents' rooms? Can residents open windows in their own rooms? Can residents lock the doors to their rooms? Is there free egress from the unit? Do residents have access to snacks and beverages at any time? Do residents have free access to outdoor areas? Does the environment afford opportunities for intimacy?

The physical environment can only provide the setting for the expression of personal autonomy. Although the setting must have the necessary features in place for such expression, these features alone cannot initiate resident autonomy. The program and policies of the facility must support and encourage the residents to express autonomy. For instance, does the programming and policies actively support residents' prerogative to personalize their rooms? Do policies allow residents to hang pictures and mementos on the wall, to lock their doors, to have access to food and drink at any time? The staff and the caregivers must reflect a commitment to the program and policies of the facility as well as to the attributes of the environment designed to ensure residents' autonomy. For example, does the staff assist residents in personalizing their rooms? Does the staff, through the articulation of programming and policies, respect residents' desires to control who or when someone comes into their rooms? Does staff encourage and assist residents in having meals whenever desired? The assessment instrument clearly reveals differences among the facilities in question. There was a high degree of agreement in rating scores among the investigators who used it, who could distinguish among facilities that were more residential and those that were less residential.

More recently, a survey of 591 licensed residential care facilities in Missouri was conducted to identify facilities that provide, through their environmental attributes and care services, accommodations comparable to exemplary assisted-living communities described in the literature (Schwarz et al., 1997). While some developers of assisted living include residential attributes in resident units, others consider these amenities a waste of money and a drain on profits. The State of Missouri is one of several states that does not have an assisted-living licensure category or program. Assisted-living facilities in Missouri currently are treated as residential care facilities, which are defined as

> Any premises, other than intermediate care facility or skilled nursing facility, that is utilized by its owner, operator, or manager to provide 24-hour care to three or more residents, who are not related within the fourth degree of consanguinity or affinity to the owner, operator, or manager of the facility.
>
> Residential Care Facility I provides shelter, board, and protective oversight and may include storage and distribution or administration of medications and care during short-term illness or recuperation.

Residential Care Facility II provides supervision of diets, assistance in personal care, the storage and distribution or administration of medications, supervision of health care under the direction of a licensed physician, and protective oversight, including care during short-term illness or recuperation. (Division of Aging, 1995)

The facilities must provide housekeeping, laundry, three meals per day, and 24-hour protection oversight. Residents must be given ten days notice of discharge from the facility, and they may be transferred only for medical reasons, for their health or welfare or that of other residents, or for nonpayment. These definitions establish standards that are broad enough to include diverse accommodations.

Using an eight-item residential index, researchers asked directors of 591 residential care facilities whether their facility provides any of the following:

1. All singly occupied units unless by choice of the tenant.
2. Private, full baths with a shower in each unit.
3. Cooking facility and refrigerator in each unit.
4. Individual temperature control in each unit.
5. Lockable door from inside and outside in each unit.
6. Option for residents to furnish their units using personal furnishings.
7. Services provided for and scheduled around residents' preferences.
8. Allowing residents to remain in the facility in times of severe illness, injury, or incapacity.

The 196 facilities that responded to the survey vary in scale and building type. These include freestanding facilities, naturally occurring communities, market-rate housing, government-subsidized senior housing, independent facilities with home health services, and nursing home wings that were previously skilled nursing care and have been "downgraded" to residential care. The results indicate that 22.5 percent (44) of the 196 facilities have seven or eight of the residential characteristics. Only 3.1 percent (6) have one or none of these attributes, and the remaining 74.5 percent (146) have two to six of the characteristics.

Only 57.7 percent of the facilities are all singly occupied units unless by choice of the tenants, and 56.1 percent have private full bathrooms with a shower in each unit. While 91.8 percent of the facilities claim that residents have the option of furnishing their units with personal items, only 60.2 percent have individual temperature control in their units, and only 13.8 percent have cooking arrangements with refrigerators in each unit. The majority provides services scheduled according residents' preferences. The basic services available include all hotel-type services (e.g., meals, laundry, housekeeping) plus scheduled and personal care, such as bathing or assistance with medications. About 86 percent of the facilities allow residents to remain in the setting in times of severe illness, injury, or incapacity.

Pearson correlation coefficients were used to assess the extent to which these characteristics tend to occur together in the same facility. There were many positive significant correlations and no significant negative correlations between characteristics. In other words, the physical characteristics tend to occur together, supporting the notion that residential care facilities have either most of the characteristics or few of the characteristics. Other findings indicate that the payment schedules of 56.6 percent of the facilities (111) vary according to residents' needs. These facilities provide services in two major forms, à la carte or buffet. In the à la carte system, tenants pay a base price, with add-ons based on services used or increments of time. The buffet provides a range of services, with the tenant picking any combination of the services that fall within the price ceiling allowed.

The study demonstrates that numerous facilities in Missouri can be described as assisted-living arrangements. However, though 86 percent of the facilities' directors assert that their facilities provide medical services for residents who suffer from severe illness, injury, or incapacity, residents cannot stay in the settings when their needs exceed the licensure regulations of the facility. According to the admission criteria for Missouri residential care facilities, tenants cannot require skilled nursing care and must be physically and mentally capable of negotiating a normal "path to safety" unassisted or with the use of an assisted device in case of emergency. Residents of these facilities may remain in the facility if incapacitated and may return to the facility after staying in a hospital if their period of incapacity does not exceed forty-five days and if written approval of a physician is obtained.

Perhaps more than any other requirement, this rule determines the fate of tenants in residential care facilities with regard to their ability to age in place. It clearly distinguishes between nursing homes and assisted-living arrangements. Though innovative providers and developers of assisted living have been responding to consumer desire to avoid placement in an institutional setting even if they require a high level of services, the admission and discharge criteria in Missouri residential care facilities prohibit them from making these choices. In addition, only a few of the reviewed communities provided residents with cooking facilities in their units. It is not clear whether this was due to operators' prejudice or to fire safety codes. Obviously, in facilities with cooking options, there should be provisions for disconnecting appliances when a resident is no longer functioning adequately to operate them safely. There is a need for a study that can explore the importance of being able to keep cold beverages, to have a cup of tea, or to cook something in the microwave and the importance of these characteristics in supporting residents' independence. Developers and environmental designers of assisted living lack critical input from the people who must live with their designs. The setting should be designed to meet residents' needs. To paraphrase W. I. Thomas, if the residents do not perceive that their needs are being met, then their needs are not being met.

It has been argued that minimum environmental standards stressing privacy, adequate space, and autonomy through supportive features should be established. "These features may be criticized as either an expensive indulgence or a dangerous innovation that combine more opportunity for accidents with less opportunity for staff surveillance. Therefore, studies of the costs, risks, and benefits of these interventions are needed" (Kane, 1995b: 181). A subsequent study was designed to address the broader research questions: What effect do environmental attributes associated with home have on residents, their families, and the staff of assisted-living arrangements? Under what conditions? In what circumstances. And why?

It is hoped that the two studies will bring to light the larger question of a flexible, outcome-oriented, regulatory framework for assisted living. Although proponents of assisted living are clear as to the general characteristics and philosophy of care, there is no agreement on the details of the legal definition, the function, the physical setting, the individuals served, or the standards of practice for assisted-living communities. As a relatively new industry, assisted living is currently not subject to federal regulatory standards. In the absence of federal licensure or reimbursement standards, each state has developed its own requirements, which have evolved in piecemeal fashion (Mollica and Snow, 1996). The need for this framework is felt by providers, regulators, and consumer advocates. "Many stakeholders fear that regulating assisted living will result in prescriptive standards that will limit assisted living's innovation and consumer orientation. Others believe that standards for assisted living are essential to protect consumers" (Wilson, 1996:13). The development of such regulations needs to be based on collaboration among consumers, advocates, providers, and regulators at the state level in the context of each state's legal and regulatory system. The regulations should respond to the characteristics of frail elders by maintaining minimum standards to ensure safety, health, and environmental attributes. The system should improve the quality of life of the population served by these facilities while providing a flexible operating system to ensure the combination of efficiency in service provision and innovation to satisfy the needs and desired accommodations of older people.

Conclusion

Assisted living represents a dynamic pattern of change in the provision of long-term care and responds effectively to the health-related concerns of older Americans. It also seems to be a cost-effective alternative to other forms of long-term care and an emotionally acceptable option for families of seniors. In its essence, assisted living is a response to the way our society medicalizes, institutionalizes, and professionalizes long-term care provision in ways not originally envisioned. The future of assisted living appears promising, but it is not without some future regulatory and marketplace turbulence.

As a place type, assisted living may be reviewed, first, from a result-driven market perspective, where the question is whether assisted living as a place type impacts the marketplace of housing arrangements for frail elders. The simple answer is that, at this particular moment, assisted living constitutes the state of the art and, as such, it sells. The market recognizes a successful building type when it achieves substitution—it succeeds in convincing people to choose a new building type over the one they now have. Clearly, assisted-living settings have achieved this objective.

When we review assisted living from a design perspective, we notice the range of environments, which vary from one-room accommodations to apartments complete with kitchens and living rooms; from places providing basic services to settings that provide multiple forms of nursing care. No wonder we find it difficult to respond. Nevertheless, assisted living as a fundamental concept constitutes an environment that carries evidence of choices for frail elders. However, the design of these settings needs to be based on knowledge of how to make human and environmental characteristics congruent. To meet these challenges, research about assisted-living settings should address the three basic questions of environment-behavior studies formulated by Rapoport (1990). The following is my interpretation of these questions, in reference to assisted living:

— What characteristics of frail elders, their families, and the staff as individuals and as members of their respective groups should influence how assisted-living environments are organized and shaped?
— How do the attributes of assisted-living settings affect users' behavior, mood, and well-being. That is, how significant is the setting? For whom? Under what conditions? In what circumstances? And why?
— Given this mutual interaction between these people and the assisted-living setting, what are the mechanisms in which they are linked?

As we continue to devise parameters for settings, services, and reimbursement rates within a changing regulatory base and evolving managed care system, let us remember one premise: Despite their sometimes damaged minds and sometimes worn bodies, frail elders want to exercise their will and enjoy the companionship of others in harmony in a place type that can nurture human dignity and feed people's enthusiasm for life.

References

Agich, G. 1993. *Autonomy and Long-term Care.* New York: Oxford University Press.

AARP. 1996. *AARP Housing Report.* Washington, D.C.: American Association of Retired Persons.

Baltes, M. 1996. *The Many Faces of Dependency in Old Age.* New York: Cambridge University Press.

Brawley, E. 1997. *Designing for Alzheimer's Disease: Strategies for Creating Better Care Environments.* New York: Wiley.

Brummett, W. 1997. *The Essence of Home: Design Solutions for Assisted Living Housing.* New York: Van Nostrand Reinhold.

Canter, D., and S. Canter, eds. 1979. *Designing for Therapeutic Environments.* Chichester, U.K.: Wiley.

Carp, F. 1987. Environment and aging. In D. Stokols and I Altman, eds., *Handbook of Environmental Psychology.* New York: Wiley.

Cohen, U., and K. Day. 1993. *Contemporary Environments for People with Dementia.* Baltimore: Johns Hopkins University Press.

Cohen, U., and G. Weisman. 1991. *Holding on to Home: Designing Environments for People with Dementia.* Baltimore: Johns Hopkins University Press.

Cummings, J., and E. Cummings. 1964. *Ego and Milieu: Theory and Practice of Environmental Therapy.* London: Tavistock.

Davidson, A. 1995. Using the environment to promote human well-being. *Journal of Healthcare Design* 7:109–21.

Division of Aging. 1995. *Long-term Care Facility Regulations and Licensure Law for Residential Care Facilities I & II, Intermediate Care Facilities, Skilled Nursing Facilities.* Jefferson City: State of Missouri, Department of Social Services.

Gowans, A. 1992. *Styles and Types of North American Architecture: Social Function and Cultural Expression.* New York: Icon Editions.

Hayward, G. 1975. Home as an environmental and psychological concept. *Landscape* 20:2–9.

Hillier, W., and J. Hanson. 1984. *The Social Logic of Space*. Cambridge: Cambridge University Press.

Jones, M. 1962. *Social Psychiatry in the Community, in Hospitals, and in Prisons*. Springfield, Ill.: Charles C. Thomas.

Kane, R. A. 1990. Everyday life in nursing homes: The way things are. In R. Kane and A. Caplan, eds., *Everyday Ethics: Resolving Dilemmas in Nursing Home Life*. New York: Springer.

———. 1995a. Autonomy and regulation in long-term care: An odd couple, an ambiguous relationship. In L. Gamroth, J. Semradek, and E. Tornquist, eds., *Enhancing Autonomy in Long-term Care*. New York: Springer.

———. 1995b. Expanding the home care concept: Blurring distinctions among home care institutional care, and other long-term care services. *Milbank Quarterly* 73:161–86.

Kane, R., and K. Wilson. 1993. *Assisted Living in the United States: A New Paradigm for Residential Care for Frail Older Persons?* Washington, D.C.: American Association of Retired Persons.

Kane, R. L. 1994. The American nursing home: An institution for all reasons. In J. Hollingsworth and E. Hollingsworth, eds., *Care of the Chronically and Severely Ill: Comparative Social Policies*. New York: Aldine De Gruyter.

Kushlick, A. 1975. *Some Ways of Setting, Monitoring, and Attaining Objectives for Services for Disabled People*. Research Report 116. Winchester, U.K.: Wessex Region Health Authority.

Lawton, M. 1990. Knowledge resources and gaps in housing for the aged. In D. Tilson, ed., *Aging in Place: Supporting the Frail Elderly in Residential Environments*. Glenview, Ill.: Scott, Foresman.

Lawton, M., and L. Nahemow. 1973. Ecology and the aging process. In C. Eisdorfer and M. Lawton, eds., *Psychology of Adult Development and Aging*. Washington, D.C.: American Psychological Association.

Lipman, A., and R. Slater. 1979. Homes for older people: Towards a positive environment. In D. Canter and S. Canter, eds., *Designing for Therapeutic Environments*. Chichester, U.K.: Wiley.

Malkin, J. 1994. The design of healing and prosthetic environments. *Journal of Healthcare Design* 6:141–52.

Markus, T. 1993. Buildings as social objects. In B. Farmer and H. Louw, eds., *Companion to Contemporary Architectural Thought*. London: Routledge.

———. 1994. Social practice and building typologies. In K. Franck and L. Schneekloth, eds., *Ordering Space: Types in Architecture and Design*. New York: Van Nostrand Reinhold.

Mollica, R., and K. Snow. 1996. *State Assisted Living Policy, 1996*. Portland, Maine: National Academy for State Health Policy.

Moore, G., ed. 1970. *Emerging Methods in Environmental Design and Planning*. Cambridge: MIT Press.

Moore, J. 1996. *Assisted Living: Pure and Simple Development and Operating Strategies*. Forth Worth, Tex.: Westridge Publishing.

National Academy on Aging. 1997. *Facts on Long-term Care*. Washington, D.C.: National Academy on Aging.

Pallasmaa, J. 1995. Identity, intimacy, and domicile: Notes on the phenomenology of home. In D. Benjamin, ed., *The Home: Words, Interpretations, Meanings, and Environments*. Aldershot, U.K.: Avebury.

Parmelee, P., and M. Lawton. 1990. The design of special environments for the aged. In J. Birren and K. Schaie, eds., *Handbook of the Psychology of Aging*, 3d ed. New York: Academic.

Pastalan, L., L. Jones, B. Schwarz, R. Sekulski, and L. Struble. 1993. Homelike attributes of dementia special care units. Poster presentation at the annual meeting of the Gerontological Society of America, New Orleans.

Pynoos, J., and P. Liebig, eds. 1995. *Housing Frail Elders: International Policies, Perspectives, and Prospects*. Baltimore: Johns Hopkins University Press.

Rapoport, A. 1990. *History and Precedent in Environmental Design*. New York: Plenum.

———. 1995. A critical look at the concept "home." In D. Benjamin, ed., *The Home: Words, Interpretations, Meanings, and Environments*. Aldershot, U.K.: Avebury.

Regnier, V. 1994. *Assisted-Living Housing for the Elderly: Design Innovations from the United States and Europe*. New York: Van Nostrand Reinhold.

Regnier, V., J. Hamilton, and S. Yatabe. 1995. *Assisted-Living for the Aged and Frail: Innovations in Design, Management, and Financing*. New York: Columbia University Press.

Robinson, J. 1993. Messages from space: Privacy and power in housing. In R. Feldman, G. Hardie, and D. Salie, eds., *Power by Design: Proceedings of the 24th Annual Conference of the Environmental Design Research Association*. Chicago: EDRA.

———. 1994. The question of type. In K. Franck and L. Schneekloth, eds., *Ordering Space: Types in Architecture and Design*. New York: Van Nostrand Reinhold.

Robinson, J., T. Thompson, P. Emmons, and M. Graff. 1984. *Towards an Architectural Definition of Normalization*. St. Paul: University of Minnesota.

Roush, D., and T. Grape. 1995. *Integrated Senior Care: Assisted Living and Long-term Care Manual*. New York: Thompson.

Rowels, G. 1987. A place to call home. In L. Carstensen and B. Edelstein, eds., *Handbook of Clinical Gerontology*. New York: Pergamon.

Schwarz, B. 1996a. *Nursing Home Design: Consequences of Employing the Medical Model*. New York: Garland.

———. 1996b. Designing long-term care settings. *Nursing Home Economics* 3:14–23.

Schwarz, B., R. Brent, S. Bloom, and M. Amor. 1997. Residential attributes in assisted living: The Missouri study. Paper presented at the EDRA 28 Conference, Montreal.

Strahan, G. 1997. An overview of nursing homes and their current residents: Data from the 1995 National Nursing Home Survey. In *Advance Data from Vital and Health Statistics* 280. Hyattsville, Md.: National Center for Health Statistics.

Tiesdel, S., and T. Oc. 1993. Architecture and people. In B. Farmer, and H. Louw, eds., *Companion to Contemporary Architectural Thought*. London: Routledge.

Vilder, A. 1977. The idea of type: The transformation of the academic ideal, 1750–1830. *Oppositions* 8:95–113.

Ulrich, R. 1995. Effects of interior design on wellness: Theory and recent scientific research. In S. Marberry, ed., *Innovations in Healthcare Design*. New York: Van Nostrand Reinhold.

Wilson, K. 1995. Assisted living as a model of care delivery. In L. Gamroth, J. Semradek, and E. Tornquist, eds., *Enhancing Autonomy in Long-term Care: Concepts and Strategies*. New York: Springer.

———. 1996. *Assisted Living: Reconceptualizing Regulation to Meet Consumers' Needs and Preferences*. Washington, D.C.: American Association of Retired Persons.

JOHN P. MARSDEN
RACHEL KAPLAN

CHAPTER 13

Communicating Homeyness from the Outside

Elderly People's Perceptions of Assisted Living

Assisted living, an emerging concept that encompasses both a housing type and a philosophy of care, has been promoted as a noninstitutional alternative that offers personal care services to mentally and physically frail older persons so that they can live as independently as possible in a homelike context. Yet, it is unknown whether assisted living is actually perceived as homelike. This is due in part to a resistance to research by the design professions. It is also due to the elusive meaning of home. The purpose of this chapter is to examine whether one aspect of assisted living—the exterior appearance—is perceived as homelike by elderly persons. A framework for studying the communication of homeyness in assisted living is proposed. Two studies that focus on the exterior appearance of assisted living in relation to the framework are also discussed. The chapter concludes with a summary of findings as they pertain to the proposed framework.

Properties of Homeyness in Assisted Living

Homeyness has traditionally been studied in the context of the single-family house. This building type has dominated middle-class consciousness as an ideal since the eighteenth century (Clark, 1986), and many people have experienced homeyness in that context. Homeyness has also been explored primarily from the perspective of traditional households (Despres, 1991). Few have addressed what home actually means to nontraditional populations, such as the elderly. As a result, research in the area of homeyness may not be applicable to settings such as assisted living, which are larger and entail group living for seniors. Moreover, physical properties that are thought to reinforce homeyness have received little empirical attention and have not been successfully integrated into theoretical perspectives, which complicates an examination of how homeyness is communicated by buildings other than single-family houses.

One study that offers a useful framework and starting point is an ethnographic research project conducted by McCracken (1989). Based on descriptions provided by forty Canadian men and women, McCracken identifies seven symbolic properties and several physical properties as defining characteristics of homeyness in the house. For the purpose of this work, only physical features relevant to the exterior envelope of the house are included.

1. *The diminutive property:* The diminutive aspect of homeyness "makes an environment more graspable, conceivable, thinkable" (171). Front doors and windows are small, proportions are manageable, and roofs are low.
2. *The variable property:* "Homeyness has a variable aspect. It appears to delib-

erately eschew uniformity and consistency" (171). There is a preference, for example, for houses made of rubble stone rather than cut stone.

3. *The embracing property:* "The embracing property of homeyness demonstrates a descending pattern of enclosure. The structure of the neighborhood, the foliage of the street and yard, the ivy of the exterior wall, the overhanging roof, the exterior wall . . . all work by graduated stages to create the sense of enclosure" (172).

4. *The engaging property:* Homeyness "appears deliberately designed to engage the observer." For example, "the wreath has something in its character that extends an invitation for interaction, promises a warm reception, represents a certain emotional tone for the interior within" (173).

5. *The mnemonic property:* "This aspect of homeyness has the effect of deeply personalizing the present circumstances" (174). "Objects are intended to recall the presence of family and friendship relationships, personal achievements, family events, ritual passages, and community associations" (173).

6. *The authentic property:* "Homeyness has an authentic aspect. . . . Homey spaces and things" are seen as "more 'real' and somehow more 'natural' than certain alternatives . . . which are the product of modern aesthetics, interior designers, show piece homes, and high status individuals" (174).

7. *The informal property:* The informal aspect of homeyness entails warm colors such as gold, brown, and green. The "exterior details of the house design are deliberately rustic, rural, cottage-like, and unprepossessing" (174).

McCracken's symbolic and physical properties provide a framework for examining how homeyness can be communicated by single-family houses in North America. When this framework is viewed in relation to the exterior of a building type such as assisted living, however, some modification may be appropriate. Accordingly, a revised framework is proposed in light of McCracken's work. Specifically, the proposed framework focuses on three overarching themes: supportive protection, human scale, and naturalness.

Supportive Protection

Three factors—familiarity, enclosure, and care—are subsumed within the theme of supportive protection. McCracken indirectly addresses the concept of familiarity under the mnemonic property of homeyness when he indicates that personalization helps to recall family associations or achievements. In the context of assisted-living housing, however, personalization to the exterior of the building is less pertinent. That does not belittle its importance; personalization is just more difficult to execute and examine in a group living arrangement. As a result, the mnemonic property is viewed somewhat differently. It is suggested that this property, through such memory-jogging symbols associated with the house as window shutters, may help to make an unfamiliar living arrangement more familiar for the elderly. This may provide a general sense of supportiveness, assurance, and protection.

A number of studies that address housing for the elderly stress the importance of familiarity in the home environment (Pastalan and Schwarz,

1993; Rowles, 1983, 1987; Rubinstein, 1989). Küller (1988) demonstrates how a collective housing unit decorated in an old and familiar style provides a much better therapeutic environment for the elderly than a geriatric hospital. Regnier (1994), Regnier, Hamilton, and Yatabe (1995), and Brummett (1994), in their investigations of assisted living, assert that designing with a familiar architectural language is important. Specifically, Regnier (1994) and Regnier and colleagues (1995) suggest using familiar residential materials such as brick, wood, and stone, wooden windows as opposed to aluminum frame commercial windows, and a sloped roof rather than a flat one. In addition, Regnier recommends observing historical and regional references to housing features. The porch of the typical midwestern house and the low-slung roof of the California bungalow are examples.

McCracken's (1989) embracing property, which stresses enclosure, may also provide a general sense of supportive protection. This need for enclosure in order to feel safe and protected is certainly not new and can be traced historically. "Many early buildings hugged the earth like a bear cub's den, designed for protection against tornadoes as well as excesses of heat or cold. Ranch houses were designed for protection against enemies and the sun, with air circulation in mind; porches were added for sitting outside and as a center for observation and conviviality. Many vernacular houses represent a safe place, almost a fortress, a reflection of a basic tribal memory of the need for security, a need that modern man, beset by different enemies, feels as strongly as his forebears" (Kavanaugh, 1983:13).

A number of investigators in addition to McCracken refer to protection in this sense in the single-family house. Wright (1954) indicates that he often provides a ground-hugging "broad protecting roof shelter" (33), with large projecting eaves over the whole building to give the dwelling the "essential look" of shelter (16). Roof overhangs also protect the walls, another enclosing element that affords protection. Alexander et al. (1977) suggest that if windows in upper stories are small, one may feel a greater sense of enclosure and safety when occupying those upper floors. Window muntins, as opposed to big areas of clear glass, may also reassure occupants that something is enclosing them. Bay windows suggest personal enclosure and imply protection as well. In addition, elements associated with the house such as front lawns and porches offer transitions between the public street and the private house, and this is connected with protection (Alexander et al., 1977).

The concept of care, as demonstrated by human attention to place, also implies supportive protection for the elderly. An environment may express care directly through the act of building, "as in the meticulous gingerbread details in the little houses at Oak Bluff on Martha's Vineyard in Massachusetts" (Moore and Allen, 1976:139). Care, however, is probably most associated with maintaining or tending to a place (Moore, Allen, and Lyndon, 1974). When the landscaping is neat, the fences freshly painted, and details like window boxes and shutters given attention, care is evident (Nassauer, 1995). These also suggest a human presence; a person has been to that place and returns often. Signs of occupancy such as open curtains, open windows, or outdoor seating also suggest human presence. Human presence, as demonstrated through occupancy and attention to details and maintenance, implies that support is nearby if needed. This may provide assurance for elderly persons, who are likely to feel vulnerable if they are dealing with age-related losses and impairments.

Human Scale

The second theme, human scale, is closely related to McCracken's diminutive aspect of homeyness. Human scale helps to make an environment more graspable and manageable. This is an important consideration for the elderly, who may be experiencing age-related sensory, physical, or cognitive losses. An environment that is, or appears to be, manageable may instill a sense of power, control, and competence in elderly persons.

Orr (1985) indicates that the spread of one's arms, the length of a stride, the size of a grip with one hand, and human height are indicators of human scale. A doorknob that can be easily grasped especially if placed at a comfortable height from the ground, a brick that can be easily held with one hand, steps that have wide enough treads and risers within a certain range, and a doorway wide enough to pass through are examples. We cannot use these features easily unless they are related to the dimensions of the human body. With respect to the overall building, Orr asserts that elements of a building that are large in relation to the body tend to make a building appear monumental. In contrast, small features such as doors, porch railings, and window muntins help to create a feeling of intimacy or diminutiveness.

This idea of human scale is particularly important when dealing with a housing type like that of assisted living, which is larger than the single-family house, and with a group such as elderly persons, who are typically more vulnerable than the general population. Regnier, Hamilton, and Yatabe (1995), in their investigation of assisted living, offer recommendations for reducing scale in elderly housing. Certain features such as porches, balconies, and dormers help to reduce the perceived mass and height of an assisted-living building. Although they do not specifically refer to human scale, they do stress that assisted living should "be perceived as small in size" (47). Similarly, Brummett (1994) proposes that an articulated building mass in the wall plane through the creation of bays and in the roof form through the use of dormers or changes in ridge lines helps to relate the building to the individual. More specifically, window openings and panes, door openings, and materials and details should be of a "human-related size and refinement" (115).

McCracken's engaging property, which stresses the welcoming aspect of homeyness, can also be included in the theme of human scale, because a building that is more manageable both visually and as a place to physically use is certainly more inviting. Orr (1985) refers to this notion when he states that "a building should be almost huggable: it should present us with a surface or surfaces that we feel we could, if so inspired, physically embrace" (54). Likewise, it appears that the building should, metaphorically, also open itself up, welcoming the observer and inviting entry. Alexander et al. (1977) indicate that a glazed entry door can provide a glimpse of what is inside a building, alleviating fear of the unknown and allowing the person approaching the building and those within to prepare for a reception. Thus, human scale can be more broadly interpreted as relating a building to the dimensions of the body in order to make it more manageable and welcoming.

Naturalness

Three of McCracken's properties—variable, authentic, and informal—appear to deal with the authentic quality, or realness, of a place. These may be combined into a third theme, naturalness. With respect to the exterior of assisted-living housing, naturalness can be interpreted as a relationship to landscape elements and the authentic use of building materials and colors.

A number of studies in the landscape-perception literature suggest that some landscape elements communicate naturalness. These studies repeatedly identify elements such as vegetation, especially canopy trees, and water (Nassauer, 1995). Kaplan and Kaplan (1982) contend that such preferred "contents" are linked to our evolutionary history and are interpreted as elements needed for survival. Nature itself is also a preferred content, and research indicates that natural environments are preferred over both urban and residential environments (Kaplan, Kaplan, and Wendt, 1972).

Building materials can be considered modified elements of nature. Wood, for instance, was once alive. Although it does not continue to grow once it is cut down, it continues to remind us of its natural origins through its appearance, texture, and sometimes even its smell. The connection between materials and nature was once particularly strong: "The materials from which a building was made came virtually from the site itself: stone was cut from local quarries and timber from neighbouring forests; brick and tiles were baked in clay from nearby pits. There was a strong link between the artifact and the earth from which it grew that was not just economic, but deeply satisfying at a psychic level too" (Materiality and resistance, 1994:4).

Color is also linked to nature. Color is integral to specific building materials, such as red brick, and their weathering qualities. In addition, color is tied to specific regions and sites. "One of the most popular in New England—then and now—is red, which was applied on the exteriors of barns and houses to help absorb solar heat. In the days before paint was manufactured, New Englanders created a mixture of rust (scraped from nails and fences), skim milk, and lime that coated the wood like a varnish" (Kemp, 1987:25).

This connection between materials, color, and nature was weakened "in the Industrial Revolution, when materials that had been common in one part of a country could be transported to another as whims of production and economics dictated" (Materiality and resistance, 1994:4). While traditional materials like wood, brick, mud, straw, and plaster were tied to the site, processed, and put together by hand, buildings now are usually mass produced and built of factory-made, factory-finished materials. The connection between materials and nature was further weakened by the advent of modern materials and construction techniques. For instance, modern materials such as reinforced concrete, steel, plastic, imitation stone, and wood laminates are usually not perceived as natural. "Steel is hard, cold, bearing the impress of the hard, powerful industrial machines that rolled or pressed it; plastic has something of the alien molecular technology of which it is made, standing outside the realm of life and, like reinforced concrete, bound by no visible structural rules" (Day, 1993:113). These modern materials are also often used in a deceptive way—vinyl siding replicating wood—which tends to corrupt the nature of materials. As a result, authenticity is questionable, and modern materials tend to "look as fake and hollow as they sound when you tap them" (116).

The Studies

Two studies focused on the exterior appearance of assisted-living facilities in relation to the proposed framework of supportive protection, human scale, and naturalness. Both studies used color photographs of existing assisted-living buildings. The first study explored elderly participants' perceptions of this housing option by requesting them to indicate how much they liked or disliked various scenes of buildings. The second study focused on the concept of homeyness, examining which physical features contributed to a homelike appearance by asking elderly participants to evaluate scenes in terms of homeyness. This section describes the method used to sample both photographs and participants and concludes with a discussion of the procedures used.

Environmental Sampling

Various assisted-living facilities were represented through color photographs. According to Robert Hershberger (cited in Eleishe, 1994), the practical and logistical advantages of using photographs to simulate environments are the possibilities of including buildings located in scattered places without having to obtain responses on-site, reducing the amount of time required of participants, focusing on specific aspects of designated buildings, and controlling for such distractions as inclement weather, seasonal differences, people, cars, signage, poles, wires, glare, and dark shadows. A number of empirical studies demonstrate that responses to photographs of environments correlate highly with responses to actual environments (Stamps, 1990).

The buildings in the photographs were freestanding. They were either remodeled or specifically designed and constructed to incorporate the assisted-living philosophy or were part of a continuing care retirement community. They were three stories or less and devoid of signs of deterioration, construction, or renovation. Single-family houses designated as assisted living for the elderly were not included. The photographs were taken from a main parking lot or street, and an effort was made to exclude people and automobiles. They were taken under sunny conditions with the vegetation in bloom and typically focused on either main entries or an expanse of the building near the main entry. It is virtually impossible to photograph an entire building and at the same time exclude parking lots and retain a sufficient amount of detail.

The buildings photographed for study 1 are in Florida; twenty-one photographs were intuitively selected. The buildings photographed for study 2 are in Michigan and Massachusetts. The Florida buildings were considered for inclusion in study 2 if the surrounding vegetation was similar to landscaping typical of the Midwest and the Northeast. For study 2, thirty-four photographs were selected, based on main entries, rooflines, and building materials; during preliminary data analyses, window treatments, massing, and landscaping were added as post hoc variables. (Degrees of variation in these features, with the exception of landscaping, were determined by a panel of six graduate architecture students at the University of Michigan. A panel of six graduate landscape architecture students at the University of Michigan judged the photographs in terms of landscape features.)

Participant Sampling

Reaching a representative sample of the older population is the most challenging problem in gerontological research (Gueldner and Hanner, 1989), for several reasons. First, a sampling frame covering a significant portion of older persons is unavailable in the United States (Herzog and Kulka, 1989), making it difficult to accurately identify potential participants. Second, certain segments of the elderly population, such as the oldest old and men, are typically excluded due to the unavailability of sufficiently large segments of these groups. For instance, there are approximately sixty-six men for every one hundred women 65 years and older and thirty-nine men for every one hundred women among those 85 years and older (Manton and Suzman, 1992). This disparity is exacerbated further in assisted-living facilities. Since the family may assume a greater role for the care of elders within certain ethnic groups, and since federal and state subsidization is for the most part lacking in assisted living, certain races and income levels are not proportionally represented. Third, sample representativeness may be jeopardized if potential participants refuse to participate. Many cite poor health as a reason for refusal (Danermark and Ekstrom, 1993). Others are protected from researchers by family members or institutional caretakers. In addition, many are unwilling to sign a consent form (Gueldner and Hanner, 1989), are unfamiliar with research and environmental concerns, are uncertain as to what participation involves, believe that they have little to contribute to research, equate research with test anxiety, and fear that participation may reveal their ignorance or cognitive impairments.

Within these limitations, seventy individuals 65 years old and older were selected for study 1. All participants lived in southeastern Michigan, either in retirement housing or in individual homes. For the second study, a hundred participants at least 65 years of age were selected from assisted-living facilities in Michigan and New York. All participants were unfamiliar with the buildings depicted in the photographs. For those living in elderly housing, the investigator met with the facility's administration in person to explain the purpose of the research and to request the cooperation of housing personnel. After permission was granted to conduct the study, a staff member familiar with the residents directed the investigator to potential respondents.

Instrument and Procedure

A face-to-face interview format was used for both studies. Directions were read aloud, and responses were recorded by the investigator. This format is considered ideal when working with older persons, regardless of instrument (Lawton, 1987). Obvious advantages include the possibility of moderating speech patterns to aid the hearing impaired, circumventing finger dexterity problems that might make completing questionnaires difficult, ensuring that instructions are understood and information is accurately recorded, tailoring the pace of the procedure according to the abilities of the participant, and establishing a rapport to facilitate cooperation. "Additionally, the one-to-one verbal format tends to be less anxiety-producing, and may even be viewed by some subjects as a pleasant visit" (Gueldner and Hanner, 1989). Nevertheless, elderly persons have a tendency to reminisce or attempt to engage the investigator in conversation, which can extend the already lengthy time required for the face-to-face format.

The interview procedure for both studies consisted of two parts: a rating scale, with responses structured through preference judgments in study 1 and a sorting task in study 2; and open-ended questions. For the first portion of both studies, participants were told that they would be looking at photographs of retirement housing whose cost and location were the same. When necessary, potential participants were assured that their memory would not be tested and that participation merely entailed their opinion; there were no right or wrong answers. Participants were encouraged to glance through the photographs first to get a sense of the range of scenes included.

In study 1, participants were asked to imagine that they were helping a close senior citizen friend or relative select a housing arrangement for seniors. Using a 5-point scale in which 1 equals "not at all" and 5 equals "very much," participants were instructed to indicate how much they would like their close friend or relative to live in such a place, based on what was shown in twenty-one scenes presented in a photograph album. A visual display card with the response options was provided.

In study 2, participants were asked to imagine that they were helping a senior citizen relative select homelike retirement housing. They were instructed to sort the thirty-four photographs into five piles, ranging from 1 ("not at all homelike") to 5 ("very homelike"). The main objective of the sorting task was to "provide a method for revealing and exploring the ways in which people naturally conceptualize and categorize their world" (Sixsmith, 1986:283). When using photographs, sorting can resemble a game board format, reducing test anxiety and the monotony often associated with surveys.

The second part of the interview procedure for both studies included open-ended questions. In study 1, participants were asked to explain why they liked and disliked their two highest rated and two lowest rated scenes, so that the investigators could gain a sense of the reasons underlying their preferences. To alleviate the confusion that might have ensued if the investigator had had to flip through the photograph album to locate these scenes, copies of these pictures were placed in front of the participant. In the second study, participants were asked to explain what led them to put each photograph they included in the "very homelike" pile and each photograph they included in the "not at all homelike" pile. The entire procedure took approximately fifteen minutes for both studies.

The Results of Study 1

The goal of study 1 was to explore the perceptions of an elderly population with respect to the exterior appearance of assisted-living housing. While people are generally unaware of their perceptions and relatively little is known about the way people perceive environments, research shows that people classify environments according to salient themes and commonalities (Kaplan and Kaplan, 1989). Preference judgments provide a useful means for discovering underlying perceptual categories, because preferences are based on perceptions. By examining preference ratings, it is possible to work backward to determine the commonalities underlying perceptions. This section begins with a description of the procedure used in study 1 to extract perceptual categories and is followed by a discussion of preference as way to explore the research results.

The Perceptual Categories

Perceptual categories were determined through a procedure called category-identifying methodology (CIM). Using preference ratings, CIM examines the pattern of responses and "extracts information about how scenes are grouped. The scenes constituting a category reflect a common perceptual theme; there is no requirement, however, that they be similar in terms of the degree of preference" (Kaplan and Kaplan, 1989:20–21). This approach allows the researcher to sample broadly and still reduce a large amount of data to a small number of categories. Common perceptual themes are determined empirically, and these can be compared to a priori hunches. As with any analytic procedure, the results are open to interpretation by others.

Factor analysis, a specific form of CIM, was used as the statistical technique. It relies on a correlation matrix and is based on the "fundamental assumption that some underlying factors, which are smaller in number than the number of observed variables, are responsible for the covariation among the observed variables" (Kim and Mueller, 1978:12). The number of underlying categories was unknown, and factor analysis was used as a means for exploring the data. Factor analysis yields a matrix with loadings that indicate the degree to which each observed variable belongs to each factor. Factor loadings are equivalent to correlations between variables and categories. When determining which scenes composed each category, several conventions were used: a minimum loading value of 0.40; eigenvalues, or the explanatory power of the category, greater than 1.00; exclusion of scenes with high loadings (>0.40) on two or more categories; and at least two scenes for each category. This produces categories that are independent, coherent, and internally strong. In general, it is advantageous to explain the maximum amount of variance with a minimum number of factors.

The statistical program used in this study was principal axis factoring, a method of initial factoring in which the adjusted correlation matrix is decomposed hierarchically (Norusis, 1994). In addition, normalized varimax rotation imposes two restrictions: the·underlying factors are orthogonal; and the first factor accounts for as much variance as possible, the second factor accounts for as much as possible of the variance left unexplained by the first factor, and so on. The analysis yielded three categories for study 1. Cronbach's (1951) alpha, a commonly used measure of internal consistency or the degree to which the items that form a factor "hang together," is between .68 and .81. The factors, or categories, appeared to focus on three physical characteristics: massing or building height, the sense of "institutional" or "homelike," and sheltered entryways.

The first category consisted of six scenes focusing on an expanse of the building near the main entry (see figure 13.1, top row). The horizontal nature of the scenes was stressed through the low pitch of the roofs and the one-story height of the buildings. In addition, there was a rhythm of small, individual, punched windows along the facades.

The majority of six scenes in the second grouping, as in the previous category, focused on an expanse of the building near the entry (figure 13.1, bottom row). An important difference, however, was that all buildings in this grouping appeared massive and imposing due to either height of building or window size. The strong vertical lines of articulations (pilasters, quoins, trim, etc.), bays, window alignment, and muntins reinforced the massive appearance. For these reasons, the second category was labeled "larger institutional."

The third category included four scenes focusing on entryways (see figure 13.2). Three of the scenes depicted a porte cochere large enough for vehicles to pass through and provide a sheltered drop-off point.

Several scenes were not included in any of the categories. In some instances, the scenes loaded on more than one dimension, and in other instances, scenes did not load on any of the categories.

Preferences

Preferences can be used to understand the perception of assisted-living housing for elderly persons. Perceptual categories, in turn, can be used to determine patterns of preference. Furthermore, an examination of the mean preference rating for each scene provides additional insight. Although many may infer that preferences are discrepant, idiosyncratic, and even frivolous, previous studies consistently show that preference is a stable and reliable measure across diverse settings and groups (Kaplan and Kaplan, 1989).

PREFERRED CATEGORIES

To determine how much each perceptual category was liked, the mean preference score was computed by averaging the means across all participants for the scenes included in the category (see table 13.1). Adopted conventions suggest that means below 3.0 were low in terms of preference and that those greater than or equal to 3.7 were high. The three dimension means were below 3.0, a value considered relatively low based on many other preference studies.

There are several possible reasons for this pattern, including type of setting depicted, use of the setting, and characteristics of the participating population. For example, Kaplan (1977), in a study of a storm drain system, suggests that ratings were low in her investigation because most of the scenes depicted places that required maintenance. In a similar manner, retirement housing may connote infirmities associated with old age and unfamiliar living arrangements for elderly participants. In addition to considering the absolute values of each dimension, it is useful to examine the ratings in relation to other category means. In this case, however, significant differences were not found among category means. In other words, while the categories represented useful perceptual distinctions, they were not distinct with respect to preferences.

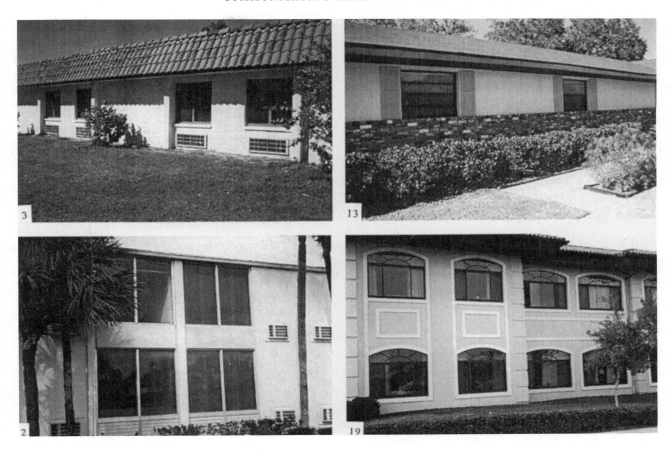

FIGURE 13.1. Examples of one-story, long view (top row) and larger institutional (bottom row)

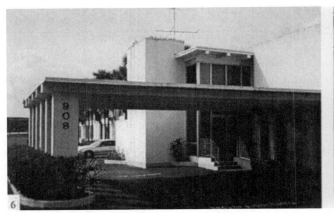
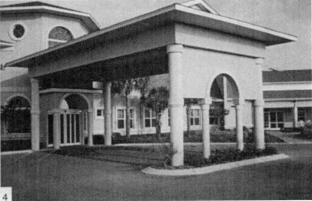

FIGURE 13.2. Examples of sheltered entries

MOST PREFERRED SCENES

A second way to understand environmental preferences involves the examination of the mean preference rating for particular scenes. Identifying characteristics that they may have in common can be useful as a basis for hypotheses for future studies. Two examples of scenes that received the highest preference ratings are shown in figure 13.3, top row. The scene on the

217

Table 13.1. Elderly Participants' Preferences for the Categories, Study 1

Category	Alpha	Rank	Mean	Standard Deviation
Larger institutional	.78	3	2.69	.33
One-story, long view	.81	2	2.72	.70
Sheltered entryway	.68	1	2.99	.37

Note: Significant differences between categories: none.

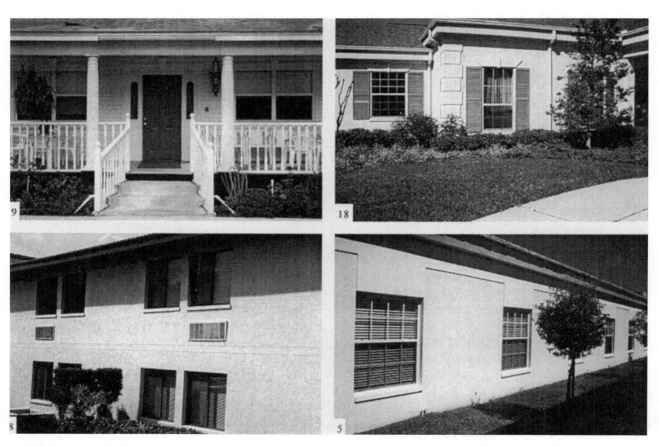

FIGURE 13.3. *Most (top row) and least (bottom row) preferred building views*

right (mean preference 3.44) depicts a one-story building made of stucco with color contrast. The green shutters are striking against the light-colored building. The quoins and lintels add some interest, as well. A substantial lawn area is also shown. The scene on the left (mean preference 3.60) also uses color contrast, the blue door emphasizing the entry. Ornamentation, such as a porch railing, window sidelights, and window trim, adds interest.

Responses to the open-ended questions revealed that these scenes were preferred because they look like a home or feel homelike, friendly, comfortable, or inviting. Often, participants were unable to explain what they meant by this. The fact that people cannot always articulate reasons underlying their preferences, however, does not diminish the strength of their preferences. Some participants were able to articulate that certain features contributed to the notion of homelike. Features of the entry such as the porch railing, the porch itself, or the front door were often cited in conjunction with homeyness. Other preferred characteristics mentioned by several participants included vegetation and building materials (tile roofs and brick).

LEAST PREFERRED SCENES

Two examples of the least preferred scenes are shown in figure 13.3, bottom row (mean preference 2.30, left; mean preference 2.04, right). In both, the windows have little ornamentation and are aligned one after the other. Window sizes are all the same. Roof pitches are low, vegetation is minimal, exterior walls are bare, and there is little color contrast.

Responses to the open-ended questions revealed that scenes that were not liked include those that evoke images of other institutional building types, such as "museum," "motel," "hotel," "gas station," "church," "nursing home," "hospital," "funeral home," "mortuary," "prison." For instance, the building shown in figure 13.3 bottom row, right, reminded many participants of a school. Once again, the majority of participants were not always able to articulate which features evoked those images. Some did refer to high columns, high buildings that might hinder accessibility and exiting, ostentation, starkness, dark colors, and lack of vegetation.

The Results of Study 2

The major objective of study 1 was to explore how the exterior of assisted-living housing is perceived by elderly persons. An overwhelming number of participants tended to view scenes as either "homelike" or "institutional." This is evident in the perceptual categories that emerged from data reduction, the preference measurements, and in particular, the open-ended responses. These findings provided a foundation for study 2, in which specific physical features that might contribute to a homelike appearance were explored. This section identifies these perceptual categories and examines the mean preference ratings for the categories and scenes.

The Perceptual Categories

As with study 1, the perceptual categories were determined through CIM, using the same factor analysis procedure and criteria. For this study, however, homeyness ratings were used as the bases for extracting categories. Factor analysis was used both as a way to explore the concept of homeyness and as a tool to confirm the homelike and institutional connotations identified in study 1. Using principal axis factoring and normalized varimax rotation, five categories were identified (Norusis, 1994). Alpha coefficients were between .66 and .81. The categories appeared to focus on entryways, massing or building height, and sense of institutional or homelike.

The first category consisted of ten scenes showing one-story buildings (see figure 13.4). All one-story buildings, except for the scenes focusing on entries and a scene included in a two-story category, formed this category. In all scenes, there was a rhythm of individual, punched windows along the facade. This was all that the buildings appeared to have in common besides the one-story building height; a variety of rooflines, building materials, win-

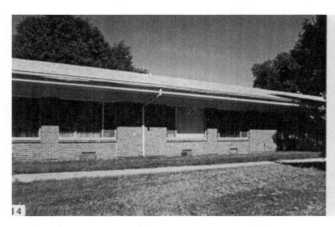

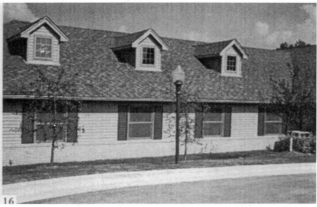

FIGURE 13.4. Examples of
one-story buildings

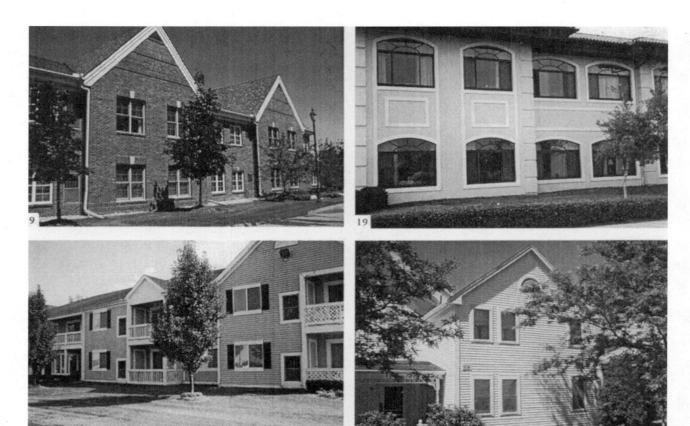

FIGURE 13.5. Examples of two-story
institutional buildings (top row) and two-
story homelike buildings (bottom row)

dow treatments, and landscaping was depicted in the scenes in this category.

The four buildings composing the second category, two-story institutional, appear massive due to building height and length of facade (see figure 13.5, top row). Windows are aligned in rows, and repetitive columns emphasize the length of the front elevation, giving the impression that the building is endless. This impression is alleviated somewhat by setbacks and

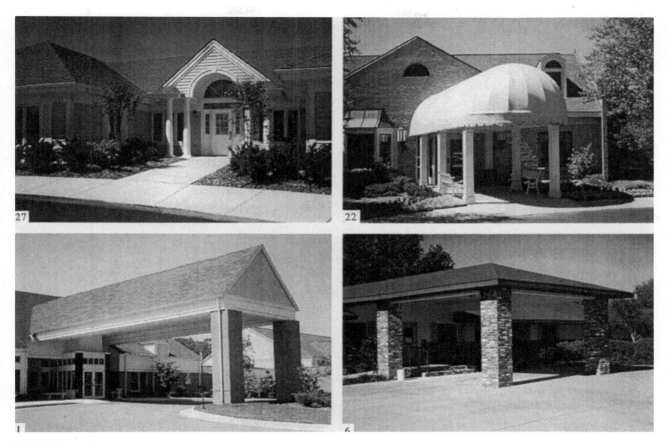

FIGURE 13.6. Examples of pedestrian entries (top row) and vehicular entries (bottom row)

gables. All buildings also appear heavy due to the brickwork and stucco. Decorative features are minimal. Trees are immature, and foundation plantings are generally lacking.

Buildings in the third category, two-story, homelike, appear less imposing and heavy due to the building materials used and the finer and smaller-scale detailing (figure 13.5, bottom row). The buildings are clad with light-colored wooden clapboard siding, consisting of narrow, overlapping boards laid horizontally. Windows are differentiated from the surrounding flat surface of the facade by lintels, sills, and casings that define the shape of the window. This is particularly evident in the building (bottom row, left) in which the window trim is white. Decorative features are the spandrel, spandrel bracket, and the turned post of the porch (bottom row, right) and the handrail, baluster, and trellis of the balconies (bottom row, left).

Four entry scenes composed the fourth category. All focus on main entries that accommodate the person traveling on foot (figure 13.6, top row); the drive or a sidewalk aligning the drive is a short distance from the front door. One scene (top row, left), includes a one-story portico with a pediment supported by columns. In another scene (top row, right), a canopy provides shelter between the drive and the front door, and a gable behind the canopy helps define the entrance. Wooden doors decorated with panels or glass, a fanlight, a transom window, and sidelights are also present. Rooflines in both scenes are articulated with dormers, gables, or pediments.

Three scenes in the fifth category depict a porte cochere—a porch roof projecting over the driveway at the entrance to the building (figure 13.6, bottom row). In one scene (bottom row, left), the porte cochere appears large enough for buses or even trucks to pass through.

Homelike Ratings

In the previous section, ratings of homeyness are used as a means to understand physical features of assisted-living housing that contribute to perceptions of homeyness. In turn, the perceptual categories that were extracted can be used to determine patterns of homeyness. Examining the mean homeyness rating for each scene can also provide insight.

RATINGS FOR THE CATEGORIES

Table 13.2 provides the mean ratings for the perceptual categories. It is apparent that these groupings were not considered particularly homelike. All ratings, in fact, were below midscale. Pedestrian entries, the category with the highest mean, was rated significantly more homelike than both vehicular entries and two-story institutional buildings. The one-story category was also considered significantly more homelike than the lowest rated two-story institutional category. While perceptually distinct, the two categories composing two-story buildings were not significantly different.

MOST HOMELIKE SCENES

Comparison of mean ratings for the perceptual categories provides a sense of the qualities that elderly persons consider homelike. Each category, however, can consist of individual scenes with quite different mean ratings. By examining the photographs that received the highest and lowest ratings in terms of homeyness, a fuller understanding can be achieved. Four examples of scenes that received the highest homeyness ratings, with means ranging from 3.36 to 3.67, suggest that lush landscaping represented through foundation plantings and wood siding or wood in combination with brick were particularly important for homeyness (see figure 13.7). In addition, the two entry scenes included in this collection depict porticos. The top-rated scenes share three other physical features besides building materials and attention to landscaping: shutters are present in all the scenes, gables or a pediment over the entrance are evident in the majority of the scenes, and the highest rated scenes are one story.

Content analysis of the open-ended responses also indicate that decora-

Table 13.2. Elderly Participants' Homelike Ratings of the Categories, Study 2

Category	Alpha	Rank	Mean	Standard Deviation
Two-story institutional	.68	5	2.07	.21
Vehicular entries	.71	4	2.10	.24
Two-story homelike	.66	3	2.73	.65
One story	.81	2	2.75	.55
Pedestrian entries	.70	1	2.97	.41

Note: Significant differences between categories: one story and two-story institutional: $p < .05$; pedestrian entries and two-story institutional: $p < .005$; pedestrian entries and vehicular entries: $p < .05$.

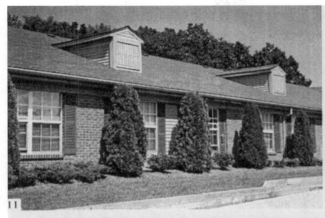
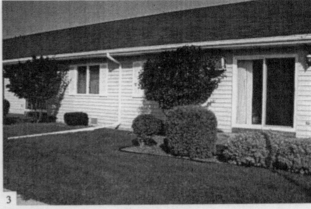
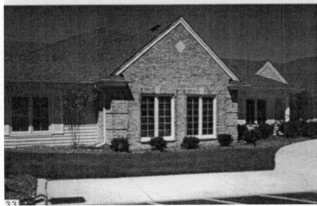
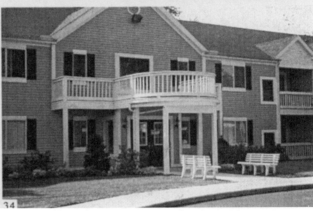

FIGURE 13.7. *Building views evaluated as the most homelike*

tive features (shutters and muntins) and entry features (porch detailing, columns, fanlight, sidelights, front door materials) contributed to perceptions of homeyness. Other physical features mentioned (but to a lesser degree than the previous characteristics) include one-story building height, light color, and roof articulation with gables or dormers. In addition, scenes that were considered very homelike were described as "cozy or comfortable," "not too overdone or grandiose," "neat and clean," "interesting," and "attractive."

LEAST HOMELIKE SCENES

The four scenes that received the lowest homeyness ratings (ranging from 1.82 to 2.05) are shown in figure 13.8. With one exception, these building are brick or stucco and are more than one story in height, making them appear rather massive. The one exception is a scene depicting a large porte cochere. Open-ended responses revealed that scenes categorized as "not at all homelike" evoked images of other building types, as in study 1. This is particularly true with the massive entries: participants often referred to motels, funeral homes, or restaurants when viewing them. In addition, buildings were described as "cold," "stark," "plain," "uninteresting," "monotonous," and "ostentatious." Some participants articulated properties that contributed to their "not at all homelike" perceptions, noting that some cover over the entry was advantageous but that entryways that were too large in comparison to the rest of the building were not homelike. Porte

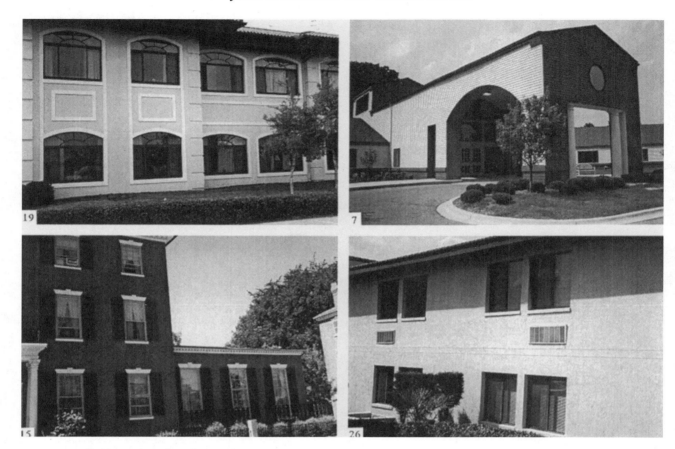

FIGURE 13.8. Building views evaluated as the least homelike

cocheres, canopies, long walks to the front door, and tall columns or non-functional columns drew negative reactions. Other features cited include two-story buildings or buildings that were too big; numerous, plain, uniform, repetitive windows; lack of landscaping; flat or low-pitched roofs; and dark colors.

Links between the Studies

Study 1 examined how the exterior of assisted-living facilities were perceived by asking elderly participants to evaluate, in terms of preference, buildings shown in color photographs. Results indicate that preferred scenes were homelike while other scenes were disliked because they evoked images of institutional buildings. Study 2 addressed the question of physical features that contribute to a homelike appearance, which was accomplished by asking elderly participants to evaluate photographs of assisted-living buildings in terms of homeyness. There were some differences between the two studies, but there were also strong similarities in terms of the categories derived from factor analyses, category ratings, and the highest and lowest rated scenes.

Despite the different questions addressed in the two studies, the perceptual categories that emerged from the ratings focused on three common characteristics: entryways, massing or building height, and a sense of institutional or homelike. These three characteristics were also evident in the analysis of the highest and lowest rated scenes and the open-ended responses.

Entryways

Entryways were a salient perceptual category. In study 1, all porte cocheres (with one exception) were grouped together, based on preferences. In study 2, entries (with two exceptions) were grouped together, based on homelike ratings. However, entries in study 2 divided into two categories, depending on whether they were small and pedestrian oriented, such as porticos and covered walkways, or large and vehicular oriented, such as porte cocheres. This may be because study 2 included a broader spectrum of entry types, including porte cocheres, porticos, porches, and covered walkways.

Since the pedestrian entries category was rated significantly higher than the vehicular entries category in study 2, the issue of human scale, one theme of the proposed homeyness framework, appears to be an important aspect of homeyness. The issue of massiveness with respect to entries was also cited often by participants in their open-ended responses. As a result, size of the entrance and its associated features, such as columns and fanlights, should be taken into consideration. The fact that these smaller entries, including porticos and porches, were more familiar housing cues than porte cocheres also suggests that certain types of entry may impact the homeyness theme of supportive protection.

Massing or Building Height

Study 1 yielded two distinct groupings, which differ in terms of massing. Scenes of one-story buildings focusing on an expanse of the building formed one category. Scenes of two-story buildings focusing on an expanse of the building formed a separate category. Responses by the elderly in study 2 showed a similar pattern; here again, scenes of one-story buildings focusing on an expanse of the building formed a category. Scenes of two-story buildings, however, formed two categories, reflecting differences in homelike and institutional character.

Whether measurements of preference (study 1) or homeyness (study 2) were employed, one-story buildings tended to be rated more favorably. In study 2, for instance, the one-story category received significantly higher ratings than the two-story institutional category. Many of the lowest rated scenes in study 2 were of two-story buildings, and open-ended responses reveal that a two-story building height contributed to perceptions of massiveness. Thus, the theme of human scale, as represented through building height and facade length, was an important factor in perceptions of homeyness.

Sense of Institutional or Homelike

In study 1, two-story buildings and large porticos were considered institutional because all the buildings appeared massive and imposing due to building height and window size. The most preferred scenes evoked images of home, as described in the open-ended responses, largely because they employed small-scale elements, many of which are decorative (tile roofs, quoins, lintels, window shutters, individual plantings in pots, and porch railings). Color contrast was often used to emphasize these decorative features.

In study 2 as well, the institutional and homelike theme was central to participants' perceptions. Two-story homelike buildings, which composed one category, appeared homelike due to detailing on a finer scale. This was exhibited, as in study 1, by decorative features such as window trim, muntins, lintels, shutters, verge or bargeboard, and balcony balusters and handrails. In addition, building materials such as wood and wood in combination with brick, which were not depicted in the scenes of study 1, helped the buildings appear less massive and imposing and contributed to a sense of homelike. As was the case in study 1, the two-story buildings of study 2 that seemed more institutional appeared massive due to height. Unlike study 1, however, in which buildings were also considered institutional due to window size, the buildings of study 2 appeared massive due to building materials, such as brick and stucco. This was not as evident in study 1, because the majority of buildings were made of stucco or brick. A larger number of structures made of wood were included in study 2, and these tended to accrue to different categories. The amount and maturity of landscaping also impacted perceptions of homeyness. Furthermore, open-ended responses revealed that starkness and uniformity contributed to institutional character.

Attention to decorative features or detailing at a fine scale provides support for the theme of human scale and the concept of care under the supportive protection theme. The fact that wood and wood in combination with brick contributes to perceptions of homeyness may be due to their human scale and their references to nature. Lush and mature landscaping also contributes to perceptions of homeyness, lending support to the theme of naturalness. As noted, human scale and naturalness are proposed as two themes of homeyness.

The findings of both studies shed light on an area that has received very little attention by the research community. Although assisted living has been promoted as a residential or homelike housing choice for the elderly, few researchers have examined how this living arrangement is actually perceived. And the question, What does home mean to elderly people? is rarely asked in the context of the exterior of the building. Yet, the exterior is the first impression one receives. In addition, many of the buildings included in the studies were probably designed by well-meaning architects relying primarily on intuition and imagination. The buildings, however, were not all well received by the research participants. This highlights the importance of public input about places like assisted-living facilities that may become home for many people in the future.

References

Alexander, C., S. Ishikawa, and M. Silverstein, with M. Jacobsen, I. Fiskdahl-King, and S. Angel. 1977. *A Pattern Language*. New York: Oxford University Press.

Brummett, W. 1994. The essence of home: Architectural design considerations for assisted-living elderly housing. Master's thesis. University of Wisconsin, Milwaukee.

Clark, C. 1986. *The American Family Home*. Chapel Hill: University of North Carolina Press.

Cronbach, L. 1951. Coefficient alpha and the internal structure of tests. *Psychometrika* 16:297–334.

Danermark, B., and M. Ekstrom. 1993. The elderly and housing relocation in Sweden: A comparative methodology. In E. Arias, ed., *The Meaning and Use of Housing*. Brookfield, Vt.: Ashgate.

Day, C. 1993. *Places of the Soul: Architecture and Environmental Design as a Healing Art*. London: Thorsons.

Despres, C. 1991. The meaning of home: Literature review and directions for future research and theoretical development. *Journal of Architectural and Planning Research* 8:96–114.

Eleishe, A. 1994. Contextualism in architecture: A comparative study of environmental perception. Ph.D. diss. University of Michigan, Ann Arbor.

Gueldner, S., and M. Hanner. 1989. Methodological issues related to gerontological nursing research. *Nursing Research* 38:183–85.

Herzog, A., and R. Kulka. 1989. Telephone and mail surveys with older populations: A methodological overview. In M. Lawton and A. Herzog, eds., *Special Research Methods in Gerontology*. Amityville, N.Y.: Baywood.

Kaplan, R. 1977. Preference and everyday nature: Method and application. In D. Stokols, ed., *Perspectives on Environment and Behavior: Theory, Research, and Applications*. New York: Plenum.

Kaplan, R., and S. Kaplan. 1989. *The Experience of Nature: A Psychological Perspective*. New York: Cambridge University Press.

Kaplan, S., and R. Kaplan. 1982. *Cognition and Environment: Functioning in an Uncertain World*. New York: Praeger.

Kaplan, S., R. Kaplan, and J. Wendt. 1972. Rated preferences and complexity for natural and urban visual material. *Perception and Psychophysics* 12:354–56.

Kavanaugh, G. 1983. Foreword. In C. Moore, K. Smith, and P. Becker, eds., *Home Sweet Home*. New York: Rizzoli.

Kemp, J. 1987. *American Vernacular: Regional Influences in Architecture and Interior Design*. New York: Viking/Penguin.

Kim, J., and C. Mueller. 1978. *Introduction to Factor Analysis: What It Is and How to Do It*. Newbury Park, Calif.: Sage.

Küller, R. 1988. Environmental activation of old persons suffering from senile dementia. In H. van Hoogdalem, N. Prak, R. van der Voordt, and H. van Wegen, eds., *Looking Back to the Future: Proceeding of the Tenth Biennial Conference of the International Association for the Study of People and Their Physical Surroundings*. Delft: Delft University Press.

Lawton, M. 1987. Methods in environmental research with older people. In R. Bechtel, R. Marans, and W. Michelson, eds., *Methods in Environmental and Behavioral Research*. New York: Van Nostrand Reinhold.

Manton, K., and R. Suzman. 1992. Forecasting health and functioning in aging societies: Implications for health care and staffing needs. In M. Ory, R. Abeles, and P. Lipman, eds., *Aging, Health and Behavior*. Newbury Park, Calif.: Sage.

Materiality and resistance. 1994. *Architectural Review* 194:4–5.

McCracken, G. 1989. Homeyness: A cultural account of the constellation of consumer goods and meanings. In E. Hirschman, ed., *Interpretive Consumer Culture*. Provo, Utah: Association for Consumer Research.

Moore, C., and G. Allen. 1976. *Dimensions: Space, Shape, and Scale in Architecture*. New York: Architectural Record Books.

Moore, C., G. Allen, and D. Lyndon. 1974. *The Place of Houses*. New York: Holt, Rinehart, and Winston.

Nassauer, J. 1995. Messy ecosystem, orderly frames. *Landscape Journal* 14:161–70.

Norusis, M. 1994. *Professional Statistics, 6.1*. Chicago: SPSS.

Orr, F. 1985. *Scale in Architecture*. New York: Van Nostrand Reinhold.

Pastalan, L., and B. Schwarz. 1993. The meaning of home in ecogenic housing: A new concept for elderly women. In H. Dandekar, ed., *Shelter, Women, and Development*. Ann Arbor, Mich.: Wahr.

Regnier, V. 1994. *Assisted Living Housing for the Elderly: Design Innovations from the United States and Europe*. New York: Van Nostrand Reinhold.

Regnier, V., J. Hamilton, and S. Yatabe. 1995. *Assisted Living for the Frail: Innovations in Design, Management, and Financing*. New York: Columbia University Press.

Rowles, G. 1983. Place and personal identity in old age: Observations from Appalachia. *Journal of Environmental Psychology* 3:299–313.

———. 1987. A place to call home. In L. Carstensen and B. Edelstein, eds., *Handbook of Clinical Gerontology*. New York: Pergamon.

Rubinstein, R. 1989. The home environments of older people: A description of the psychosocial process linking person to place. *Journal of Gerontology* 44:545–53.

Sixsmith, J. 1986. The meaning of home: An exploratory study of environmental experience. *Journal of Environmental Psychology* 6:281–98.

Stamps, A. 1990. Use of photographs to simulate environments: A meta-analysis. *Perceptual and Motor Skills* 71:907–3.

Wright, F. 1954. *The Natural House*. New York: Horizon Press.

CHAPTER 14

Designing to Meet the Needs of People with Alzheimer's Disease

J. DAVID HOGLUND
STEFANI D. LEDEWITZ

A good house is a created thing made of many parts economically and meaningfully assembled. It speaks not just of the materials from which it is made, but of the intangible rhythms, spirits, and dreams of people's lives. Its site is only a piece of the real world, yet this place is made to seem like an entire world. In its parts it accommodates important human activities, yet in sum it expresses an attitude toward life.

Charles Moore, Gerald Allen, and Donlyn Lyndon, The Place of Houses

Most of us feel we are kings or queens of our castle and the masters of our destiny. We make daily choices that mold our lives and the lives of those around us. We modify the environment to accommodate our needs and desires and to reflect the lifestyle we have chosen. Our homes offer us a friendly and familiar haven, secure and private from the rest of the world. For older people with declining mental competence, however, home may not have a physical manifestation but may inhere rather in the continuity of the rhythms and patterns of life. For people with Alzheimer's disease, bricks and mortar may meet the temporal need for shelter, but subtle design qualities can restore their dignity and encourage freedom (Cohen and Weisman, 1991). A good house encourages spontaneity, creative pursuits, and joy yet acknowledges declining physical and mental competence by accounting for physical and psychological barriers.

The discussion in this chapter has several basic premises:

— Good design makes a difference in the quality of a person's life and the individual's ability to master the environment.
— The built environment has a real and lasting emotional and physiological effect on its inhabitants.
— Good care and good staff are the cornerstones of programs for people with Alzheimer's disease, but the physical setting expresses an attitude about the residents that can have a significant influence on the program's success.
— Residential, nonmedical settings are the most appropriate environments for people with Alzheimer's disease, particularly those in the early and middle stages of impairment.
— Purpose-built settings offer the most opportunities to realize specific programmatic goals and ideas.
— The environment can reinforce individuality by avoiding prescribed routines.
— Designing facilities for people with increasing cognitive impairment is relatively new; there are no proven rules. The environmental setting must al-

low for flexibility in ideas and programs, establishing a framework that is adaptable to new ideas.

These premises reflect the belief that good design can have a therapeutic effect on the behavior and quality of life for residents with Alzheimer's disease.

In 1988, Presbyterian SeniorCare, in Oakmont, Pennsylvania, approached Perkins Eastman Architects to research and design a residential, assisted-living alternative for thirty-six people with Alzheimer's disease and related forms of dementia. The owner provided the intriguing opportunity to investigate other models of care and explore existing research findings, to develop and design such a residence, and to conduct a multiyear evaluation of the facility, staff, residents, and families. The residence, Woodside Place, has been open since 1991; the three-year research study was completed and published in 1996. This chapter explores the key environmental design concepts in the Woodside Place model, identifies specific findings from the research study, and develops recommendations for further design exploration. In the following pages, we offer a brief background on the initial research and design process that led to Woodside Place and review the nine key design issues and the recommendations of the research team's evaluation. The chapter concludes with lessons learned and their application to other facilities now in design or operation.

Planning for Woodside Place

Woodside Place (named after Dr. Isaac's facility, Woodside, in Birmingham, England) has become a national model for environmental design and programmatic care. The project began modestly in 1987, however, as an opportunity to fill a perceived gap in the continuum of services offered to the elderly of western Pennsylvania. The client was concerned that residents with dementia were being inappropriately placed in nursing home settings with inadequate programmatic support. Institutional environments did little to support their remaining cognitive abilities and, in fact, became a major hindrance to their residents. Confusing layouts, repetitive, undistinguished elements, and safety hazards contributed to behaviors that had to be "managed" (Calkins, 1988).

The client placed great importance on the physical environment as an integral part of an appropriate care program for people with Alzheimer's disease. In fact, the design explorations went hand in hand with the evolution of staffing and services. The Woodside Place design process offers numerous insights into how management, operational, and care goals were included in design concepts and then translated into the actual building components. Design, by its very nature, is not a scientific process; it is a balance of many criteria and goals, with compromise as an inherent part of the decision process. Compromise comes from many sources—conflicting goals, in which the greater good reigns, such as spacious living spaces that compromise cost-effectiveness and codes that may limit the variety of options or operational goals. It is difficult to relay all the design decisions integral to creating Woodside Place—some are applicable to a wide range of facilities, while some are specific to Woodside Place.

From the outset, the development team wanted to explore a residential alternative to caring for people with Alzheimer's disease, in the hope that it could provide a higher quality of care at less cost per day. It was also hoped that savings in initial capital costs could be achieved due to less stringent code requirements and less restrictive licensing standards. A major goal was to remove all institutional routines, allowing residents, to the greatest practical extent, to choose when to eat, bathe, and go outdoors. To facilitate residents' independence, the facility would have to be designed to ensure staff of residents' security, in outside spaces as well as inside. It was also intended that the facility would support informal interaction between staff and residents in lieu of the formal hierarchical patterns of traditional nursing homes. Early financial projections, as well as research into other facilities, set the facility size between thirty and forty residents, but the architectural program was made more complex by the desire to accommodate the respite needs of family caregivers in the community and a full-time day care program. Another ambitious part of the design agenda was the goal of using the built facility as a laboratory for measuring the success of the program and environment. In the hope that the facility would be worthy of replication, it was to be designed as a self-contained, freestanding building, despite its proximity to buildings on the campus on which it was to be constructed.

Our team's research into environments for people with Alzheimer's disease and related dementias found few built facilities or programs and even less documented research (Lawton, 1987). Initial investigations uncovered numerous articles about experiences with Alzheimer's disease patients in nursing home settings, with anecdotal design information about how an existing facility was adapted to ease behavioral issues caused by the physical environment (removing doors, disguising objects). There was very little written design information based on new ideas or new facilities. This is due in part to the newly emerging recognition that Alzheimer's disease and related dementias present specific program and design challenges. Unlike other diseases and chronic conditions, no medical interventions can stabilize the condition or increase the quality of life. In fact, several studies show that drug therapies actually increase unconventional behaviors and create complementary problems of incontinence, lack of appetite, and muscular degeneration.

The most useful resources, interestingly enough, were in publications during our initial research, and the most innovative facilities were just opening. These resources, such as Calkins's *Design for Dementia* (1988) and the architectural research work of Cohen and Weisman, of the University of Wisconsin at Milwaukee (Cohen and Weisman, 1991; Cohen et al., 1988), are invaluable tools for assessing the design options explored in other facilities. Perhaps the most valuable research was the site visits to several United States and European facilities:

— The residence in Gardiner, Maine, by Yankee Healthcare offered design criteria as well as staff and programming insights from their initial months of operation.
— The Corrine Dolan Center, in Chardon, Ohio, challenged many of our initial premises because of its more radical programmatic and unconventional architectural direction.
— The John Douglas French Center, in Los Alamitos, California, was less

useful because of its skilled care orientation, whereas our team's orientation was more residential.

— The Woodside facility in Birmingham, England, by Dr. Bernard Isaacs was more useful from the standpoint of his decade of experiences in programming, staffing, and reducing drug therapies than for environmental design principles.

— The Lefroy Hostel for Elderly Persons, in Australia, was extremely valuable because it was the only facility that had operated long enough for a postoccupancy evaluation and a critical commentary of their successes and failures.

Although there were a vast number of other facilities for persons with Alzheimer's disease, these were, for the most part, converted nursing homes with special staffing and program goals. While many offered creative ideas, they did not offer the critical interplay between programs, care goals, and environmental design that our team was seeking.

The three-year evaluation of Woodside Place, begun in 1991 (Silverman et al., 1996), was designed to examine the impact of a complex group of organizational, programmatic, and environmental factors on resident health and social experience, staff performance, and family caregiver satisfaction. These factors were measured using structured interviews, rating scales, ethnographic research, and systematic observation of resident behavior. The data collection included a baseline assessment of residents upon entry to the facility and follow-up assmentments at two, six, twelve, eighteen, and twenty-four months. Assessment instruments included scales designed to measure residents' severity of dementia, behavioral pathology, and functional and mental status. Residents' physical health was monitored through a review of their charts to note use of medical services, number of falls or injuries, number of days bedridden, and type and number of hospital visits.

To obtain a view of the social experiences of the residents and their use of the environment, an ethnographer observed their daily life and activity patterns and their interaction throughout the research period. In addition, computer-assisted observations of residents' behavior were made at defined time sequences during the first and second years of the evaluation. For a period of approximately six weeks during each of the three years, trained observers also mapped the location and activity of everyone in the facility, including residents, staff, and visitors. Care attendants from all shifts were interviewed twice during the evaluation, using a semistructured format. Family caregivers were interviewed at baseline and at two follow-up periods, at six and eighteen months. All administrative and supervisory personnel were interviewed five times, at six-month intervals. Interviews with the architect occurred twice during the study. Cost and fee data were obtained from accounting records and also from facilities similar to Woodside Place.

To understand better the benefits of Woodside Place as an alternative to nursing home placement for persons with mild dementia, a comparison group of residents was identified at a nursing facility on the same campus and under the same administration. At the time of the study, dementia residents were integrated into the population of the nursing facility. In the last year of the study, a special care unit for dementia residents was opened in the nursing facility, and an abbreviated evaluation was performed to compare with the two full-scale studies. Residents in the nursing facility were selected to be similar to Woodside Place residents in terms of mental status, health, and demographic characteristics, so that differences in outcome could be attributed to differences in program and environment. Operational and ethical constraints limited the selection of study participants, so there were differences among the groups in average age, length of institutionalization, mobility, and other factors. The number of participants—fifty-nine at Woodside Place, thirty-four at the traditional nursing facility, and eighteen in the special care unit—was also too small to allow for much generalization. Because of these limitations, the study was structured primarily as an extensive case study of Woodside Place itself and only secondarily in terms of comparative outcomes.

The Design of Woodside Place

Woodside Place is composed of three houses, each home to twelve people. The houses are physically connected to a central common area (see figure 14.1). The building is sited in a three-acre, secure, wandering garden, in which each house has a private courtyard. Each house has eight private rooms with half baths, two couples' rooms, a living/dining room, a kitchen, and a residential bathroom with shower. The common area contains a great room as its centerpiece, with sitting areas, craft room, music room, and entertainment (television) room. The central building also has a kitchen for meal preparation plus storage, mechanical, and administrative areas. On the exterior, the building is composed of several residential-sized volumes that conceal its overall size (23,000 square feet) and has gabled roofs and horizontal siding. The interior design borrows from Shaker and other simple residential motifs, using wood trim, bead-board paneling, decorative fixtures, and recessed lighting. The carpet, the wood-grain sheet vinyl, and the wall covering were selected to add to residential warmth and comfort.

It is the purpose of this section to focus on design issues that should be considered in the design of a facility for people with dementia (see figure 14.2). The nine design issues are acknowledging privacy and community, flexible rhythms and patterns, small group size, caregiver and family relationships, engaged wandering, alternative wayfinding systems, independence with security, focused and appropriate stimulation, and residential qualities. We examine these issues in the context of our observations at Woodside Place and the research study (Silverman et al., 1996) and offer design recommendations that respond specifically to the topic discussed.

Acknowledging Privacy and Community

One of the most profound findings from the Woodside research is the sense of community that was formed. Residents freely socialize among houses, forming friendships and associations. They use the common areas of the building as if they are front porches or a town square. Some residents also indicated a concern for the privacy of their house by requesting that the front door be locked at night. Residents who were mapped exhibited a number of societally normal behaviors: territoriality, repetitive walking patterns, display of homemaking skills or offering hospitality. These patterns imply a recognition of the public and private realms among some residents. While not all residents acknowledge it, the hierarchy of public and private spaces

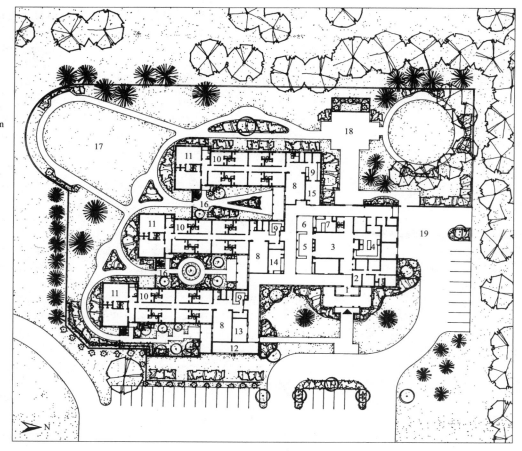

Woodside Place

1. Entry
2. Administration
3. Great Room
4. Main Kitchen
5. Library
6. Sitting Area
7. Country Kitchen
8. Living Room/Dining Room
9. Pantry
10. Single Bedroom
11. Double Bedroom
12. Quiet Room
13. Music Room
14. Arts & Crafts Room
15. Entertainment Room
16. Secure Courtyard
17. Secure Wandering Area
18. Patio
19. Service Yard

0 10 30 50 ft.

Site Plan

PERKINS EASTMAN ARCHITECTS PC

FIGURE 14.1. *Floor plan at Woodside Place, Oakmont, Pennsylvania*
SOURCE: *Perkins Eastman Architects, P.C.*

within the building appears to reinforce appropriate behaviors. Each house developed its own character around the personalities, backgrounds, and cultures of its residents and care attendants. The kitchen in each house became the social center and tends to be the locus of homemaking and other domestic activities. The common areas accommodate other public behaviors, such as social walking (strolling arm-in-arm), watching (with many residents sitting in "their" chairs), and visiting.

The research at Woodside Place confirms the desirability of a high proportion of single rooms with private bathrooms. Both staff and family members express satisfaction with the privacy of dressing and bathing spaces. Respect for residents' privacy is consistently practiced by staff but sometimes is violated by other residents. Residents in single rooms have the option of being alone in their bedrooms, but they choose to spend less than 10 percent of their day there. In general, they frequent spaces occupied by others, such as the main corridor and spaces overlooking circulation areas. More socializing occurs in the main corridor than elsewhere in the facility.

Social life, a high priority among family caregivers, occurs through both formal, staff-organized activities and informal, resident-initiated activities. Residents spend three times as much time socializing as residents of the nursing facility, participating to varying degrees in the social life, depending on their personality and level of impairment. Residents exhibit consid-

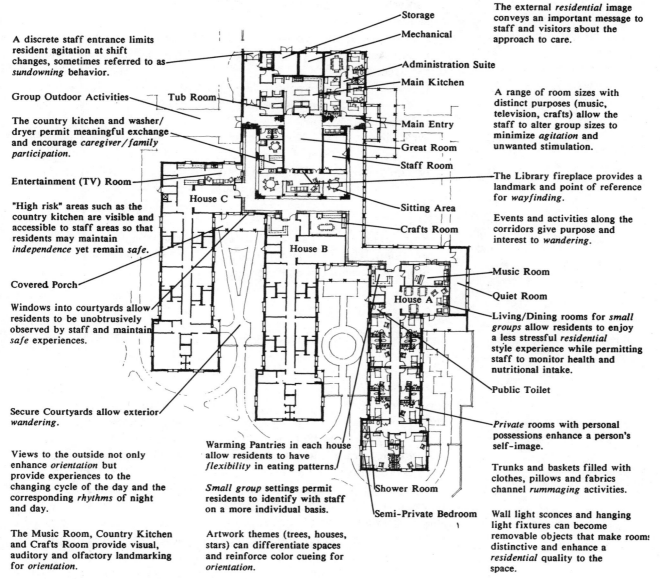

A discrete staff entrance limits resident agitation at shift changes, sometimes referred to as *sundowning* behavior.

Group Outdoor Activities

The country kitchen and washer/dryer permit meaningful exchange and encourage *caregiver/family participation.*

Entertainment (TV) Room

"High risk" areas such as the country kitchen are visible and accessible to staff areas so that residents may maintain *independence* yet remain *safe.*

Covered Porch

Windows into courtyards allow residents to be unobtrusively observed by staff and maintain *safe* experiences.

Secure Courtyards allow exterior *wandering.*

Views to the outside not only enhance *orientation* but provide experiences to the changing cycle of the day and the corresponding *rhythms* of night and day.

The Music Room, Country Kitchen and Crafts Room provide visual, auditory and olfactory landmarking for *orientation.*

Tub Room

House C

House B

House A

Warming Pantries in each house allow residents to have *flexibility* in eating patterns.

Small group settings permit residents to identify with staff on a more individual basis.

Artwork themes (trees, houses, stars) can differentiate spaces and reinforce color cueing for *orientation.*

Storage

Mechanical

Administration Suite

Main Kitchen

Main Entry

Great Room

Staff Room

Sitting Area

Crafts Room

Music Room

Quiet Room

Public Toilet

Shower Room

Semi-Private Bedroom

The external *residential* image conveys an important message to staff and visitors about the approach to care.

A range of room sizes with distinct purposes (music, television, crafts) allow the staff to alter group sizes to minimize *agitation* and unwanted stimulation.

The Library fireplace provides a landmark and point of reference for *wayfinding.*

Events and activities along the corridors give purpose and interest to *wandering.*

Living/Dining rooms for *small groups* allow residents to enjoy a less stressful *residential* style experience while permitting staff to monitor health and nutritional intake.

Private rooms with personal possessions enhance a person's self-image.

Trunks and baskets filled with clothes, pillows and fabrics channel *rummaging* activities.

Wall light sconces and hanging light fixtures can become removable objects that make rooms distinctive and enhance a *residential* quality to the space.

FIGURE 14.2. *Design goals at Woodside Place*

erable diversity of social roles and greater role continuity than is typically found in an institutionalized setting. Cognitive decline tends to reduce resident's participation in social interactions. Some residents are also limited in their ability to engage in community life because the facility's daily programming is not adapted to their social and emotional needs. Inadequate integration of informal, everyday, resident activities with the staff-led activities program limits the full realization of social life and functioning.

Based on this research, several key points should be considered in the design of a facility:

—Provide private bedrooms with private bathrooms, which contain at least a toilet and a sink. Consideration should be given to a shower. (Some accommodation for shared rooms should be made for couples or people who choose to share. One shared room for every ten private rooms should be sufficient.)

—Provide private zones, preferably private bedrooms, in which residents may choose to be alone and to keep important personal items that help them feel secure.

—Provide a hierarchy of public and private spaces. Avoid inappropriate adjacencies, such as bedrooms opening off living rooms, which may confuse the expected behaviors.

—Maintain privacy and dignity by differentiating and locating public circulation away from private residential hallways and by locating and designing private rooms and bathrooms such that obtrusive visual observation is minimized. This is particularly important since certain customarily modest behaviors may not be followed (residents may undress or use the toilet without closing the door).

—Provide appropriate bathing facilities within the private zone of the house (or room). It is unfamiliar for residents to leave the privacy of their bedroom, go through common areas and into a public zone, to find the bathing room.

Flexible Rhythms and Patterns

Avoiding rigid schedules and substituting small-group activities for flexible eating patterns contributes to a noninstitutional environment (Cohen et al., 1988). For people with dementia, it is particularly important to offer a setting that conforms to their needs and preferences, rather than forcing conformance. Rigid programming, even with the best intentions, can lead to catastrophic reactions and negative adaptive behaviors. Programmatically, the key is to allow residents the flexibility to evolve their own daily routines, from which a consistent and familiar individualized framework for daily living can be established. Creating engaging activities, rather than forced interaction, is also important. To achieve these goals there must be a strong operational focus on supporting staff and informing families. The building should accommodate a wide range of lifestyles, create opportunities for a variety of daily activities, support personalized attention by staff, and provide clues to encourage appropriate behaviors.

The limit on flexibility at Woodside Place is not in the physical environment but in the staff's capacity to manage it, due to the amount of time needed to respond to individual needs. The houses provide places for residents to eat at various times and to have snacks on their own schedule, although actual flexibility depends on care attendants' approach to regulating diet. The residents' access to food is an ongoing source of conflict. Bedrooms with private bathrooms facilitate flexible sleeping times, and the house kitchens provide a place for residents to spend time with a care attendant at any time of day or night.

Along with flexible schedules, the design of Woodside Place provides opportunities for a diversity of roles. Continuity of social and emotional roles, such as friend, listener, leader, or nurturer, is pronounced, while continuation of roles that require more technical or specialized skills, such as prior occupations, is less common. Housekeeping and typically female roles are more easily maintained than are roles that require more public or outdoor environments. Casual seating places, such as porch rockers, a kitchen counter, or chairs at a window, offer appropriate settings for friendly conversation, while other small group spaces are used for impromptu visiting or social gathering. The key issues to maintaining flexible rhythm and patterns are listed below:

— Provide for flexible mealtimes so they can be enjoyed as residents desire. This means providing preparation space that is not on an institutional schedule as well as refrigeration and warming capabilities. Provide cooking facilities so that staff can meet residents' eating requests or requests for alternative selections.
— Separate activity areas from resident rooms so residents can sleep or nap without interruption.
— Create a variety of settings, making a deliberate effort to include different room size, orientation, character, and degree of stimulation.
— Reinforce seasonal and daily rhythms by providing easy views to the outside so residents can see whether it is day or night, summer or winter. Traditional institutional environments typically have little relationship to the outside, and the interior environment is always artificially lit. Confusion over day and night cycles is typical.
— Integrate structured activity programs with informal activities initiated by residents or staff. Provide space in the residential kitchens for informal activities (coffee, craft activities, puzzles, folding laundry).
— Explore new settings and activities, both informal and formal, that reflect residents' prior lives and roles—not just homemaking but situations such as office or workshop.

Small-Group Size

In traditional nursing care environments, people with dementia are sometimes overwhelmed or distracted by large numbers of people or large spaces. Behavioral disturbances commonly occur at mealtimes, when residents with dementia may be surrounded by as many as fifty or sixty other people in a large dining room (Calkins, 1988). Staff members report that persons with dementia are more successful in coping with smaller groups, no larger than six to eight persons. Smaller groups at meals or in programmed activities can be accommodated in smaller spaces, which are less noisy and less visually distracting. A residential facility, in contrast to an institutional setting, offers a more familylike environment, with both smaller groups of people and smaller spaces. A facility that houses more than twelve persons should be organized into smaller clusters, or houses, for six to ten residents. Each cluster would contain small group spaces, such as a living room and a dining room, as well as residents' bedrooms. In addition, the facility might provide several common rooms, or gathering spaces, sized to accommodate six to ten persons.

There is, of course, a noticeable range in the need that persons with Alzheimer's disease have for stimulation and the tolerance they have for the level of activity around them. Some large-group activities, such as watching a performance or sharing a holiday dinner, can be enjoyed by as many as thirty to forty residents. Some residents seek activity among a large number of persons, while others are comfortable only in a sheltered setting, with no more than a few familiar persons. A residential facility should provide,

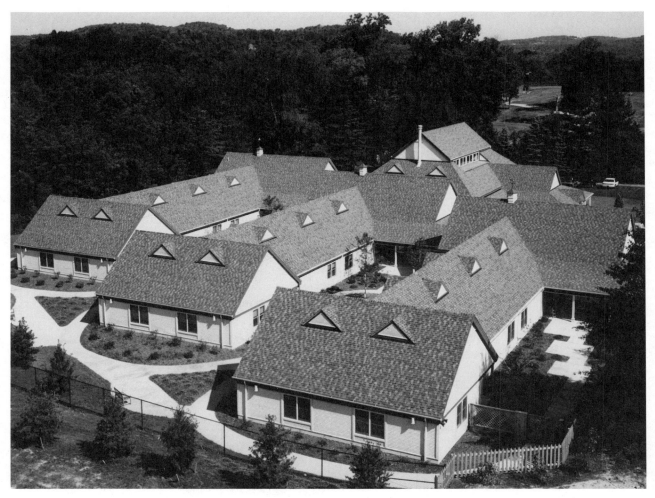

FIGURE 14.3. *Aerial view at Woodside Place* SOURCE: *Photograph by Robert Ruschak*

in addition to small-group spaces, a variety of settings that enable residents to find the scale of social engagement they prefer.

The three houses of Woodside Place are a major organizing feature of the facility, a frame of reference for staff and visitors (see figure 14.3). Residents identify with their houses, and some even exert territorial control over their house by trying to keep "outsiders" from entering. Small-group spaces, both inside and outside the houses, provide for a variety of small-group activities. Many of these spaces, however, have not been used for the purpose intended. In part, this is because of the unanticipated emphasis on large-group functions in the activity program and in part because the rooms accommodate uses other than those intended. The music room, for instance, is also used for morning gatherings, spiritual services, family visits, and staff meetings. Toward the end of the study, with the effects of the progress of the disease apparent among residents, small activity spaces became increasingly important and more frequently used.

Observations and recommendations from the research include

— Keep units to a size to house no more than forty-five residents, a size that operates economically and serves residents' needs in a comfortable and intimate setting.

—Arrange clusters or houses to accommodate no more than ten persons.

—Provide small-group spaces in each unit. Provide visual separation from other spaces so that residents vulnerable to distraction can be comfortable in a limited social environment.

—Create other spaces for small groups that offer distinctive attractions, such as a large window, a fireplace, or special seating. Some spaces should be less enclosed than others, offering a place from which to watch other activity.

—Provide several rooms that residents can associate with different experiences; multipurpose spaces may be confusing because residents do not know how to alter their behavior appropriately to respond to changing uses.

—Do not design space specifically for one activity; it should be able to be adapted to other uses, since it is likely that the use of rooms will change over time in response to changing resident needs or as the management style of the facility evolves.

—Select furnishings to accommodate clusters of three to eight persons. Tables that can expand or be combined are useful.

Caregiver and Family Relationships

The primary caregiver in a residential facility, a trained member of the staff, plays a very important role in the quality of a resident's life. The quality of care is, of course, a function of the philosophy and management of the facility, but it may be affected by the design of the physical environment (Lawton, 1970). Similarly, interactions between residents and their family, essentially a matter of habits of personal relations, may also be influenced by the surroundings. The environment in many care facilities presents an obstacle to attentive and effective care. Long corridors can discourage frequent contact, lack of sufficient private space for dressing or bathing can lead to conflict, inappropriate seating arrangements can make casual conversation difficult.

The environment not only can help the care staff improve their efficiency, it can also communicate a shift in philosophy of care. When the staff workplace is located within the residents' living space rather than at a station at the end of a corridor, the value of interpersonal relationships between caregivers and residents is reinforced. The caregiver's place is with the resident, rather than with the charts, records, or medications.

The design of the workplace itself is also important to the nature of the relationship between caregivers and residents. The traditional nurse's station is separated from residents by a high transaction counter and is especially uninviting for residents in wheelchairs. In a residential facility, the work space should become part of the residents' environment and should not isolate the caregiver in a space from which residents are excluded. The work space might be as simple as a desk in a corner of the residents' living room or a seat at the kitchen counter. A locked drawer can accommodate the need for keeping records both accessible and secure. Medications, supplies, and records not needed on a regular basis can be stored in a locked room elsewhere.

Care staff in a resident-oriented facility find their role challenging and the work stressful. Staff involvement with residents with dementia is far more demanding than the role of nursing assistant or attendant in a traditional nursing facility. The level of stress reported by Woodside Place staff was greater than anticipated in the planning stage and was reflected in a desire for a staff room with more amenities. The evaluation showed how important it is to provide the care staff with a relief space, where they can take a break and return refreshed to their work. A well-designed and considerately furnished space can convey to the staff an appreciation for their importance to the lives of the residents and for their professional contribution to the quality of the facility.

The quality of the physical environment of the facility communicates the respect and dignity accorded to both staff and residents. It is also an attractive feature for family members, who are an important part of residents' lives. The aesthetic quality of a facility—it's visual harmony, peaceful ambiance, and warmth and welcome—is noted and appreciated by family visitors. They also enjoy settings that enable them to participate in familiar activities with their relatives, whether that might be sitting on the porch, making coffee, or watching television. Some family members experience difficulty in parting, particularly when their leaving is highly visible to the resident, and they would use an alternative exit if it were available.

Care attendants at Woodside Place report that they experience both a high level of stress and a high level of satisfaction with their job. Their satisfaction comes from their sense of helping and caring, from their ability to communicate with residents, and from their social relationships with them. They find it particularly satisfying when residents express affection for them or when residents or family members show appreciation for their work. However, watching residents' decline or dealing with their resistance are major sources of stress. The house organization reinforces relationships between house residents and house care attendants, as intended, generally leading to positive staff-resident relationships. On the other hand, perceptions of contested or inadequate space, such as sometimes occurs in house kitchens, increases staff burden and stress. The inadequacy of the staff room contributes to these feelings.

As expected, family caregivers experience a considerable amount of stress and depression just before placing their family member in Woodside Place. However, six months later, both the perception of burden and the symptoms of depression drop slightly and remain constant for the next twelve months. Overall, family caregivers are extremely satisfied with Woodside Place (82 percent rated the experience as excellent). They are most enthusiastic about the quality of life and also express their satisfaction with the overall environment, freedom of movement for the residents, types and quality of the activity, and quality of care and extra attention given. At Woodside Place, family caregivers tend to visit more frequently than in the traditional nursing facility and are more often in the common spaces than in the bedrooms or houses. In fact, family caregivers report "walking" as the most common activity during their visits to Woodside Place and are frequently observed in the common corridor or in the yard with their relative—and sometimes with other residents as well.

The design of the facility affects the relationship of staff and families to the resident in many ways, from details of furnishings to overall spatial organization. Some of the specific pointers that emerged from research at Woodside Place are

—Integrate a staff work station into each unit as part of the residential furnishings (desk) or equipment (kitchen counter). Locate it near the main circulation path in the unit, where the residents and caregiver can enjoy casual interaction and participate in everyday activities. Provide a lockable file drawer at the work station.

—Design the work station as a social seating area, in which residents can cluster comfortably with the caregiver. A table or counter that the residents can share is desirable for common activities.

—Furnish suitable, close-at-hand, storage for supplies (laundry machines, linens, a well-equipped janitor's closet) that caregivers need on a regular basis, to minimize trips out of the unit.

—Create a separate staff room that has a comfortable yet professional ambiance. Provide a conference/lunch table, shelves and equipment for resource material, and a pleasant outdoor view. Lockers and bathroom facilities should be nearby.

—Create an esthetically pleasing environment in which a variety of homelike settings can be enjoyed by residents and family members. Provide visitors with the option of an unobtrusive way out of the facility.

Engaged Wandering

Wandering—that is, movement without apparent purpose—is a common behavior among people with Alzheimer's disease. Little is known about the physiological reasons for this behavior (Coons, 1988). Rummaging, another common behavior, involves the apparent search for personal items. It may be that these two behaviors reflect boredom or anxiety as well as loss of memory. People with dementia may simply be searching for familiar places or objects, without a specific location or item in mind. When questioned, many Alzheimer's patients may respond that they are looking for "home," although they cannot describe it. Wandering and rummaging may also result from an internal restlessness and a need for movement and exercise. In general, people in the early stages of Alzheimer's disease are more physically active and tend to be more mobile than is common in later stages.

In institutional settings, wandering is frustrating for staff because of the security issues that arise when residents are unobservable. Rummaging is viewed as an inappropriate behavior because people may enter other residents' rooms and rearrange or remove personal objects. Physical restraints, locked doors, and other features that limit movement are sometimes used to restrict residents' activities; drugs are commonly used to control such behaviors and to sedate residents. There is no question that wandering is accompanied by risks and that it may not always be viewed positively. However, the benefits of wandering—improved muscle tone, increased appetite, and enhanced social opportunities—are significant.

The environmental design implications are numerous. Since wandering and rummaging are not curable aspects of the disease, the designer should channel these behaviors into appropriate activities, which must be considered safe by the staff and satisfying to the residents. If one assumes that wandering is in part a response to a random search for the familiar, then the environment should offer orientation cues, or objects may be deemed lost. Since wandering actually provides self-managed, healthy exercise, the environment should enhance walking in both interior and exterior places. In-

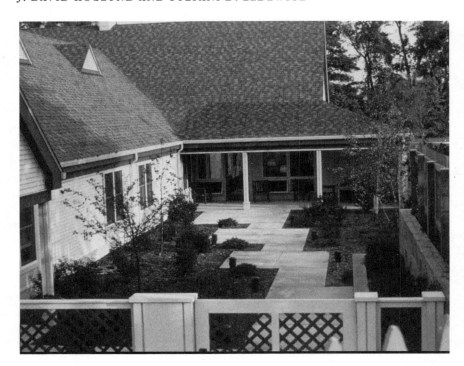

FIGURE 14.4. *Courtyard at Woodside Place* SOURCE: *Photograph by Victor Regnier*

sofar as wandering and rummaging may also be a response to boredom, the program should incorporate activities along the wandering path.

Designing the wandering path should be viewed as a major opportunity for innovation. Although some facilities strongly endorse loop walking paths to eliminate dead ends (which can lead to frustration), such paths can also lead to almost catatonic behavior or repetitive cycling, without apparent purpose. One should also not assume that wandering should be limited to corridors; creatively weaving rooms into the wandering path can facilitate orientation and provide activity spaces as destinations for socializing along the path. It is important that the path appear distinctive, with transitional changes in texture, lighting, and acoustics that may help make physical segments memorable and the actual activity of walking more enjoyable.

Wandering at Woodside Place is integrated into everyday life. The main corridor, or wandering path, is the most heavily occupied space in the building. The corridor connects and is open to major activity spaces, separated only by a low counter, columns, or a change in flooring. The areas visible from the path are the great room, the library, the country kitchen, the television room, the crafts room, the music room, the three houses, and the exterior courtyards (see figure 14.4). The corridor is used by some residents for continuous circling but is more frequently used for general circulation and socializing than for wandering. Residents, staff, and visitors often engage in social walking (walking and talking with others). The most intensively used segment of the corridor is along the front windows, where chairs lining the path are frequently occupied. Both walkers and watchers have opportunities for greeting and conversing with others as well as engaging in nearby activities. Social interaction in the corridor is the highest

Issues that should be kept in mind when designing the wandering path include the following:

— Loops of circulation should be created to provide walking circuits. Many intersecting loops are preferable to a single loop.

— Avoid dead ends, which can lead residents to a destination without an obvious choice of what to do next. Specifically, avoid locked doors at the ends of corridors.

— Remember that walking may include people who shuffle and who have gait difficulties, making them prone to falling. Minimize flooring changes, particularly from carpet to vinyl.

— Since residents can easily become disoriented, provide recognizable cues that lead them back to an area that may be more secure and familiar. Visible connection to destinations is important.

— Incorporate both interior and exterior wandering areas. Temperature, sunlight, and breezes can reinforce daily rhythms and patterns and are likely to assist in orienting people to place and time.

— Keep in mind that residents typically watch the floor as they walk and that sharp contrast in color or light value may cause them to perceive nonexistent steps or changes in depth. High-contrast spots in the flooring may appear to be items that need to be picked up. The use of a consistent material and color can keep people in a continuous path. The use of contrasting finishes can provide visual and auditory cues that residents have entered a different zone or place.

— The scale of circulation paths should be kept small and residential, but there should be room for seating, especially near intersections and entrances to houses or other rooms.

— Minimize the number of choices a resident needs to make along the way, or mark certain predetermined choices with landmarks. Also, provide a hierarchy of walking places; some may be through public areas, which offer one range of experiences; others may be through more private areas, which would be available for wandering only at certain times.

— Provide safe experiences along the wandering path so that the staff feels comfortable when residents are out of view. Consider using security systems that can monitor and control door activity, so that residents cannot go into secure yards or gardens in inappropriate weather without the staff being notified. Minimize the use of security systems as a means to limit resident access.

— Make objects that may be searched for directly visible. Use open wire baskets and similar storage systems. Provide appropriate places for rummaging, where it is not destructive to personal belongings.

Alternative Wayfinding Systems

Cognitive impairment, by its very nature, challenges the usefulness of common wayfinding, landmarks, and cueing strategies. The concept of wayfinding is based on the ability to connect objects and sensory stimulation with orientation to place (Weisman, 1987). Our firm's informal research and that completed in the Woodside Place study show little support for cognitive environmental mapping by residents. In fact, experience has taught us that some of the most subtle cues, such as color changes, are lost even on staff and families. According to Zeisel (1997), "For people with dementia the concept of 'wayfinding' needs to be thought of as 'place knowing.' People with dementia know where they are when they're there; they only know

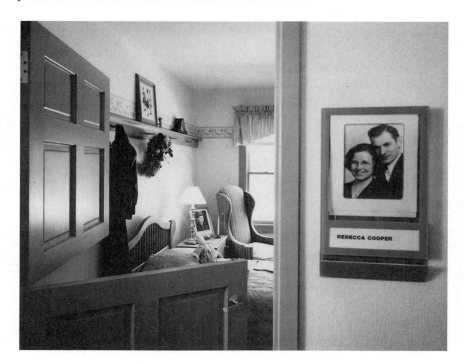

FIGURE 14.5. *Resident room from hallway at Woodside Place*
SOURCE: *Photograph by Robert Ruschak*

where they are going if they see the destination; and they realize where they were going when they arrive."

For this reason, conventional signage, color coding, and differentiation of finishes, flooring, hardware, and lighting do not provide perceptible cues for most people with dementia. A visual connection between landmarks and residences may provide clear destinations, but it may not be the destination sought. Landmarks and sight lines do, however, seem to hold the most hope for environmental wayfinding and cueing. In fact, in the Woodside Place research, the effectiveness of environmental cues was very difficult to evaluate without experimental techniques that were considered too disruptive for the study. The value of specific features, therefore, could not be ascertained, but overall wayfinding patterns were documented. Not surprisingly, residents with lower mental status were generally less spatially oriented. But at least half of Woodside Place residents were typically able to find their own bedroom, although they tended to be more successful at finding their way once they were in their house than they were at finding their house. The visibility of the house entrance (good sight lines) seemed to affect residents' wayfinding. The residents of the house that is less visible from the common spaces were more likely to be found in the wrong house.

Residents seemed to respond better to people as orienting cues than to the built environment. They often looked for their care attendants, rather than colors or objects. Personalized cues such as photographs or a stuffed toy animal were also more likely to be recognized than colors or other abstract symbols (see figure 14.5). The implications for design, while still inconclusive at this point, are challenging:

—Reinforce visual connection between the path (or hallway or corridor) and
   important destinations. Residents may not be aware what they are search-

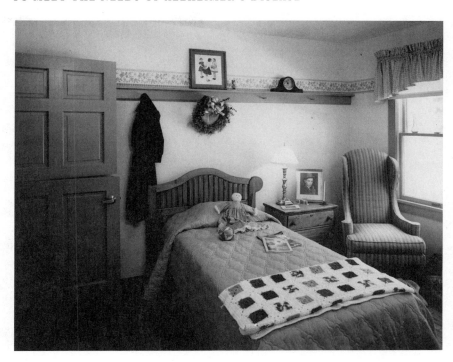

FIGURE 14.6. Resident room at Woodside Place SOURCE: Photograph by Robert Ruschak

ing for, but once they can see an activity or into a room, they may choose to join in.

— Provide flexibility so that visual connections can be controlled. Dutch doors, which can be open, closed, or half open, and interior windows that can be curtained are good examples.

— Arrange public and shared spaces as a continuous progression so that, as the resident moves through the building, there are inviting opportunities for social engagement.

— Use landmarks and objects that will attract a resident's attention.

— Create visual cueing for important activities. For instance, design bedrooms so there is clear visual connection between the bed and bathroom (specifically the toilet). Arrange this view so that bathroom activities remain private and are not obvious from other public spaces or hallways.

— Use objects that are important and memorable to each resident as a way of marking the entrance to their room. For some, it may be photographs of themselves; for others, it may be a familiar piece of clothing. Consider adding personalization opportunities (plate shelf, deep windowsill, or window seat) to the unit or house entries (see figure 14.6).

— Design room signage or memory boxes at bedroom doorways to provide personalized cues for the residents.

Independence with Security

Independence is a major design issue for facilities and services provided to the elderly. Independence is an important quality to society as a whole because it is associated with strength, self-reliance, and leadership. For the frail elderly person, the aging process leads to a gradual decrease in independence and a constant adaptation to maintain whatever qualities of independence that can be maintained. For the elderly person with Alzheimer's

245

disease, independence becomes a more elusive quality (Calkins, 1988). Physical measures to make the environment accessible only answer a small part of the issue, especially since the current Alzheimer's population is largely ambulatory and physically healthy. Offering choice is important in maintaining independence, but for those with dementia, choices must be restricted in order to limit catastrophes. Maintaining continuity of lifestyle is clearly important because it reinforces behaviors and patterns important to the individual. Also, the environment can support an individual's abilities and enhance those skills that remain. Complicated procedures, confusing directions, or too many choices can lessen a person's independence and self-esteem.

Safety in care settings always seems to become the antithesis of independence. Management and staff concerns for residents' physical well-being can limit the range of opportunities offered. It is important to create an environment that is responsive to staff concerns for safety while maintaining residents' opportunities for self-determination. Careful planning can balance independence and safety by creating a hierarchy of spaces at varying levels of risk. In spaces where staff are usually present, activities perceived to be higher risk can be incorporated, because staff can be either directly involved or discreetly observing the activity. As residents move away from the staff center, access should be limited to progressively lower risk activities.

Woodside Place was created based on the belief that the environment could have "acceptable risks" and that the environment could adapt to each resident's particular abilities. A hierarchy of surveillance was created by placing staff work stations in the houses and providing numerous views to the outdoor areas. The design does not, however, use medical model planning concepts, in which all areas can be seen by a central nurse's station and outdoor areas can only be accessed with staff accompaniment. The design affords security with flexibility by providing keyed shutoffs for major appliances, programmable door locks for exits, and secured storage and locked cabinets for harmful products. These devices allow staff to meet individual needs by adapting the environment to remove potential risks (Hall and Buckwalter, 1987).

The research results from Woodside Place are fascinating in regard to safety issues. Residents' safe use of the kitchen and kitchen appliances exceed anyone's expectations, with the most problematic episode resulting in only a melted coffeemaker. After the first year of occupancy, the courtyard gates were removed to allow residents free access to the entire secure garden. The incidence of residents falling does not exceed that of a traditional nursing home (in which reduced ambulation and restraints are more common); in fact, injuries are less severe than in nursing homes, presumably because of the use of carpet to cushion falls and residents' better muscle tone because of their activity.

In general, the research findings indicate that Woodside Place provides adequate security with a higher degree of independence than at a traditional nursing facility. Although there have been occasional technical problems with the electronic security system and several residents have tried to leave, there have been no serious injuries or safety problems. The electronic lock system, which was designed to allow for emergency exiting, was modified after the front door failed to lock; backup alarm systems were added.

Residents have access to all areas of the facility other than service and administrative spaces, an independence of movement greatly appreciated by residents' families. Some staff members are uneasy at not being able to monitor residents at all times, but they seem to have accommodated to residents' movements.

Allowing risk taking requires the participation of management, staff, and families. If quality environments are to be created for people with dementia, we need to remove unnecessary restraints and create safe conditions through unobtrusive surveillance and through features that are not visible and thus do not encourage use. Careful attention to other simple design decisions—such as good lighting, nonskid floors, carpeting, handrails, locks on drawers—contributes to a safe environment that does not diminish an individual's dignity or independence. The solutions range from planning and design to simple technology:

— Organize the building so that high-risk areas (such as kitchens and outdoor areas) are visible or accessible from areas where staff are commonly present.
— Secure only doors that lead to high-risk places, such as mechanical rooms, commercial kitchens, rooms storing cleaning chemicals, and unsecured outdoor areas. Design these doors to be unobtrusive.
— Restrict access to areas or equipment (storage, bathtubs) that may be hazardous. Provide staff-controlled power switches so that equipment is controlled without requiring rooms to be restricted. Provide keyed electric outlets for kitchen equipment.
— Provide a secure outdoor area with appropriately designed six-foot-tall fences and allow free access from the interior into the safe yard. Select garden plants to be nontoxic, with leaves that are not abrasive or sharp edged.
— Use carpet wherever possible to limit falls from slippery floors and to cushion falls when they occur.
— Provide good lighting levels. Provide night lighting at resident bathrooms
— Provide windows that open, but restrict the opening to eight inches or less.
— Provide handrails on at least one side of major inside walking paths.
— Provide locks on cabinet drawers and on doors that contain potentially harmful products, but allow access to other cabinets.

Focused and Appropriate Stimulation

A lot has been written in the mental health fields about too much or too little environmental stimulation (Lawton, 1981). In the field of designing for people with dementia, the goal is a constant and careful balance that attempts to offer interest and raise curiosity without becoming distracting or stressful. There is no easy formula for finding this balance. What one individual may find stimulating, another may find banal. Even an individual's need for stimulation varies over time.

Catastrophic reactions such as aggressive behavior or inappropriate emotional outbursts may indicate that the individual is unable to cope with environmental demands. Such behaviors may also occur when a person feels overwhelmed and confused or when a particular learned pattern has been disrupted. Overstimulation from activities, noise, and the movement of people may also cause this behavior.

247

Sundowning, a common behavior, is similar to the increased physical and vocal activity that animals, such as birds, have at dusk. Several resources discuss the increased activity level in the late afternoon among residents with Alzheimer's disease and the related agitation that comes from this behavior (Calkins, 1988). While the source of the term is unclear, writers have linked it to the historical term *sundowner*, a person who hopes to obtain food and lodging after it is too late to perform work. The specific references to Alzheimer's disease are obscure but seem—from staff reports—to be connected with increased restlessness at the end of the day. Since there appear to be no documented studies of this phenomenon, one explanation offered is that sundowning occurs at a time when people in their past have traditionally left one place (work or school) to head for home. A second possibility is that in many institutions, staff shift changes near the end of the afternoon may cause people to become agitated as the familiar face prepares to leave and is replaced by a new, unfamiliar, and therefore frightening face. Some restlessness may be attributed to an innate internal rhythm that searches for a change of setting or to a basic physiological response to the onset of evening and the end of daylight. Sundowning behavior is uncharacteristic at Woodside Place, although other facilities report disruptive behavior attributed to sundowning.

Creating a balance between too much and too little sensory stimulation is always challenging. An environment that is soothing, calm, and not agitating to all of the residents may also be institutional, stark, and lacking in clarity. The place may feel cold, with nondescript rooms. One must also remember that declining sensory information, a result of the normal aging process, may also mute subtleties in the environment; slight changes in color may not be discernible to the aging eye. It may prove more advantageous to offer the same information passively through the channels of different senses (redundant cueing) rather than aggressively through one sense. This approach may prove successful in view of the inevitable variation in the cognitive abilities of the residents. Color coding, for instance, is too complex for most residents to understand, but when accompanied by images as well (such as blue stars or red sailboats) it may make the information more salient. However, most environmental cueing is too subtle for most people with dementia; there appears to be little connection between an image (such as a blue star) and its meaning (my room).

The research did not attempt to quantify the level of environmental stimulation, but the facility is generally described as "quiet" or "calm" by visitors. Activity and noise level varies from room to room; the most active spaces are house entries and kitchens and the great room when group activities are taking place; the quiet spaces are the bedroom wings and the little-used music and oasis rooms. Noises commonly heard in long-term care facilities are absent: there is no electronic paging system, and carpeting muffles the movement of people and carts. The most significant sources of noise and distractions are the television sets in house living rooms and the TV room; the sets are often left on for long periods, including mealtimes and times when no one is in the room. However, the TVs are not associated with any specific behavior disturbances.

One indication of little environmental stress at Woodside Place is that residents commonly choose to be in the more stimulating spaces, such as the main circulation path, where people tend to gather in groups or move about and converse with a variety of people. Many residents participate by watching others. The only places where disturbances are noted on a recurrent basis are at doorways, particularly at the front door and the entrance to one of the houses. The front door has become more of a gathering place for residents than was intended. Being able to watch people coming and going seems to attract residents; others seem to enjoy visiting the administrative offices adjacent to the entrance. Occasionally, a resident attempting to open a door that is either locked or difficult to open stands at the door rattling the hardware until someone either opens the door or interests the resident in a different activity.

The design implications are numerous, ranging from the size and locations of rooms to the color of the walls, the lighting sources, and the print on the wallpaper. The following points are offered as a range of design issues to address when confronting the issue of stimulation:

— Provide rooms that comfortably accommodate small groups of six to eight people. Such rooms allow the staff to plan activities that can be shared by small groups without creating overstimulation from interactions among the residents of the group.
— Provide rooms with auditory privacy so that noise from one activity is not distracting to participants in another. Use carpet where possible, because it reduces unwanted noise and reverberation and eliminates glare from floor surfaces.
— Be aware of the confusion that can occur for residents who use rooms for a variety of activities. A resident who knows a particular room to be a dining room with certain expected behaviors and patterns (such as quiet) may find it difficult to understand that it is now acceptable to perform activities such as exercise and dancing.
— Provide a staff exit/entrance away from the public front door so that their leaving, which may cause feelings of despair and abandonment, is not readily apparent to the residents. Channel late-afternoon activities into dinner preparation, freshening up, or other appropriate late-day events. Orient some rooms to the west to gain from sunsets. (Rooms that face east may also gain from their sunrise orientation.) Provide TV rooms for watching the news and kitchens for preparing dinner.
— Provide views to the outside from all places so that residents can experience the changing rhythm of the day.
— Consider the front entrance an important place of arrival for families who may visit after work but a different place for residents, who should be prevented from observing people approaching the entrance. Screen the front entrance from residents' view by providing a vestibule or lobby between the front entrance and the residential entry door. This will allow deliveries, visitors, and others to come and go without having to enter the resident's domain.

Residential Qualities

While there is almost universal support today for a residential environment for people with Alzheimer's disease, there is very little agreement as to what residential environment means (Cohen and Weisman, 1991). Rural, subur-

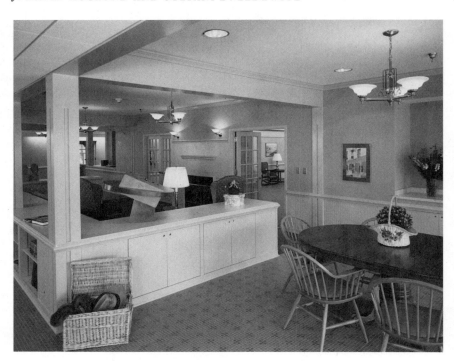

FIGURE 14.7. *Fireplace room at Woodside Place* SOURCE: *Photograph by Robert Ruschak*

ban, and urban locations all affect the way we perceive "residential," and many dementia facilities are much larger than a single-family home. Including "homelike" qualities in the design of the building touches on many issues, ranging from overall size and appearance to use of interior and exterior materials to the purpose, scale, and detailing of rooms. Lighting, finishes, and furniture are also key to evoking residential imagery (see figure 14.7).

Providing supportive care settings with a residential appearance has gained significant support. The size and physical arrangement of the facility has a lot to do with whether it is perceived as an institution. The design—that is, the finishes, furniture, windows, exterior materials—conveys a great deal about the character of the facility. A noninstitutional image can convey a pleasant experience to family and visitors, encouraging more involvement between families and residents. A domestic quality can also be conveyed by the organization of staff and management. Environments that appear overly structured, with nurse's stations, staff in nursing uniforms, and numerous charts and carts, reinforce institutional patterns of compliance and uniformity.

The domestic qualities of the environment are particularly important for people with dementia. Cognitive losses obscure orientation to time and place. A residential environment does not replicate an individual's home but rather maintains connections to that which is familiar and comfortable. Kitchens with residential appliances will probably seem familiar, whether or not the room is like the one residents are used to. Floor and wall finishes should replicate those commonly used in homes even while incorporating technological improvements in materials (moisture-resistant fabrics, solution-dyed carpets, and vinylized wall coverings).

250

The exterior image is equally important in establishing a familiar, noninstitutional appearance. The repetitive, almost monolithic character of many care settings separates them from the community. It is important to focus on those elements that most convey residential images, consistent with the size of the facility. Smaller facilities may use such single-family home imagery as pitched roofs, horizontal siding (or stucco or brick), and small-scale windows and doors. Conceptualizing the facility as a house, a country inn, or a hotel can be helpful in establishing the appropriate imagery.

The research shows that visitors and staff perceive Woodside Place as residential, but that term is used broadly and includes references to a "large house," a "country house," a "country inn," and a "hotel." Family caregivers rate it at 4.8 points of a possible 5.0 in response to the question, How residential does Woodside Place seem to you? They note that the facility has a pleasant, cheerful atmosphere, a decor that is pleasant and homey, with good places to talk with their family members and with others. Residents' rooms are considered especially successful, and the house kitchens and fireplace seating area are also well liked. Spaces in the house are used for such typically residential activities as eating, preparing food, sitting on the porch, watching television, and housekeeping.

In terms of the psychological dimension of home, residential quality is a function of privacy and autonomy. (Privacy is discussed in a previous section.) Residents demonstrate autonomy by making their own "home improvements." The best example is moving chairs to create a front porch effect along the front windows and outside the craft room. Residents express a sense of belonging and ownership in relation to Woodside Place, but they do not refer to the facility as home. They speak of going home *from* there. House kitchens and the gatherings that take place there haved a very homelike feeling (see figure 14.8). The environment is especially well suited to a lifestyle based on the traditional homemaking role that women in our society have occupied. Most of the residents of Woodside Place occupied this role during their lives and seem to find the environment comfortable and familiar.

A residential environment requires careful attention to the overall design and detailing:

— Subdivide the building volume into smaller elements so that the exterior does not appear monolithic or institutional.
— Organize spaces like other residential prototypes such as houses, inns, hotels (i.e., typically, when you enter, you do not walk past bedrooms to get to the living room).
— Conceptualize rooms and spaces as they are in a house. Living rooms (not dayrooms), bedrooms (not private or semiprivate rooms), family rooms or dens (not lounges), and bathrooms (not toilets) all add to the ambiance.
— Avoid hard finishes, which are typically found only in institutional settings: vinyl tile, ceramic tile, sheet vinyl, plastic laminate, stainless steel, metal doors. If these materials are used, use them in limited quantities in appropriate locations: sheet vinyl in kitchens, plastic laminate countertops in kitchens.
— Locate spaces carefully so that the necessary operational equipment— carts, fire alarm panels, nurse call stations—is hidden from view.

251

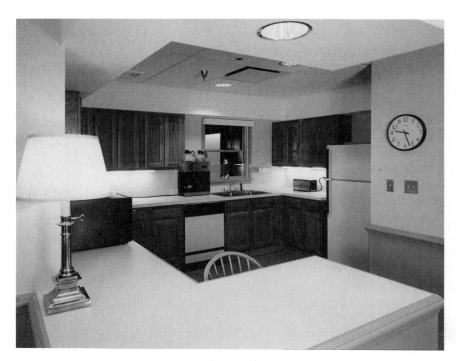

FIGURE 14.8. *Staff work space in house kitchen at Woodside Place*
SOURCE: *Photograph by Robert Ruschak*

—Select furniture that is familiar and comfortable. Careful selection and placement of furniture can permit more use of nonmedical, designed furniture. Some specially designed geriatric furniture, while meeting hygienic and physical comfort requirements, are ugly. Fortunately, there are better choices. Check furniture for stability (especially tables and chairs) when used for support of resident movement.

—Treat surfaces the way they would be in a home setting. For example, windows typically have fabric curtains or valances to soften their appearance.

—Use light sources that are residential; 2-foot × 4-foot fluorescent lights are not residential in appearance and are not good sources of lighting because of their glare. If fluorescent lighting is used for energy efficiency, incorporate it into discreet lighting sources, like coves or concealed uplights. The new full-spectrum fluorescent lamps can be used in most sconces, downlights, and pendant ceiling fixtures.

Learning from Woodside Place

The research, both formal and informal, shows that issues such as staffing levels and staff work spaces, visibility of the front entrance, and use of tub and showers proved more challenging than envisioned. While the building met with enthusiastic response from operators, staff, and families, the experience at Woodside Place clearly teaches a number of important lessons about what not to do. Perkins Eastman Architects has developed a number of innovative environments for people with Alzheimer's disease since Woodside Place opened. Experience at Copper Ridge, in Sykesville, Maryland (completed in June 1994) and Asbury Place in Mt. Lebanon, Pennsylvania (completed in July 1997) highlight planning and design issues that were resolved in ways different from Woodside Place and that incorporate lessons learned from the Woodside Place experience.

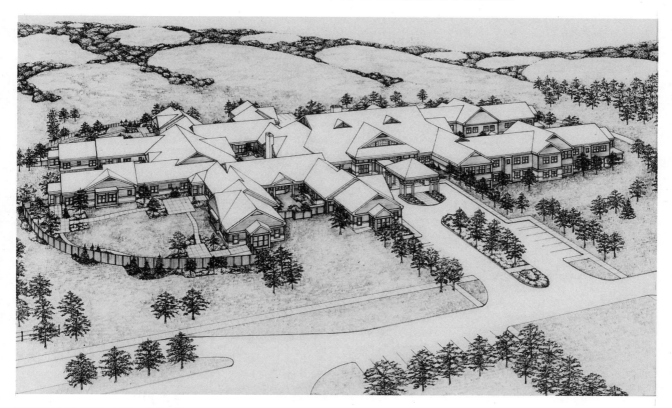

FIGURE 14.9. *Copper Ridge, Sykesville, Maryland*

Copper Ridge

Copper Ridge is a continuum-of-care setting for people with Alzheimer's disease (see chapter 9). It offers adult day care, sixty assisted-living units (like Woodside Place), and sixty-six nursing care beds (see figure 14.9). Developed by Episcopal Health Ministries to the Aging, the project was meant to provide a noninstitutional alternative to the traditional nursing home while offering a range of support services broader than that offered by Woodside Place. The assisted-living unit was conceptualized as three houses, each with two wings of ten rooms, for a total of sixty rooms, surrounding a courtyard and shared public spaces (see figure 14.10).

Asbury Place

Asbury Place was developed by United Methodist Services to the Aging as a further refinement of the Woodside Place concept (see figure 14.11). The advisory team consisted of the Woodside administrator and members of the Woodside Place research team and the Woodside chief executive officer, whose father had been a resident of Woodside Place. Asbury Place, which contains forty rooms, combines concepts from both Woodside Place and Copper Ridge. Opened in the summer of 1997, Asbury Place offers a unique opportunity for follow-up research to inform both the design process and to measure outcomes from design changes incorporated after Woodside Place.

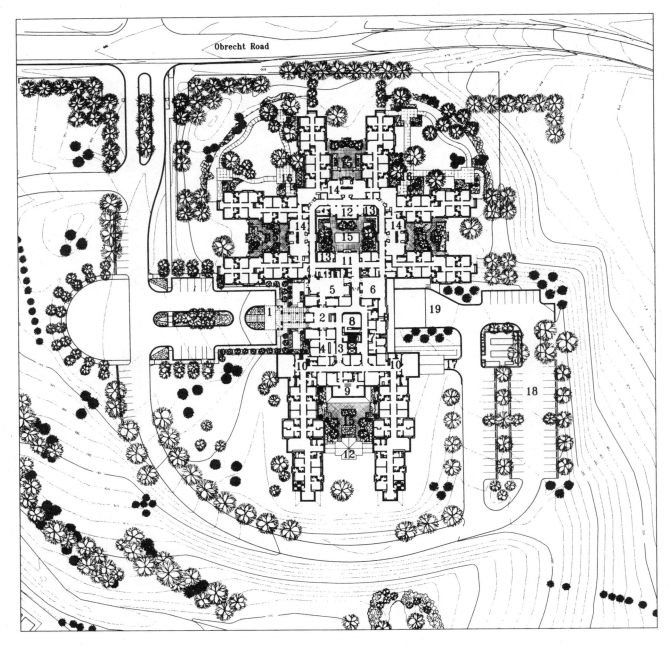

FIGURE 14.10. *Main level site plan at Copper Ridge*

Legend

1. Entrance Drop-Off
2. Entrance Lobby / Reception
3. Elevator
4. Administration
5. Adult Day Care
6. Multi-Purpose Room
7. Medical / Dental Suite
8. Coffee & Gift Shop
9. Occupational & Physical Therapy
10. Comprehensive Care Resident Wings

11. Living Room
12. Garden Room
13. Activity Room
14. Domiciliary Care Resident Houses
15. Secure Courtyards
16. Secure Wandering Garden
17. Health Care Pick-Up
18. Staff Parking
19. Service Area

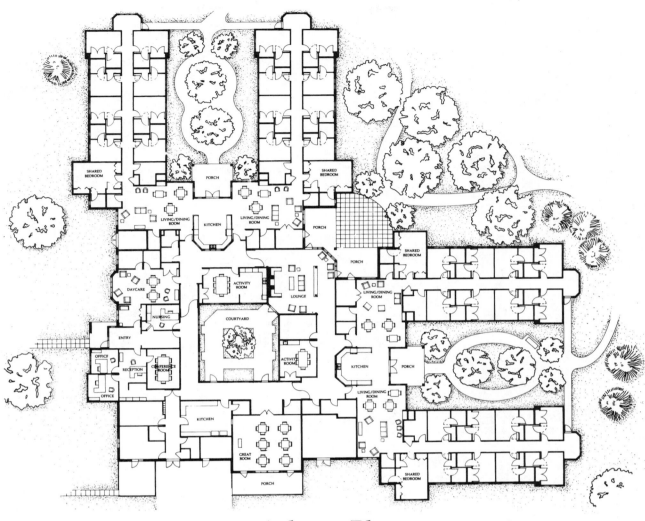

Asbury Place

FIGURE 14.11. *Floor plan at Asbury Place, Mount Lebanon, Pennsylvania*

Interpretive Findings

The Woodside Place research and other informal observations yield a vast amount of design information, ranging from overall organizational issues to detailed findings specific to Woodside Place. The information falls into three broad headings: size and spatial organization, staff work space, and product use. All of these reinforce the importance of the nine design issues and their interdependence.

Size and Spatial Organization

Woodside Place, as a thirty-six-bed facility, is sized to meet a range of resident needs yet remain intimate and friendly. The research shows a significant formation of community and friendships at Woodside Place. Copper Ridge, with sixty residents, tests the outer boundaries of size and, in fact, is exploring ways to create two separate environments (for forty and twenty

255

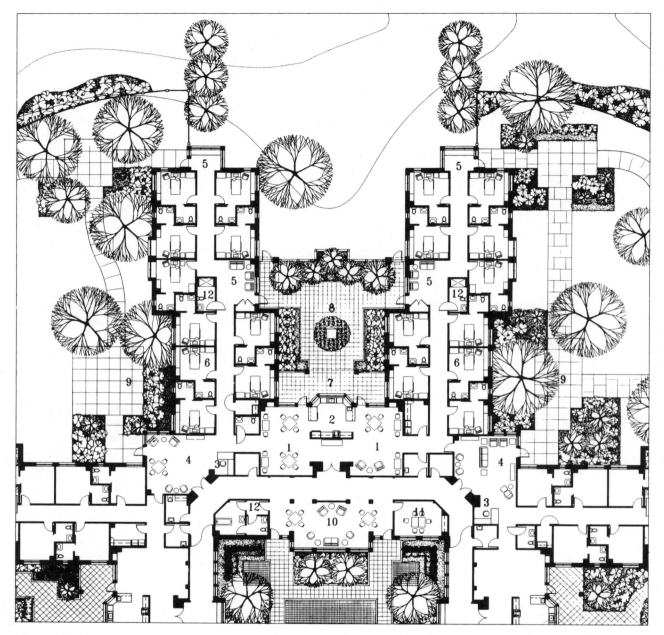

FIGURE 14.12. *Detail plan of assisted-living unit at Copper Ridge*

Legend

1. Dining Room
2. ADL Kitchen
3. Nurse Alcove
4. Den
5. Sitting Area
6. Private Resident Room
7. Porch
8. Secure Courtyard
9. Secure Wandering Garden
10. Garden Room
11. Activity Room
12. Tub & Shower Room

residents) in its assisted-living unit (see figure 14.12). The houses of twelve residents at Woodside Place have proven manageable for staffing, but they are not as desirable as houses with eight to ten residents. The research also shows that Woodside staff have extremely high job satisfaction because of their ability to bond with a small group of residents, yet they have very high job stress levels because they sometimes feel alone and unsupported in the house where they work. Refinement of the Woodside Place model at Copper Ridge and Asbury Place uses two wings of ten residents, joined to form a "house" of twenty residents, allowing staff to share responsibilities between wings.

The concept of organizing the building as houses (or wings), with a common activity area, is supported by the research in the way it reinforces public and private zones and allows residents to choose to participate or to withdraw from the community aspects of group living (Silverman et al., 1996). Refinements in Copper Ridge and Woodside Place focus primarily on rethinking activity spaces and where they are located. The great room at Woodside Place is strategically central to the facility and is incorporated as a part of the wandering path. Recommendations from research and staff are to retain its purpose but to enclose it for more focused and private activity. Music has become a key large-group activity in the great room, and the music room was converted to other purposes. The TV/entertainment room no longer serves this function, because all of the house living rooms now share TVs; the room has been reconceptualized as a den for small group and private family activities. Traditional arts and craft activities are becoming more integrated into household activities at the kitchen table; however, providing a central location for more involved projects still seems warranted. The country kitchen of Woodside Place is replaced in the later projects by an activity room that families can use for private meals and parties (see figure 14.13). The involvement of residents in meals and cooking has been moved to the house kitchens, where it normally belongs. Providing natural light and exterior views to the outside from these activity rooms has proven to be extremely important. The research did not confirm the hypothesis that views would lead to higher levels of agitation and reduced focus; in fact, the opposite is true (Silverman et al., 1996).

Secure outdoor space is the highest rated feature at Woodside Place, although the need to provide secure courtyards separate from the larger garden was, in the end, not required. Copper Ridge was designed before this finding came to light, and its courtyards were not connected to the wandering gardens. Based on observations at Copper Ridge, we believe that not linking all of the outdoor spaces is a significant missed opportunity. Apparently, the experience of the wanderers is oversimplified by a simple loop design with only one entrance or exit to each of the courtyards. Some of behavioral patterns at Woodside Place are missing at Copper Ridge, which may stem from reducing the use of outdoor space.

The design of residents' rooms at Copper Ridge was refined to introduce residential amenities, such as wainscot and built-in window seats (see figure 14.14). The window seat uses minimum floor area and adds seating for visitors, storage, and a homelike feature to the rooms. Lighting and furniture were selected to meet the functional criteria and contribute to the residential ambience.

Staff Work Space

Interaction between residents and staff exceed most of the expectations set during the design process. The concept of clustering the residents with staff (as in the house) provides a base of security and familiarity for residents. For staff, it provides the opportunity for more personal relationships with residents and an increased sense of responsibility for their well-being. While the research supports the basic concept of having staff space in house kitchens, we now know that the kitchen must be larger, with areas set aside for staff that are not seen as meal preparation areas by residents. At Asbury

257

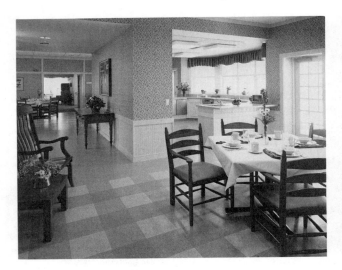

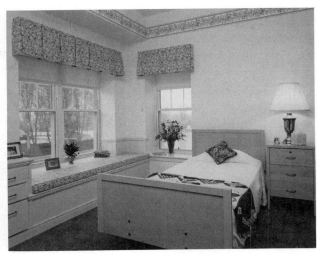

FIGURE 14.13. *Activity room at Copper Ridge* SOURCE: *Photograph by Curtis Martin*

FIGURE 14.14. *Resident room at Copper Ridge* SOURCE: *Photograph by Curtis Martin*

Place we not only increased the size of the kitchen but also provided space for a table that can be used for informal coffees or laundry folding without impacting the staff work area.

Woodside Place explored a number of ways to help people with orientation, ranging from landmarks to sensory cues (fabrics, floor coverings, etc.). The most significant wayfinding device at Woodside Place was discovered to be staff themselves. At Asbury Place the kitchens are visually connected to the common areas through bay windows for the staff person working in the house. The hope is that the visual connection between residents and staff will assist with orientation and that the possibility for unobtrusive surveillance will help staff feel more secure in their responsibilities for residents' safety.

Woodside Place was planned with open work stations for staff and private, enclosed workrooms and conference spaces. The staff workroom, located in the center of the common area, never worked as a place for staff retreat: attendants felt they needed to leave the room for breaks, since the room did not fulfill this requirement. Copper Ridge and Asbury Place both provide staff lounge spaces outside of the active resident areas of the building. In the case of Asbury Place, an outdoor smoking porch and space, totally free of the facility, is provided.

The overall quality and quantity of resident to staff interaction can be significantly enhanced by allowing for unstructured activities in which staff lead "normal" activities within the houses. For some residents, leaving their own houses can be anxiety provoking, so their activities need to grow out of the natural day's rhythm: coffee at the kitchen table, setting up for dinner, doing laundry. Structured activity programming can provide a framework for the day, but allowing time for direct care staff to initiate informal activities and respond to initiatives of residents enhances the interaction. The Woodside Place research strongly supports a more integrated activities program and recommends an environment that could adapt to music, crafts, and exercise outside of rooms purposefully set aside for them (Silverman et al., 1996). At Asbury Place, each kitchen contains a large table for informal activities. At Copper Ridge, dens are provided between houses to provide space for unstructured events.

Product Use

Woodside Place has been in operation for more than five years, yielding a number of insights into the use of products and their location within the facility. Products like the wood-grain sheet-vinyl floor, the plate shelf in resident rooms, and the open basket storage systems in the closets have proved successful applications and have been replicated in other facilities. The Dutch doors at resident rooms, photographic display boards, and contrasting toilet seats (black seat on white toilet) have been replicated based on anecdotal support by staff and families rather than direct research results. Other items such as showers, therapeutic bathers, and toilet fixture locations have been totally rethought in later facilities.

The biggest area of redesign is in the bathing and bathrooms. Copper Ridge and Asbury Place use the same approach as Woodside Place in providing a private bathroom (without a bathing fixture) for each resident room. The research indicates that this is the minimum requirement and that, perhaps, showers should be included with the rooms to meet the wide variation of resident needs. If a shared bathing room is provided, it should be located close to the center of the house (as at Copper Ridge and Asbury Place) rather than at the end of the house (as at Woodside Place). If baths are closer to the center of the house, staff can more closely monitor their use and obtain assistance from other staff if needed. The research also recommends that showers have no perceptible lip, or edge, and that conventional residential bathtubs be provided for use by some residents. Locating bathtub facilities within the privacy of the house encourages use and eliminates the conflict over bathing in an area of the building that may be perceived as public. The therapeutic bather at Woodside Place was significantly underused, partially because of its location but primarily because of its appearance. The dilemma is how to provide bathing options for people when a conventional bathtub is not accessible or convenient. Some tubs look less frightening than others and can provide the option for three-sided access. Manufacturers have been working to resolve a range of design and technical issues.

Communication systems raise a number of issues as well. Clearly, traditional nurse call systems do not serve this population well and are not warranted (Silverman et al., 1996). Communication systems, however, are useful for staff to reach each other and can be simply accommodated through traditional house phone systems with local paging options or more sophisticated pocket pager/beeper systems and cellular phones. Security systems (and there are numerous ones) that notify staff when someone has left a specific area can be useful, but the first line of security should be an appropriately planned environment. Woodside Place, Copper Ridge, and Asbury Place share the same concept that unlocked exits should lead to other safe, secure areas (whether inside or outside). Minimizing the number of doors that need to be locked and alarmed is important, and locating them inconspicuously is paramount. Unfortunately, the front door to Woodside Place is visible from the inside, and arriving visitors attract significant attention. By locating the entrance so that visitors can enter (such as at Asbury Place) and visit the administration area before entering residents' domain is important. Screening the view and pulling activity generators away from major entrances simplify security systems.

The Future

It is impossible to relay all of the discovered issues and observations learned from Woodside Place. Copper Ridge and Asbury Place benefit from the experience of the Woodside research, and the next generation of facilities will learn from them. Structured research and informal observations are an important part of informing the design process, so that the next group of residents are better served by what we have learned.

The design of special care settings and programs for people with Alzheimer's disease is a very young industry. The first group of national models—Corrine Dolan, Gardiner Maine, and Woodside Place—have been open only a few years. New programs and buildings are opening with regularity, some building on these first national models, others exploring new issues and approaches. It is important that new facilities have postoccupancy evaluations so that new concepts and ideas that work can be shared. It is rare to have an extensive research study such as was conducted at Woodside Place, but even informal observations are helpful in improving the design process.

If we want our assisted-living residences to be "a good house" for people with dementia, then we must use the environment as a prosthetic device to support people and their quality of life. We can never really know how people with cognitive impairments view their world. The hope is that, at some level, they feel reassured, comfortable, unthreatened, and interested. If housing supports the intangible rhythms of people's lives, then special settings for people with dementia should be a stage for their hopes, their dreams, and their realities.

We end this chapter with a look at a Woodside Place resident, Pauline (Silverman et al., 1996):

> While . . . "travels" around Woodside Place occupy a good portion of Pauline's days, she also likes to talk about other trips she has taken in her life and those she hopes to take in the future. While . . . Pauline has lived in a number of different places and also liked to travel, it is difficult to tell how many of the trips she recounts are "memories" and how many are "dreams." In fact, Pauline includes Woodside Place as part of her travels. She does not consider herself to be living there, but rather talks about it as a place she visits for varying lengths of time. Sometimes she seems quite content and interested in her visit; at other times she is quite frustrated by the length of her stay and indicates that she is anxious to get home: "I've been here long enough!" At all times, like an experienced traveler, Pauline wears or carries her all-weather coat and has her purse stuffed full of items she might "need later," including extra food saved from the previous meal. In a way, Woodside Place has become another stop on her frequent travels.

References

Calkins, M. 1988. *Design for Dementia: Planning Environments for the Elderly and Confused.* Owings Mills, Md.: National Health Publishing.

Cohen, U., and G. Weisman. 1991. *Holding on to Home: Designing Environment for People with Dementia.* Baltimore: Johns Hopkins University Press.

Cohen, U., G. Weisman, V. Steiner, K. Ray, J. Rand, and R. Toyne. 1988. *Environments for People with Dementia: Case Studies.* Washington, D.C.: Health Facilities Research Program, AIA/ACSA Council on Architectural Research.

Coons, D. 1988. Wandering. *American Journal of Alzheimer's Care and Related Disorders and Research* 3:31–36.

Hall, G., and K. Buckwalter. 1987. Progressively lowered stress thresholds: A conceptual model for care of adults with Alzheimer's disease. *Archives of Psychiatric Nursing* 1:399–406.

Lawton, M. 1970. Ecology and aging. In L. Pastalan and D. Carson, eds., *Spatial Behavioral of Older People.* Ann Arbor, Mich.: Institute of Gerontology, University of Michigan.

———. 1981. Sensory deprivation and the effect of the environment on management of the patient with senile dementia. In N. Miller and G. Cohen, eds., *Clinical Aspects of Alzheimer's Disease and Senile Dementia.* New York: Raven.

———. 1987. Environmental approaches to research and treatment of Alzheimer's disease. In E. Light and B. Liebowitz, eds., *Alzheimer's Disease, Treatment, and Family Stress: Directions for Research.* Washington, D.C.: National Institute of Mental Health.

Silverman, M., E. Ricci, J. Saxton, S. Ledewitz, C. McAllister, and C. Keane. 1996. *Woodside Place: The First Three Years of a Residential Alzheimer's Facility.* 2 vols. Oakmont, Pa.: Presbyterian SeniorCare.

Weisman, G. 1987. Improving way-finding and architectural legibility in housing for the elderly. In V. Regnier and J. Pynoos, eds., *Housing for the Elderly: Design Directives and Policy Consideraction.* New York: Raven.

Zeisel, J. 1997. Presentation at the Sixth National Alzheimer's Disease Education Conference, Chicago.

DANIEL J. CINELLI

CHAPTER 15

Place Makes a Difference
A Case Study in Assisted Living

Most well elderly persons in this country have housing options suited to their individual needs. Home health care, senior centers, and programs such as Meals on Wheels, older adult day care, or intergenerational day care enable elderly persons to continue to stay at home. However, when the time comes for them to move out of single-family residences into what we define as the typical and logical setting, the decision becomes difficult—for two reasons. First, because the population is delaying this step, the generation that is now stepping over the threshold is more frail and acutely needy than ever before. Second, the choice traditionally has been limited to an apartmentlike setting with remote community services or an institutionally rooted skilled care or long-term care setting.

New housing options are being developed in response to the changing needs of the elder care consumer. This chapter describes the process of designing an assisted-living addition for Heritage Village, an existing intermediate and sheltered (personal) care community in northeastern Illinois.

The History of Heritage Village

Originally named Heritage House, Heritage Village once was the only retirement home of its kind in Kankakee County. Founded in 1970, this private-pay retirement home catered to the financially successful elderly residents of the area. The facility, with an excellent reputation, ran at full occupancy for many years without any marketing effort. As the elderly population grew more frail, the retirement home added a licensed health center. And as the community continued to age in place, Heritage Village found it necessary to convert into a licensed, sheltered (personal) care facility. Until the late 1980s, Heritage Village had little competition and was unaware of the many changes occurring in the senior living marketplace throughout this country and abroad.

Kankakee County, located about fifty-four miles south of Chicago, is a community in transition. The business and industrial base still includes agriculture, with a revived industrial and manufacturing presence. The Kankakee County population, now approximately 133,000, includes a growing number of senior citizens. Estimates show that by the year 2000, the population aged 65–74 will increase by 8,500–9,000, while the 75–84-year-old group will increase by approximately 5,500–6,000 residents.

With new housing options being planned and built in the Kankakee region, Heritage Village decided it was time to reevaluate their position. Early in the spring of 1992, the administrator called OWP&P Architects to submit a proposal for performing a long-overdue update of a campus master plan. When the architects toured the property, it became apparent that the board of trustees and some department heads still viewed Heritage Village as an independent-living facility with supportive care. The trustees felt that the wealthy farmer whose bequest established Heritage House intended it to be a retirement community, and that was what they had. All they had added was an "infirmary-type health center."

The architects, however, thought that the home had become industry blind and that it was truly a long-term care facility, with some 1960s residential undertones. The trustees were initially taken aback by these comments. However, after they learned what other facilities had to offer in the range of housing and service options, delivered in a wide variety of cost and image models, they realized that their facility was on the acute-care end of the spectrum. Therefore, they directed their consultants to plan a campus that would slide their facility back along the continuum to a more residential model.

The first suggestion was to develop single-family, single-story, attached townhouses targeted to a younger population than the current facility allowed. It soon became apparent that the trustees faced a bigger problem than redefining their facility's niche in the continuum. They held a wide array of preconceived ideas for the future, ranging from trailer-sized homes to 3,000-square-foot villas. Clearly, since the trustees had no unified vision, this ambiguity would project itself onto the facility as well as potential residents. Before going any further, the sponsors had to develop a vision of what Heritage Village was and what it should become.

Developing the Strategic Vision Statement

The development of a strategic vision is the essential first step in an effective strategic planning process. A well-developed vision statement represents consensus among the board of trustees, management, and key staff members and provides the framework for future activities. The board of trustees of Heritage Village knew it needed to upgrade its current facility and expand its services. Before initiating feasibility work and facility development, the trustees committed themselves to a process that would inform them about the local market and major industry trends, challenge historical assumptions, and consider the new programming and positioning of Heritage Village.

In addition to visiting leading elder care organizations, the trustees held a series of five meetings to develop the strategic vision statement. At the first meeting, an outside consultant presented an overview of industry trends. At the second and third meetings, the trustees were asked to respond to questions based upon the consultant's knowledge of the marketplace and its review of Heritage Village. The discussions addressed eight key issues:

1. The organization's basic purpose and objectives
2. Its possible responses to major market conditions
3. Its target markets
4. Its current and future programming and services
5. Its required organizational structure
6. Its basic values and desired image
7. Its desired future market position
8. Its understanding of the required resource commitment

Additional meetings were held with staff, residents, residents' children, social service agencies, health care affiliates, and potential residents. These meetings helped to gain concurrence by questioning and refining the mission.

At the fourth and fifth meetings, the trustees reviewed the findings of the vision survey, leading them to conclude that there was a strong need to re-define existing programming, to create new functions, to upgrade current facilities, and to determine the market demand for new and expanded services in the continuum. They also agreed that it was important to create a unique, well-defined housing niche, to maximize the independence of existing and future residents, and to enhance marketing and public relations efforts.

The approved Heritage Village strategic vision statement provided the direction for all programming, facility renovation, and future development: "It is envisioned that the organization will serve the changing needs of an elderly population in a unique and upscale environment. This is to be realized in the development of facilities and programming for the well-functioning independent older adult. This refinement and expansion of services is to be done concurrently in the development of appropriate facilities and programming to meet the needs of the current client population requiring more assisted or supportive care."

The trustees also asked the consultants to design and carry out a study to determine the market demand and qualifying characteristics of a potential assisted-living facility and to measure, secondarily, the potential for independent-living apartments (congregate), single-family attached duplexes, and a dedicated Alzheimer's/dementia unit. The fieldwork was not intended to provide a full market, program, and economic feasibility assessment but to offer a reasonable assessment of the value of these programs and to identify space and campus land use for future development.

For purposes of this study, assisted living was considered a housing option that serves as a bridge between independent living and traditional nursing homes. The initial step in the research methodology was to develop the general characteristics of the program and the following definition of assisted living, which was used in surveys of potential applicants:

> Assisted living serves a less independent population in which the individual is more frail and needs some form of daily living assistance (i.e., bathing, dressing, cooking). Each activity that requires assistance in daily living is often referred to as an ADL. Assisted-living units are normally efficiency apartments with a mini-kitchen. Rental payment includes all meals, 24-hour personal care assistance, and weekly maid service. Facilities often provide appropriate social activities, programming, and transportation. Residents in assisted-living units include those who take their own medication. Units can rent from $1,200 to $1,800 per month.

Using this definition, the consultants studied market demand based upon age-specific (75+), geographical-specific, income-qualifying, and need-specific (assistance with two or more ADLs) criteria. Other tasks included evaluating current and planned providers of assisted living, both direct and indirect; holding qualifying meetings with Heritage Village administrative and clinical staff; and holding focus group meetings with volunteers at Heritage Village, two groups of age-qualifying community members, representatives of elder care organizations, and potential referral sources. The outcome of the survey indicated that there were two assisted-living facilities (totaling sixty-eight units) in the market area, one sponsored by a local hospital with a strong market reputation. Therefore, the potential market area was defined as the entire Kankakee County. Using various population-based methodologies, market demand was estimated to vary from zero to forty-six units (low to high, with conditional assumptions). Heritage Village decided to serve existing residents in the new assisted-living facility and to position a potential assisted-living project as a middle-income arrangement with corresponding design and programming.

Based upon market research results and further discussions, the trustees decided to move forward with the assisted-living project. This decision was dependent upon a commitment to reposition the entire Heritage Village program by modernizing and upgrading current facilities. A group-living model, such as a cluster of single-family, attached, four-to-five-bedroom units, or various sized studios and one-bedroom suites, also would be investigated. The consultant's report recommended starting with a small assisted-living project (ten to thirty units) designed with midrange price points. Heritage Village wanted a unique physical environment to distinguish it from the competition, the newest of which was a hotel-like product with sixty identical small studio apartments and one common dining and living zone. The trustees and the new administrator, who had joined the team while the study was under way, wanted their residents to have more options. They asked the consultants to find innovative ways to reference the homes from which the residents came.

Before the consultant and the owner developed the specific assisted-living concept, the trustees directed the team to create a master plan for Heritage Village to address the needs of the most acute component of the resident continuum by creating a new wing of high-skilled care and completely renovating the midlevel skilled (sheltered) care wings. These areas needed revised and new programs and the infrastructure and space for them to succeed.

The team segmented the continuum into shareable and nonshared support programs. Each of the three programs—assisted-living, high-skilled, and midlevel skilled care—needed separate areas for dining (specialized meals), bathing, nursing, medication, and housekeeping. However, it also was possible to create or restructure some shareable spaces to allow all levels of the continuum to commingle. These shared spaces were referred to as "neutral space turf," wherein any of the residents, as well as outside members of the community, could share in some of the nonskilled care services. The goal was to ensure a seamless transition at all levels of care. These neutral spaces also played an integral role in the specific design concept for the assisted-living addition.

Lifestyle Options: Choice Making, Community, and Privacy

Family members living in single-family housing traditionally enjoy a number of options, which Chermayeff and Alexander (1965) discuss in terms of community versus privacy. The ability to make a distinction among private, semiprivate, semicommunal, and communal spaces is the core of successful personal and family relationships. Why should we lose this ability to choose when we become frail and elderly?

Typically, one of the differences between a congregate facility and skilled care is that, in the former, the resident can choose from among studio, one-bedroom, and two-bedroom units, whereas in skilled care the only choices are the bed by the window or the bed next to the bathroom.

In congregate living, residents can rise from their beds at their leisure, have breakfast in their own units, get ready for the day, then go to the store, the community's town center, or their neighbor's apartment. In contrast, at many skilled care facilities in the United States, residents are awakened between 5:00 and 6:30 in the morning, are bathed and dressed, and then are put back to bed. Later, they are wakened again and shuttled to a community dining room for a mediocre breakfast. Residents in these environments feel they have suffered a major loss in their ability to make choices. The lifestyles to which they are accustomed have been replaced by an institutional model.

The basic philosophy of some newer assisted-living facilities is to allow residents, no matter how frail they might be, either mentally or physically, to be involved with many levels of individual choice pertaining to communal living or privacy. This is accomplished by creating many environmental and programming choices. One of the premises for applying this new philosophy at Heritage Village was driven by comments from a number of residents. They wanted the designers to create a microvillage that would allow them to continue to experience choice making. Could they experience all four major components that make up a microvillage—private, semiprivate, semicommunal, and communal spaces or zones—in one environment?

Home: The Private Zone: Most residents who move into a retirement setting come from a home experience, whether an apartment or a traditional single-family home. If the new setting is shared, private zones begin in the bedroom and bathroom area. Even in the smallest private studio apartments, two other components can be added: a kitchen area and a living area for private dining, leisure, and entertaining. Most assisted-living facilities have dining programs that allow three meals a day. However, residents have voiced their desire to retain vestiges of a kitchen, which they feel have some cognitive connection to remaining independent. The kitchen might consist of a small countertop refrigerator with an integral freezer large enough to contain a pint of ice cream. The ability to get up in the middle of the night and enjoy some juice or ice cream gives residents the feeling that they remain in control of their life.

Household: The Semiprivate Zone: The household dynamics of a typical nuclear family allow members to care for others and to be cared for. However, the size of the family typically is much different from that of a retirement community, in which developing meaningful relationships with 150 people can be unfamiliar and very difficult. Most congregate facilities have apartments and community spaces for communal gathering, but rarely are these intimate spaces, except in a group home. Grouping several homes together allows them to have smaller spaces, more in scale with the family setting. These areas may be as simple as a small living room or breakfast room, in which residents can wear housecoats or robes and enjoy a simple breakfast. This smaller scale interaction allows residents to look after each other and to develop camaraderie and a sense of group preservation. It has been proven that residents who are declining mentally and physically have been supported, both holistically and physically, longer in small-scale group home settings than in larger congregate models. The ratio of optimal home units to household areas depends on a number of conditions. Socioeconomic, ethnic, rural versus urban setting, pricing structure, and culture help determine not only the desirable ratio but also the components and size of the households.

Neighborhood: The Semicommunal Zone: In urban areas, single-family settings may be arranged into neighborhoods and supported by small-scale congregating centers, such as groceries, laundromats, diners, and clinics. Similarly, the creation of a neighborhood center within an assisted-living facility allows the frail resident to continue to experience this familiar range of lifestyle choices. Group spaces may be as simple as a community kitchen, the residential laundry area, and the card area or as elaborate as a formal dining room, living room, and staff-supported finishing kitchen. The optimal ratio of household settings to neighborhood support space and the scale and complexity of the services offered are based on the same conditions as the household ratio.

Village: The Communal Zone: In any community, the village or town center has several reasons for existence. First, it serves as the gateway or portal, setting the standard for visitors and citizens. It also is the center of government transactions and civic functions and serves as the location for certain commercial and religious institutions. In an assisted-living community, the creation of a small-scale village center is encouraged to reflect the micro environment.

Establishing Programming and Design Criteria

Wanting to create a new image, Heritage Village was very receptive to new ideas and strategies for the assisted-living project. The design process began with tours of existing facilities, talking to residents and staff, and studying the latest trends in assisted living. The focus groups then established the desired image, defined as a comfortable, informal, lodgelike environment.

Four main design objectives were established to emphasize an independent residential environment, promote passive and active interaction, create options and choices, and ensure safety:

1. The apartments should be organized into two distinct neighborhoods joined by a town center, to enhance the development of private, semiprivate, and public spaces.
2. Residents and visitors should enter the building into a warm, inviting living room with a fireplace.
3. Prairie-style design, relating to the existing campus, should be used to evoke a residential image. The exterior of the new building uses the typical

strong horizontal lines, deep roof overhangs, corner windows, and the earth-tone color palette of this design idiom.

4. The prairie-style design should be continued throughout the interior.

The programming concept was to foster freedom of choice, independence, and personalization, both physically and psychologically. Private, semiprivate, semicommunal, and communal spaces were to be established, relating to the natural progression and psychological association of the home environment. These concepts were used as tools to create spaces, including dining, grooming, recreation, and contemplation areas. The success of the physical environment created is dependent on the staff supporting the program concept.

Finally, the consultant presented three conceptual layouts for consideration: a traditional double-loaded corridor, a cluster household, and a neighborhood/street concept. With client input and the consultant's recommendation, the neighborhood/street concept was chosen.

The Design Solution for Assisted Living

The design scheme embraces the philosophy that all of us, as we age and as our frailty increases, should continue to have the ability to make choices about the way we live. Heritage Village allows residents to live in a microvillage that offers options and choices that are apparent in the architecture as well as in the programming of the facility.

At approximately 23,000 gross square feet, Meadowview Lodge at Heritage Village consists of twenty-six assisted-living apartments with support spaces for residents and staff. With an average gross area of 890 square feet, the apartments include four studios at 390 square feet; twenty one-bedroom units at 525 square feet; and two two-bedroom units at 810 square feet (see figure 15.1).

Private Spaces

In their private spaces, residents have a choice of several sizes of living units, all having the core elements of any home: kitchen, living room, sleeping room, and bathroom. Flexible floor plans allow for a variety of furnishing options. The kitchenettes have an accessible sink and storage cabinets and space for a small refrigerator and microwave. Bathrooms feature residential cabinets with cultured marble lavatories, raised residential waterclosets, roll-in accessible shower stalls, and epoxy-coated residential grab bars. Shared patio and gardening areas, accessible from each apartment, offer residents views and access to the outdoors (see figure 15.2).

Neighborhoods

The neighborhood/street concept organizes the living units into two wings. In each neighborhood, units are arranged on both sides of a twenty-six-foot-wide internal "street." Placing skylit living islands and activity centers in the street was designed to promote passive and active involvement and to foster social interaction among residents. Options include a bathing room with whirlpool tub, dressing area, linen storage, and accessible restroom; craft room with display and storage space; resident laundry room with tables and chairs for socializing; and card room/private dining room with a full resi-

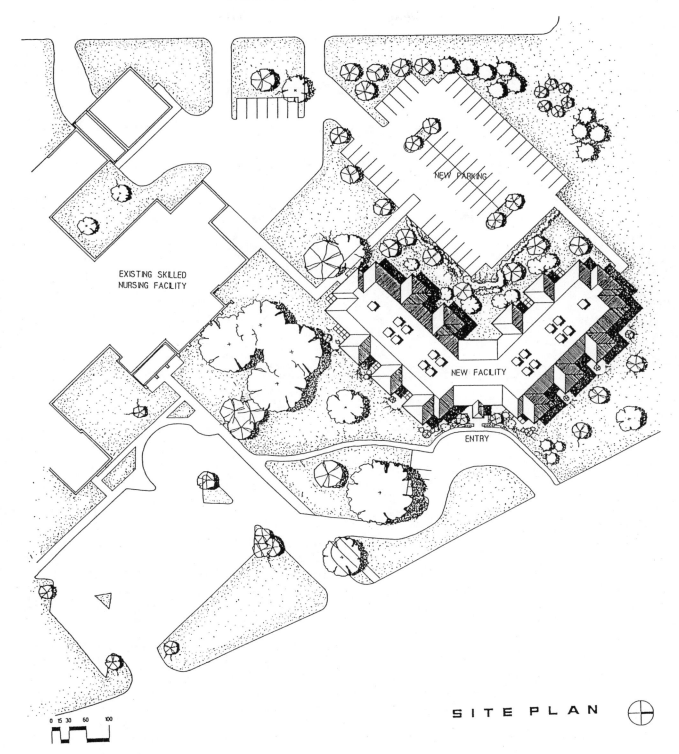

SITE PLAN

FIGURE 15.1. *Site plan at Meadowview Lodge at Heritage Village*
SOURCE: *Drawings by OWP&P*

dential kitchen. Smaller living and lounge areas—each with its own character—are located outside of every four to six apartments along the street (see figures 15.3 and 15.4.).

Numerous design solutions create a residential character and improve wayfinding for residents and visitors alike. Each street has a different theme

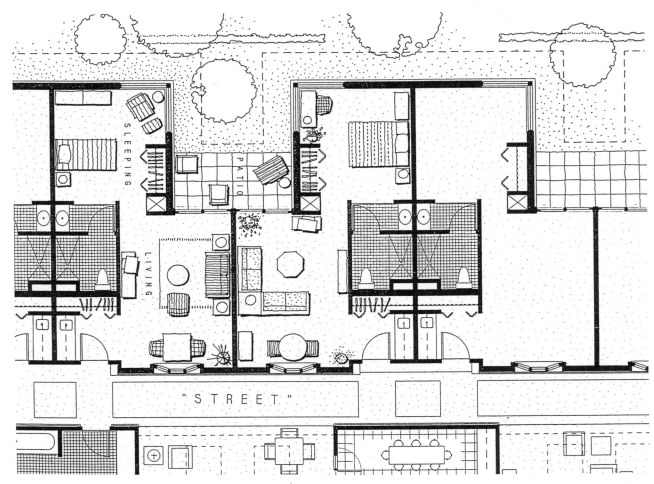

FIGURE 15.2. *Unit floor plan at Meadowview Lodge*
SOURCE: *Drawings by OWP&P*

and special core activities, with noticeable difference in carpeting, wallcoverings, and furnishings. Apartment entrances are recessed, providing space for a personalized package and display shelf at each unit.

At the main entry, guests and residents pass through a vestibule into a reception area and living space featuring a fireplace (see figure 15.5). This comfortable area provides views of the entry and the outdoors, into the dining room, and down the streets. At the concierge desk, staff offer services and assistance to residents and at the same time monitor safety and security throughout the facility. An adjacent office and exam room accommodates more services. The sense of security is strengthened for residents by apartments with internal and external views, which permit them to survey their environment visually.

Communal Spaces

In the semicommunal and communal spaces, a variety of living and dining spaces offer choice and foster independence. For example, residents can eat breakfast in their apartments looking out their bay windows, enjoy lunch in the living islands, or cook their own meals in the fully equipped card room kitchen. The main dining room, in the town center, can accommodate thir-

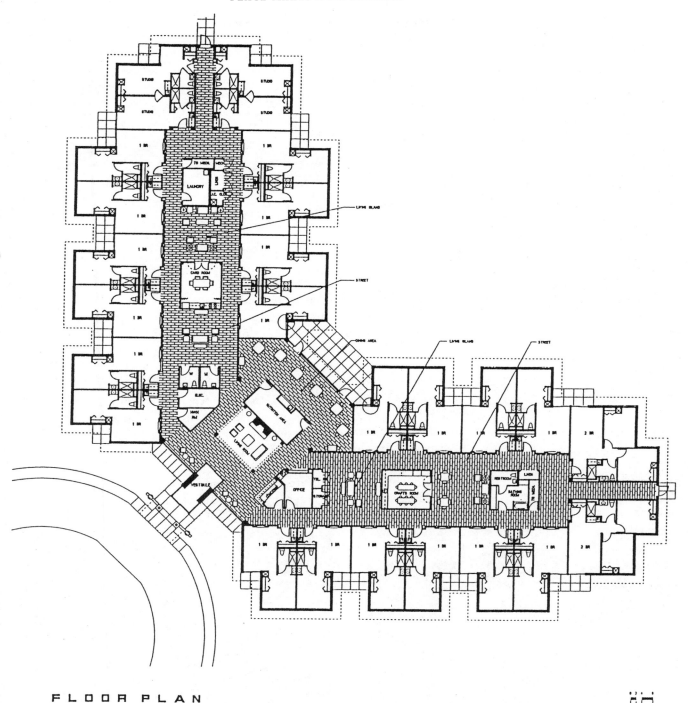

FLOOR PLAN

FIGURE 15.3. *Floor plan at Meadowview Lodge* SOURCE: *Drawings by OWP&P*

ty residents and their guests. A serving counter with a sink, coffeemaker, refrigerator, and dish and glass storage allows residents to get refreshments
whenever desired. An accessible outdoor dining terrace provides another
dining option.

As mentioned previously, some shared spaces were created as part of the
master plan. These include a greenhouse, coffee shop, chapel, multipurpose
rooms, kitchen, dietary room, laundry, and administrative offices. Without

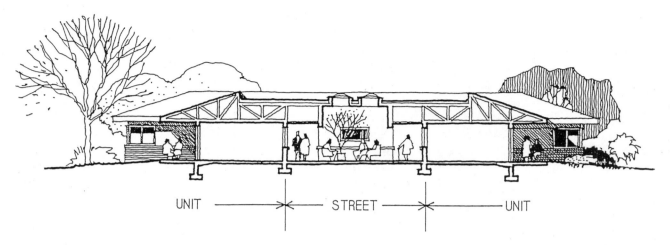

UNIT ———→← STREET ———→← UNIT

SECTION

FIGURE 15.4. *Section drawing of Meadowview Lodge*
SOURCE: *Drawings by OWP&P*

the integration of the master plan, the assisted-living component would have needed to create these village components. As it turned out, these village spaces were able to do double duty for all residents of the facility (see figure 15.6).

Marketing Issues

The success of an assisted-living community depends on properly positioning and marketing the product. It is also imperative that a plan is formulated early in the process and that the community's vision be its guide. Heritage Village positioned itself with a physical design distinct from the competition. It wanted to present itself as a unique and beneficial alternative to living at home. Heritage Village had to evaluate what the marketplace's knowledge and perception of assisted living was.

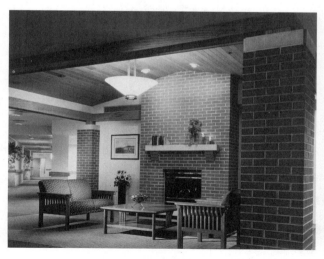

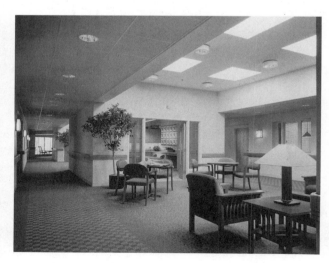

FIGURE 15.5. *Living room entry at Meadowview Lodge* SOURCE: *Photograph by Steve Hall*

FIGURE 15.6. *Living island at Meadowview Lodge* SOURCE: *Photograph by Steve Hall*

Assisted living is both a market-driven and a need-driven product. As a need-driven product, the need for assisted living is usually initiated by a sudden physical malady. With a market-driven product, some potential residents take time to shop around and weigh the pros and cons of competing facilities. This is why it is important to constantly monitor the competition as well as changes in the marketplace. In the Kankakee marketplace, the consultants identified three categories or perceptions of assisted living: (1) a medical model, offering personal care or sheltered care, (2) a hospitality model, with a double-loaded corridor and two models of small hotel rooms, and (3) a residential model in a congregate setting. The more social and residential the assisted-living model is perceived to be by the potential (market-driven) consumer, the more capital-intensive the marketing effort is. Meadowview Lodge is a high-end residential model, making it additionally costly. Meadowview Lodge had slow marketing success in its first year of operation. One reason is that the facility waited to market itself within the community. With major competition, it had to be positioned so that people perceived it as a more desirable and economical place to live.

In the second marketing phase, Meadowview Lodge invested time and money in a new marketing campaign. It hosted a series of luncheons with local people involved in estate planning, advertised in all of the penny-saving magazines and local weekly papers, and advertised on radio stations with audiences in two age ranges, 45–51 years and 75–85 years. The campaign marketed the facility's complete spectrum of services.

Meadowview Lodge was completed in November 1995. The facility was planned to be at full occupancy in one year but was only 35 percent occupied by that date. In marketing an assisted-living facility, timing is everything. Clearly, the strategic marketing plan should be developed very early in the process.

Future Flexibility and a Revised Strategic Plan

Because of the trustees' uncertainty about the assisted-living market in this location, Meadowview Lodge was designed to be easily converted into a sheltered care or Alzheimer's facility. This added significant costs to what could otherwise have been an unlicensed building.

County growth has not been reflected in the town of Kankakee, nor is it expected to be in the near future. At the time this chapter was written, the facility was struggling with several options. One option is to become a strategic alliance partner with a health care provider that does not have an assisted-living facility as part of its continuum of care and to create a joint marketing synergy with the county's elderly consumers. Once the alliance has been established, it could move out into the new growth areas and create satellite assisted-living group homes, which could act as geriatric feeders for the nursing home. Another option is to market the assisted-living facility as a congregate elderly facility and see if the residents will accept an aging-in-place concept.

In the future, once occupancy is sustained, it is the intention of the facility to expand the continuum of care to reach the broader community. A simpler version of an assisted-living program may need to be created for the more rural areas of Kankakee. This program would be combined with independent duplex cottages, which would act as satellite campuses for the nursing home and alliance health care system. At this point, the trustees have simplified their strategic plan to read, "To provide, through multiple levels of service, housing, and health care needs for seniors sixty years and older on a private pay basis."

Preliminary Postoccupancy Comments

To understand the strengths and weaknesses of Meadowview Lodge, interviews were conducted with the chair of the board of trustees for Heritage Village, the marketing and admissions manager, past and present administrators, and some residents of Meadowview Lodge. The interviews took place one year after the facility was completed. Client representatives who were interviewed included the chair of the board, the administrator, and the assistant administrator. "It's the best that I have seen anywhere," exclaimed the chair of the board, who was directly involved in the research, the preliminary market study, the design, and the construction of Meadowview Lodge. The marketing and admissions representative noted:

> The market is tight. It's not just us—it's everybody. We have people who have been in their houses for thirty to fifty years. It's a tough move for people. Many people in this area grew up in their houses and inherited them from their parents. They don't want to give it up. If they can stay, they will stay. I thought that we would fill the assisted-living component in one year. It now looks more like two years. But we remain optimistic and dedicated to the decision that this market needed this type of assisted-living.
>
> I think that the first impression that people get when entering the building is that of a bright, warm, and welcoming space. It is unique. They love it. I think people are expecting a nursing home, and when they walk in and they see how warm and inviting it is, they are surprised. The street concept really aids in creating this unique setting.
>
> When potential residents see the prices, they are initially concerned. Although in terms of value for the dollar, when they look at competitors' prices and look at ours, they can start to see the added features.

When asked to comment on the success and nonsuccesses of the Lodge, she said,

> The bathrooms are a great success. They have no thresholds, still look residential even with the added space for accessibility. And the extra towel racks were a great idea. Our competitors have something that they need to step over, and the grab bars are made of stainless steel. They look more institutional. Ours [epoxy-coated white] are more residential.
>
> Also, in the suites, we have windows and sliding glass doors so they can actually go outdoors. I don't know that people actually do go outdoors. It's just knowing that they have the option. Some people open the doors for fresh air. They have light that's bright and a feeling that they have their own private garden.
>
> We have residents here who receive home health services. Because our facility is residential-based care, they can have direct contracts with home health agents. We have one resident whose husband is taking care of her,

supplemented by additional home health services. So the couple can stay together.

In retrospect, I would have liked to have seen oak trim around the windows and also have each apartment look a little different, almost like row houses. I wish that I put doors in each private unit dividing the bedroom and the living room.

The past administrator, who helped plan the facility but who left before it opened, noted: "I think that we got full buy-in from everybody involved, except the head of nursing, who believed that the assisted living should have been designed as a medical model."

By November 1996, the facility was only 35 percent occupied. More than half of the residents had lived before their move within a thirty-mile radius. Almost all of them had at least one child or other relative living in the area. The residents' favorite room in the building was the living room at the entry foyer, with its fireplace and its lodge aesthetics. From the central location "you can see down both corridors, mail area, and dining rooms." In their own apartments the residents especially liked the bathrooms and the flexibility they have in extending their living rooms to the living atrium in each neighborhood. While the living rooms in the individual apartments allow entertainment of two to three guests, the common living area allows for accommodation of several guests.

Some of the residents commented on the pedestrian streets, stating their appreciation for the feel of these areas. They said that the streets give them options for both social interaction and privacy. They found that in inclement weather the spaces serve as nice indoor places with the qualities of the outdoors.

The following are some of the expressed concerns:

— At the time of the survey, approximately one-third of the residents used their cars on a regular basis. Clearly, provisions for parking were underdesigned, because it was not expected that any of the residents would drive.
— No operable windows were provided in the dining room. "It gets uncomfortable at times. And it needs larger overhangs to provide seating areas outside when it rains or on a sunny day." Operable windows would have allowed natural ventilation, although that typically throws off the HVAC system balance. A larger overhang should have been investigated to reduce glare from the western exposure.
— There is excessive splashing from the funneling of rainwater from the roof valleys onto the individual resident patios. Gutters were value engineered out of the project due to cost.
— There is no climate control in individual apartments; there are complaints that units are too hot or too cold. An original four-pipe HVAC system, which would have allowed different exposures of the building to draw on either chilled or hot water as needed, was value engineered out of the project.
— Only one person used the bathing and spa room on regular basis at the time of the survey. Residents and staff thought it was a waste of space and money. Since all of the units have only showers, and the potential resident

focus group came from older single-family homes with full baths, the team decided that the bathing room was a nice compromise. Time will tell whether residents will use the amenity as they age in this place.

—The biaxial symmetry of the facility influences wayfinding. With each wing being a mirror image of the other, it is very difficult for residents who are mildly impaired to distinguish the difference between them. One solution could have been to create a niche at the front of each wing and treat each neighborhood corridor with different architectural appointments. Such theme zones would announce a different character for each of the wings. Inside the neighborhoods, it would have been helpful if each unit had a unique treatment. This could have been as simple as a window box or different colored shutters around each bay window. If the budget was of little concern, possibly each wing could have had a different floor plan configuration to better distinguish between the parts of the interior space.

—There seems to be agreement that residents should live in a homelike environment, but achieving this in a large, multiple-use setting is difficult. Meadowview Lodge took most of its homelike cues from the staff. Much of the dialogue revolved around a "lodgelike feeling" that, in most cases, does not reflect the scale of the homes from which most residents came. Also, the two parallel corridors that flank the living island do not suggest a typical home setting. If individual rooms had been shifted to the outside walls and the kitchens opened to the central areas, a sense of homelike might have been better achieved. The scale and the intimate corridor could have contributed to this atmosphere.

—In buildings with steep roofs it is always tempting to raise the base of the roof truss to increase the ceiling height in the interior space. Meadowview Lodge is composed of a series of tall living-island areas outfitted with typical residential furniture. If these areas had been furnished in outdoor fashion, such as solariums or enclosed streets, the definition of these spaces might have been better defined. "Utilizing the metaphor of the street as a connecting linkage between units and common spaces has interesting design possibilities" (Regnier, 1994:54).

—The building is fully sprinklered and complies with BOCA 1993. Accordingly, a one-hour separation was required between the apartments and the corridor street. Because of this separation, the frames of the doors and windows had to be constructed of hollow metal instead of wood, and the glazing in the windows had to be wire glass (see figure 15.7.). Wood and plain tempered glass could have enhanced the residential imagery of the building. Also, a one-hour separation was needed between the structure and habitable spaces. Because of these requirements, double ceiling construction was needed to enclose mechanical and electrical equipment, greatly increasing the cost of the project.

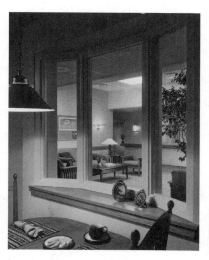

FIGURE 15.7. *View out of apartment at Meadowview Lodge*
SOURCE: *Photograph by Steve Hall*

Conclusion

Assisted living, a national trend in housing for elderly persons, will continue to flourish and expand to meet the needs of consumers in this market. However, care providers cannot allow the government to mandate the style in which this sort of care is delivered. The danger is that the government will do to this industry what it did to the nursing home industry, and we will be obliged to provide products and programs that will not meet residents' expectations. The problem is that we cannot totally refrain from regulating care without subjecting vulnerable elderly people to dangers or risks. The real question is whether we can regulate the industry to protect the quality of care without stifling creativity and innovation.

Heritage House is an example of a facility built in a nonlicensed environment, using common sense and consumer input as guidance. However, there is a need for a dialogue among architects, providers, and residents to determine what the users expect from this type of living and care. Furthermore, residents, providers, designers, and regulators must work together to meet the needs of older Americans.

References

Chermayeff, S., and C. Alexander. 1965. *Community and Privacy: Toward a New Architecture of Humanism.* Garden City, N.Y.: Doubleday.

Regnier, V. 1994. *Assisted Living Housing for the Elderly: Design Innovations from the United States and Europe.* New York: Van Nostrand Reinhold.

CHAPTER 16

Hospice
A Case Study Making a Difference

GREGORY J. SCOTT
MARTIN S. VALINS

*If architecture was to be described as music,
then at best it would follow the classic jazz format
with the composer (architect) setting out a structure
and allowing the opportunity for the players (clients/users)
to float in and out of the melody (building)
with individual expression and freedom.*

*Inspired by address by John O. Yoder,
AIA RLPS seminar, Summer 1996*

This chapter is part analysis, part history, part storytelling, part envisioning a future. This is deliberate. The chapter aims to reflect accurately and appropriately the complexities and subtleties of rationalizing the human experience and potential that we call an assisted-living environment. The authors are in no doubt that late twentieth-century humankind is witnessing the unfolding of a potential human tragedy, that of a society not yet equipped emotionally, spiritually, and certainly not financially to absorb the latest influx of a new culture—its aging citizens.

Introduction to the Case Study

The benefits of providing residential settings for the elderly frail have become apparent to both consumers and providers of care, so the concept of assisted living is beginning to challenge other care programs. Care for people with dementia is now increasingly recognized as a psychological, not a medical, program. Results in postoccupancy evaluations of the Woodside Place residential Alzheimer's facility (see chapter 14) reinforce the notion that carefully designed residential settings actually support and enhance opportunities for therapeutic programs of care.

As with environments for people with dementia, inpatient hospice programs have more to do with care and support than with medicine. Thus, the assisted-living concept has begun to move into the hospice environment. The result is a radical volte-face from traditional nursing home design parameters. As a result of intensive programming and research into the essence of hospice, a stand-alone hospice building in Lancaster County, Pennsylvania, is offered here as a case study in innovation, design, and programming that not only embraces but also moves forward the debate from the residential model toward a therapeutic setting for care.

Another very important care model that has traditionally been placed in the medical camp is the inpatient hospice. This chapter, therefore, combines both theory and the practice of an inpatient hospice building, detailing the architectural and, more importantly, the behavioral objectives for this hospice project, which is to be known as the Essa Flory Hospice.

While we recognize that this book's focus is on assisted living, the project now known as the Essa Flory Center is relevant to the field of debate in contemporary supportive environments for people, old and young, frail and sick, cognitively alert and impaired. The hospice project represents the triumph of ideas over the closed spheres of thought within the regulatory framework of health and long-term care design. The Essa Flory Center came about because it broke the rules. Its creative palette was outside the box. It is not so much an environment tailored to a hospice as a homelike setting allowing private individuals choice and dignity in a setting that happens to accommodate an inpatient hospice program. The hospice project is both a nursing home and an assisted-living facility, and yet it is neither. Nonetheless, its relevance is universal.

An inpatient hospice environment currently (1996) comes under the Pennsylvania code for a licensed nursing home. New licensing codes to address the specific requirements of hospice are currently being formulated and will eventually distinguish hospice settings from nursing homes. Within the limited language of categorization, hospice would not traditionally fall within the category of assisted living. Yet the vision of Hospice of Lancaster County is "to make the highest quality palliative and supportive care available to all terminally ill persons, their families, their caregivers and others affected by death and dying in our community. Hospice advocates effectively for patient comfort, dignity, and choice." Hospice allows an individual in a terminal condition to let go of curative medical programs and allow the condition to run its course. Paradoxically, the focus of hospice is not dying but quality of life.

The hospice project challenged many of our preconceptions not only about hospice but also about all caring environments. Hospice respects the choice of an individual to live in dignity, whatever the complexities or condition of that individual. Somehow, in the overregulated climate of the United States, even the notion of an assisted-living environment brings with it some stripping away of choice, rights, risks, and thereby dignity.

The Trouble with Categorization

Professionals in the field at times speak with an almost callous shorthand, describing formats, solutions, and environments to house people in need of care, a code that very few people outside the consulting or development field come across. Boardroom discussions, conferences, papers, and regulatory data talk of SNFs, ALUs, CIUs, ILUs. They mean nothing, because they mean nothing to the residents and their families who look to the professional world to provide supportive mechanisms, services, and accommodation. It is a language of detachment, which enables the professional world to generate large numbers of books, conferences agendas, and clever rhetoric without ever having to "play a note." There are, in fact, no skilled nursing facilities (SNFs), no assisted-living units (ALUs), no cognitively impaired units (CIUs), no independent-living units (ILUs). There are only homes where people live, where they spend their time, where they rest, play, love, work, and sleep.

The question is not whether we should build more nursing homes or assisted-living communities. That is the trouble with categorization; it focuses on how to arrive at solutions through a narrow, predetermined conduit of ideas. The key to creativity is the ability to think outside the box, to break down the barriers of the status quo if something is not working. Like Alice, we have to go through the looking glass to create a new language to respond to our aging population, a language of care and compassion.

The Torch Is Passed

The next generation of care housing, particularly for older people, will differ in many ways from what is now accepted as the norm. User expectation will become higher, more diverse, and more articulate as the market begins to benefit from consolidation of experience and wider choice. Future residents will be increasingly from the baby boom generation, which has become accustomed to improved housing, education and health care in comparison with preceding generations. They will expect the comforts and necessities of our consumer age. Furthermore, the demographic profile of these residents will shift toward the older segment (80+ years) of the elderly population.

Assisted living has attracted so much attention partly because it is so much better than everything else currently offered in the retirement field. Whether current programs of assisted living will be suitable for future generations is another matter entirely. Assisted living is not necessarily the wave of the future; it is just better than what we have at present. Current retirement communities, including assisted living, are no more than a mirror reflecting our current generation of elderly people, who were born approximately at the beginning of the century. It cannot be taken as a given that these communities will be what future generations will be looking for. While many consumers of retirement housing and services were able to reap the benefits of a life of caution and saving, these virtues do not typify the baby boom generation, for which high spending and high debt are more common. It could be that the needs and requirements of the coming generations of elderly people may well render a large proportion of the current building stock in the retirement field redundant.

While demographics point to increasing numbers of elderly people, these numbers cannot be automatically translated into an increasing demand for elder housing. A new pattern has appeared over the last ten to fifteen years, wherein entrants to retirement housing arrive at the door much older (80+ years). It is expected that this trend will be sustained. This is explained in part by increasing numbers of middle-income Americans arriving at their retirement years fitter and more active than ever before. The average 65-year-old may no longer be considered old, with middle age now stretching to the eighties and beyond. This is pushing the perceived need to move to a retirement community further up the age wave.

Other factors will also come into play that may affect future markets for retirement housing.

— The suburbanization of the United States and the breakdown of the extended and even the nuclear family means that an entirely different set of values relating to home and community are being formulated for future older generations.

—Any revision to Medicare and Medicaid programs will place a greater emphasis on the need for supportive and affordable options for those who cannot afford to buy into a retirement community. At present, one option is to seek the catchall Medicare program of nursing home placement. As an inefficient consumer of tax dollars, this option is already being phased out under state case-mix programs.

—Those who have the economic wherewithal to choose may benefit from an increasing array of support programs that allow people to age in their own homes.

—The concept of work has radically changed over the past twenty years. With this change in work pattern, the very concept of retirement is also changing. Current retirement and assisted-living environments are primarily inhabited by female European Americans aged 80+ years, whose primary occupation has been the care and rearing of their family. Their role accomplished, the concept of retirement is often a very tangible and welcome chapter in life. Compare this to the inevitable increase in white-collar seniors, to whom the term *retirement* may not apply. A business person, teacher, or scientist might see retirement as a change from a primary career to an opportunity to begin or continue a field of research and study. Information technology will make it increasingly possible for people to continue their professional or business affairs outside of the office environment. Is this not a renaissance (rebirth) rather than a withdrawal (retreat) from active participation in the real world that the term *retirement* unfortunately implies? Existing culture, programs, and environments of even contemporary assisted-living communities are geared to the traditional concept of retirement. It is uncertain how such environments will address these new concepts in post-primary-occupation lifestyles.

—A major icon of late twentieth-century suburban humankind, the jogger, is the quintessential symbol of the desire to maintain fitness and avoid aging. That does not necessarily imply that the once tranquil setting of assisted-living programs with walking paths will be overrun by octogenarian joggers and rollerbladers. Its significance is more symbolic, implying that baby boomers do not accept aging easily.

—As a solution for the future requirements of current middle-income, middle-aged Americans, assisted living will probably still fall far short. The bridge to the future in assisted living may have to involve throwing overboard late twentieth-century concepts of retirement based on essentially nineteenth-century patterns of work and domestic values and, instead, take onboard the concept of work and the continuation of our integration into the community well into our older years.

Environmental Precedent

Searching for meaning in assisted-living environments is difficult when compared with other contemporary models of care. The two great professions of health care and architecture each have their own histories of achievement, scientific and technical advances, and a desire to improve the human experience. The interface between the two professions, occurring in the design and use of buildings that accommodate and facilitate the delivery of care, can generate a dynamic fusion in the pursuance of professional excellence. History has taught us, however, that this interface can also lead to a clash between two established cultures. During the latter part of the nineteenth century and for the majority of the twentieth century, the hospital became firmly established as the main focus of the medical environment and, therefore, has been the focal point of dialogue between architecture and health care.

If we wish to envisage a new language and a new meaning for care programs and environments, we have to return to the early and fundamental principles of the human condition. Perhaps the nursing home was no more than a detour to satisfy a set of circumstances that may no longer apply. If a new language of care, support, and environmental design is to evolve, we may need to reconnect to our ancestors' understanding of the power of nature and its healing qualities and our ability to harness the earth's natural energies, such as sunlight, water, and wildlife.

In designing the Essa Flory Hospice, there was little precedent on which to base a design. Instead, the client and its design team relied rather heavily (and somewhat courageously) on intuition, compassion, and a knowing far more connected to the noble concepts of ancient healing than to contemporary ideas of institutional care.

Case Study: Hospice

In approaching the project to design an inpatient hospice environment, the architects Reese, Lower, Patrick & Scott, Ltd. (RLPS) were challenged even before stepping into the interview room as part of the client's (Hospice of Lancaster County) selection process. RLPS had never designed a hospice environment before. It was and remains a comparatively new building type in the United States. The architects' field, and their experience in care environments, lay in long-term care and retirement communities. The hospice patient would be at the terminal stage of an illness or condition. The experience of the environment that the designers were looking to help create might well be the last in the patient's life.

These thoughts did not come through rational debate or discussion in the formal setting of an architect's office. They came at night, alone, in that state between consciousness and sleep; a parallel, perhaps, between life and death. This same realization of the passage from life to death gripped the design team as they read about hospice and listened to the staff at Hospice of Lancaster County express their experience and vision before the formal interview.

Because of the life safety and licensing requirements for medical supervision, it would be necessary for the hospice building to be designed and constructed under the regulatory framework of a licensed nursing home. Hospice of Lancaster County was adamant that its building should strip away any notion of a nursing home, characterized as an environment driven by codes and regulations. It has to be stated, however, that codes and regulations rightly protect and enforce certain life safety requirements. But there is little mention in the codes of the quality of life that a resident can expect. The architects needed to sweep away regulations, reimbursement procedures, even the words *nursing home* and imagine what type of environment would best serve those in need of support during their final days of life. It would be a place of contemplation and companionship, a place of light and warmth, a place of love and hope, a place of peace, of music, of memories, of laughter. It would also be a place to cry, to be alone, to do as one chooses, and to say good-bye.

In understanding that the anticipated average length of stay for the in-patient unit was to be approximately ten days, the design team realized that this would be a building with no seasons. Its environment would need to be blissful 365 days a year. Statements like "It's beautiful here in the fall" would not do. Time is condensed from the long-term care spectrum of two to four years to a few days.

At their interview, the architects noted the challenges of this building type because of critical spiritual needs. They had become sensitive to the demands that a hospice program faces, and they would require ingenuity, creativity, and faith for the task ahead. The board of Hospice of Lancaster County selected RLPS as its architects. The architects were honored to be part of the team and at the same time were humbled by the task.

Project Data

The following are the data gathered by the design team:

NAME: Hospice of Lancaster County Essa Flory Center
LOCATION: Lancaster County, Pennsylvania
COMPLETED: May 1996
LICENSED: Skilled care; C.O.N.
NUMBER OF BEDS: twelve private
CONCEPT: Cluster design (two of six beds)
BEDROOM SIZE: 400 square feet
OXYGEN: Concentrators
ASPIRATOR: Portable
KITCHEN: One country kitchen per cluster
LIVING ROOM: One per cluster
ATTACHED GARAGE: Yes
LAUNDRY: Yes
MEDITATION ROOM: Yes
RESOURCE LIBRARY: Yes
CHILDREN'S AREA: Yes
HOME CARE: Yes, seven teams maximum
BEREAVEMENT SERVICES: Yes
ADMINISTRATION SERVICES: Yes
DEVELOPMENT PROGRAM: Yes
NUMBER OF STORIES: Inpatient, one; administration, two
CONSTRUCTION: Noncombustible metal frame with wood truss roof
EXTERIOR MATERIALS: Brick and stucco
SPRINKLERED: Yes, inpatient only
AREA: Total, 31,794 square feet; administration, 16,662 square feet; inpatient, 15,132 square feet
CONSTRUCTION COST: Total, $3,391,644; site, $270,716; general, $2,431,248; HVAC, $404,400; electric, $285,680
COST PER SQUARE FOOT: $106.85

Project Background and Design Concepts

Hospice is a model of care designed to support the physical, psychosocial, and spiritual needs of people at the end of their lives. Its goal is to allow the dying process to unfold with a minimum of discomfort while maintaining the individual's dignity and quality of life. The design process for a new, short-stay, freestanding, inpatient hospice care facility involved listening, learning, and above all being sensitive to the unique needs, requirements, and philosophy of hospice and the people it serves. The notion of balancing mind, body, and spirit at this critical stage of life was seen as paramount in the design concepts for this unique building type. Hospice was envisioned to celebrate and embrace the qualities of life, nature, and family.

The goal of "look like, act like, feel like home" was established at the onset of the project. The main entrance welcomes and receives patients and visitors (see figures 16.1 and 16.2). Building masses form a compact cluster of elements, connected by a loggia, that shape two integrated landscaped courtyards. In silhouette, the extended roofline seems to touch the ground, settling comfortably with the agrarian landscape of Lancaster County. Although patient rooms are arranged in a linear format, they are accessed by a sequence of spaces that link one public area to another in an unconventional manner (see figure 16.3). Through variations in width, height, lighting level, and floor material, the corridor becomes seamless and virtually invisible. Much like a residence, the corridor or hall connects a series of rooms unobtrusively, providing views and daylight into internal spaces. In each patient room, an environment was created to accommodate various activities in a number of configurations controlled by the occupant, including soli-

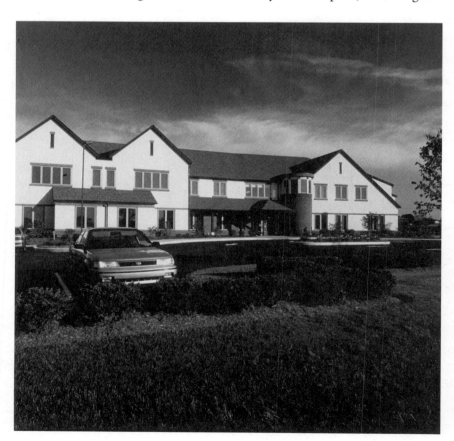

FIGURE 16.1. *Main entrance at Essa Flory Center, Lancaster County, Pennsylvania*
SOURCE: *Photograph by Larry Lefever*

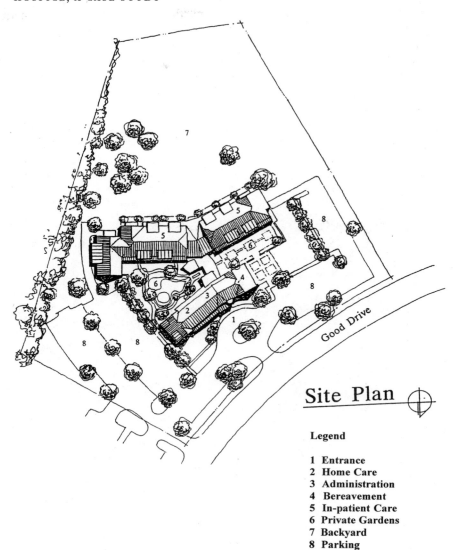

Site Plan

Legend

1 Entrance
2 Home Care
3 Administration
4 Bereavement
5 In-patient Care
6 Private Gardens
7 Backyard
8 Parking

FIGURE 16.2. Site plan at Essa Flory Center SOURCE: RLPS

tude, receiving guests, having intimate discussions, dining, sleeping, napping, viewing the out-of-doors, and accessing a private terrace. Views from the bed were carefully considered as to how light enters the room (see figure 16.4).

The rooms are oriented and trellised to provide direct sunlight when it is most pleasant and to avoid harsh afternoon glare. Each patient room allows easy outdoor access not only for family members but also for patients who are bed bound. The bed can be moved outdoors, giving dying patients something that is important to them but rarely possible (see figure 16.5). Each of the two clusters of six rooms share a country kitchen, a living room, and a bathing area (see figures 16.6, 16.7, and 16.8). The living rooms and open kitchens encourage social interaction, both among families and between families and staff. The opportunity to connect with and support one another is appreciated by hospice families. Therefore, kitchen areas, because they are welcoming and inviting, are well used.

285

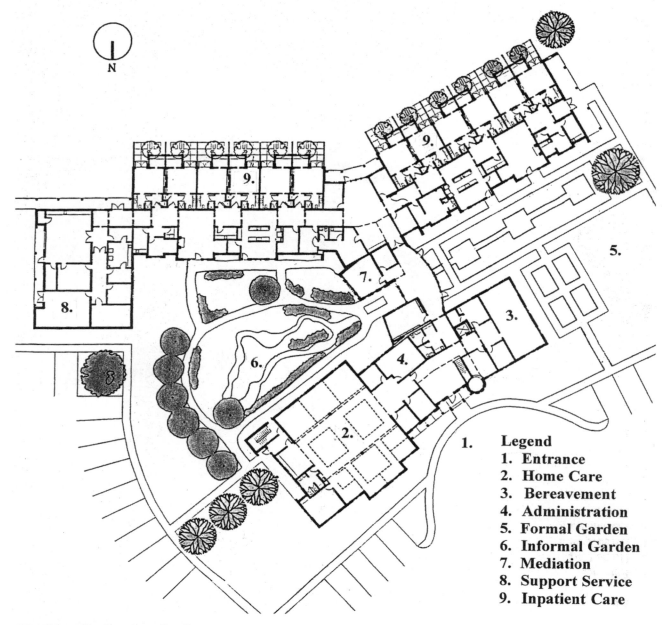

FIGURE 16.3. *First-floor plan at Essa Flory Center* SOURCE: *RLPS*

Careful attention was given to issues of dignity, independence, choice, and control. Service-related functions, from equipment servicing to the way a body is removed from the premises, were separated from patients' private spaces. Although the facility is licensed as a skilled care facility, the owner and the architect worked throughout the design process to create a building that provides a positive experience for every day of every month of the year (see figure 16.9).

At the outset, the desired outcomes were established to meet the goal of "look like, act like, feel like home."

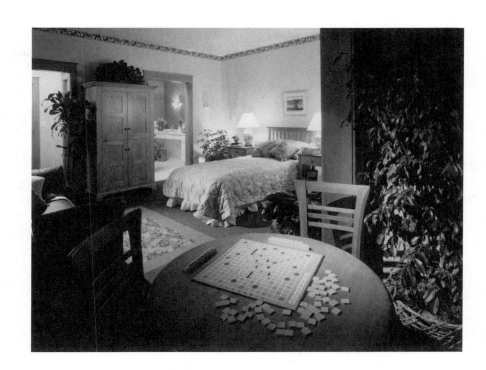

FIGURE 16.4. Guest room at Essa Flory
Center SOURCE: Photograph by Larry Lefever

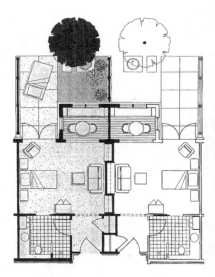

FIGURE 16.5. Guest room floor plan at
Essa Flory Center SOURCE: RLPS

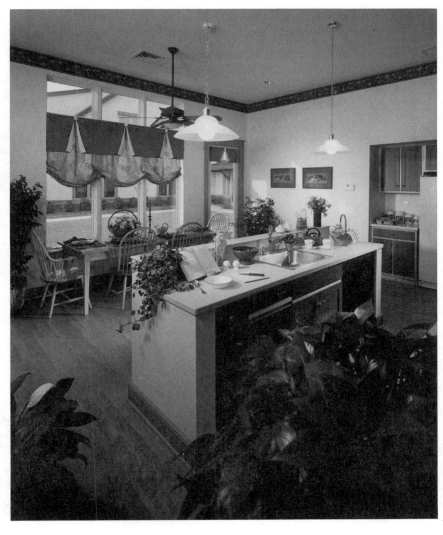

FIGURE 16.6. Country kitchen at Essa
Flory Center SOURCE: Photograph by Larry Lefever

287

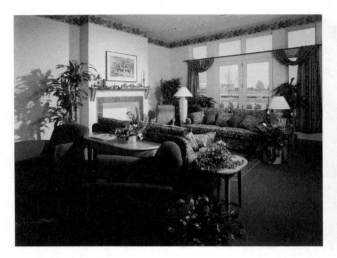

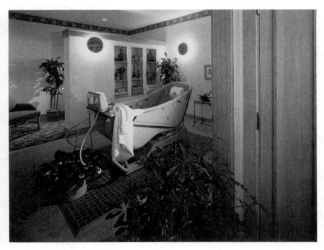

FIGURE 16.7. *Living room at Essa Flory Center* SOURCE: *Photograph by Larry Lefever*

FIGURE 16.8. *Spa area at Essa Flory Center* SOURCE: *Photograph by Larry Lefever*

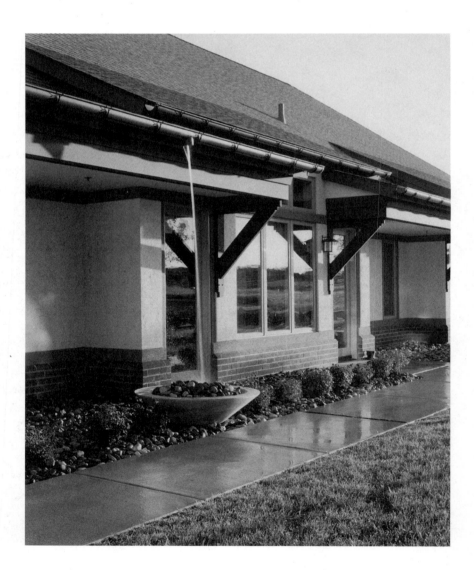

FIGURE 16.9. *Rain water flowing into receiving bowl at Essa Flory Center* SOURCE: *Photograph by Larry Lefever*

288

— Use of the outdoors: This goal requires easy access to the outside and a building design that allows both choice and independence for those using the inpatient area. Each patient room should allow easy outdoor access not only for family members but also for patients who are bed bound.

— Social interaction in a homelike atmosphere: Living rooms and open kitchens encourage social interaction, family-to-family and family-to-staff.

— A comfortable place for children: Children are visible daily and are clearly comfortable being included rather than excluded. Living rooms and small play areas allow children close proximity to loved ones yet provide space and diversion. Children freely go in and out of patient rooms as desired.

— Options for entry and exit: The building entry and exit was a critical design point. The main entrance is designed to make the building feel, from the moment of a person's arrival, like a comfortable home. The home care staff, the largest staff component, have a separate entry area, which keeps the main entrance free of excess activity and traffic. Administrative staff have easy access to many building points, permitting comfortable, operational oversight. Families enter through the front door and are personally welcomed, just as one would be at home. Patient discharge, whether to home or by death, can be equally well accommodated.

— The invisible corridor: Corridors are often one of the most difficult challenges facing designers. Previous notions of corridor design was abandoned in favor of a sequence of spaces that link one public area to another in an unconventional manner. Much like a residence, the corridor or hall connects a series of rooms unobtrusively.

Conclusion

The Essa Flory Center challenges the very notion of assisted living as a building type and, instead, holds the promise that caring environments can be built within the framework of the following universal design parameters:

— Use of daylight
— Connections with nature
— Choice and control
— Privacy and independence
— Dignity
— Appropriate sensory stimulation
— Recognition of the role of the family

Architecture is, above all, something we feel. It is the fusion of art and engineering. Good design takes time and patience. The clock is always ticking in the boardroom of decision makers, yet, fast architecture like fast food has only superficial value. For hospice, the time frame was set by the client communicating its needs to the design team. Further, the design had to put aside preconceptions of design for care and think outside of the box.

The administration of the hospice made the decision to place all the team players around one table. The playeres included the architect, the interior designer, and the general contractor. The strategy ensured that all players agreed with the concept of hospice, and each played a role in the design process.

289

The following is a provider's description of this hospice's value to a dying resident, written just a few months after the opening.

In a hospital room, a life is ebbing away. The medical team has worked hard, but there was now little to be done. The family gathered to be with their loved one before he died. Aware that the Essa Flory Hospice was now open just a short distance from the hospital, the decision was made by the patient and family to move into the hospice. He did not want to die in an institution. It was not possible or practical to return home.

From the antiseptic clinical environment of the hospital, he arrived in a room of soft sheets, daylight, and the smell of fresh flowers. He had arrived at hospice. There was a sense of relief that this would be the place to rest and to spend his last few hours or days. It looked like and felt like home. Sweet relief. His last minutes of life on this earth passed peacefully and with dignity at the Essa Flory Center, in Lancaster County, Pennsylvania.

Further Reading

Beresford, L. 1993. *The Hospice Handbook*. Toronto: Little, Brown.

Carey, D. 1986. *Hospice Inpatient Environments*. New York: Van Nostrand Reinhold.

Gibson, K., D. Lathrop, E. Stern, and E. Mark. 1991. *Carl Jung and Soul Psychology*. Binghamton, N.Y.: Harrington Park Press.

Hayflick, L. 1994. *How and Why We Age*. New York: Ballantine.

Kubler-Ross, E. 1969. *On Death and Dying*. New York: Macmillan.

Kus, R. 1995. *Spirituality and Chemical Dependency*. Raleigh, N.C.: Sacred Heart Church, Diocese of Raleigh. A monograph published simultaneously as *Journal of Chemical Dependency* 5 (2).

Munley, A. 1983. *The Hospice Alternative: A New Context for Death and Dying*. New York: Basic Books.

National Hospice Organization. 1995. *The 1995–96 Guide to the Nation's Hospices*. Arlington, Va.: National Hospice Organization.

Stoddard, S. 1978. *The Hospice Movement: A Better Way of Caring for the Dying*. New York: Stein and Day.

Emerging Themes, Further Reflections

BENYAMIN SCHWARZ
RUTH BRENT

This final chapter is written to amalgamate the diverse chapters and to engender thoughts for emerging themes and further reflections. In this epilogue, the concepts, themes, and practices associated with assisted living are arranged within five basic properties frequently used in assessing assisted living: the nature of the setting, the range of services, the characteristics of residents, the business relationships, and the philosophy of care (Nemeth and Roush, 1994). These headings cover a range of issues raised in this collection of writings. Each of the following sections has two parts: a short presentation of key concepts and themes that emerged from the chapters in this book; and diverse reflections airing issues and questions concerning this model of housing and care for frail elders. Due to the nature of assisted living, the issues are intertwined, and efforts to separate them from each other are impractical.

The Setting

Assertions and Imprints

Three underlying premises appear to be undisputed in reference to assisted living: the emphasis on consumer values, on residential settings, and on care services to facilitate aging in place. The availability of services is a strong motivation to move into a congregate housing arrangement. Clearly, to be market competitive, both the setting and the services must be consumer friendly. Yet, the setting is a crucial component in distinguishing between the medical model, associated with the institutional environment, and the social model, analogous to the residential milieu.

The common belief, shared by advocates of assisted living, is that the setting should be as homelike as possible. Accordingly, assisted-living settings are characterized by their efforts to assume residential appearance and a small scale (see chapters 1, 2, 12, 13, and 14). While the size of a facility depends on site constraints, program orientation, and business goals, most newly built, freestanding, assisted-living facilities include forty to eighty residential units, which typically contain living spaces, private bathrooms, kitchenettes, storage spaces, and laundry appliances (see chapters 1, 2, 4, 12, 14, and 15). The common spaces usually include dining areas, activity areas, and supporting service spaces such as kitchens, examination rooms, central bathing facilities, and laundry rooms. Environmental design is a significant factor in the current discourse about assisted-living settings, because it is hypothesized that providing long-term care in a residential model promotes therapeutic goals such as autonomy, independence, privacy, dignity, and free choice (see chapters 1, 4, 6, 9, 12, 13, 14, 15, and 16). The effort to humanize environments for frail elders through residential design is coupled with the search for the meaning of home and for the attributes of homeyness, both of which take on a considerable role in refining the concepts of present and future assisted-living settings (see chapters 4, 6, 7, 10, 12, 13, and 14).

Although thirty-one states have taken steps to implement an assisted-living policy, and thirteen others have instituted a process to study the issue (Mollica and Snow, 1996), currently there is no national definition of assisted living with respect to licensure or construction codes and regulations (see chapters 1 and 12). The variations in licensure across states and the multiple models of assisted living further confound the debate and add to the confusion of the product line (see chapters 1, 3, and 12). While regulations in some states still prevent the delivery of skilled care in noninstitutional settings, increasingly, as more states regulate assisted-living arrangements, similar services can be provided in various environments. Assisted living is based on a philosophy of care that can be transferred to many care settings, as demonstrated by the various environments presented in this book: free-standing arrangements (see chapters 11, 13, and 15), communities for cognitively impaired persons (see chapters, 7, 8, 9, and 14), residential or congregate care centers (see chapter 10), and hospice environments (see chapters 4 and 16).

Commentary

A growing understanding of the characteristics of frail elders has led several industrialized nations to develop housing arrangements purposely built for older people with diminishing capacities and increasing needs for care. For several years, the focus in the United States has been on the generation of purpose-built settings that combine shelter with services for specific groups of older persons. The long-standing supposition has been that, as people become frail, they will move along the continuum of care and the analogous housing types. However, the recent emergence of assisted living and other new housing arrangements for frail older adults has changed the status quo in the field. Assisted living promotes the breakdown of the continuum of care. Hereafter, frail elders in a variety of settings can receive health, social, and personal services that were once available almost exclusively in institutional environments (Pynoos and Liebig, 1995). The blurring of distinctions among institutional care and other long-term care services (Kane, R. A., 1995) affords frail elders a broad set of choices in diverse settings because the services are not linked to a specific environment. Consequently, residents of independent-living apartments or licensed board-and-care homes do not have to be removed from their dwellings because their disabilities exceed the legal capacity for services licensed for those housing arrangements. The new models, nonetheless, compel care providers to articulate their service programs clearly in order to attract an appropriate resident population. At the same time, they must balance their location on the continuum of care against the need to support the aging in place of their resident population. The implications are epitomized in the task to maintain flexibility to accommodate a broad range of needs in supportive environments.

The expansion of assisted living has led to multiple models of service delivery that have been developed to meet the care needs of specific groups of residents. Still, the numerous variations on the typical model share a similar philosophy, and the diversity is considered by many to be one of the great assets of the industry.

The issue of multiple models of assisted living is directly connected with building codes and licensure regulations. As a relatively new model of care, assisted living is not governed by federal standards. In the absence of federal codes, each state has developed its own set of requirements that affect the cost and construction of settings. In some cases, due to its noninstitutional housing character, assisted living has been allowed to develop under state regulations for board-and-care arrangements. Most states, however, recognize that residences for frail or cognitively impaired elders must ensure high levels of fire safety and rigorous compliance codes. Supporters of assisted living fear that regulating this model will result in prescriptive standards that will limit assisted living's innovation. Furthermore, the concern is that, as state regulatory agencies realize that a number of physically and cognitively frail persons in these settings are nonambulatory according to life safety standards, they may enforce stricter codes, which will result in more nursing-home-like institutional environments. The impact of such a move may interfere with the noninstitutional character of assisted living and consequently may both reduce the variety of solutions and constrict consumer choice (Regnier and Hoglund, 1995).

Beyond the minimum life safety standards, regulations for minimum environmental standards in assisted living have been developed in several states. Regrettably, only few state licensing agencies require that sponsors provide accommodations that emphasize privacy and autonomy-enhancing features such as spacious living areas with private bedrooms, private bathrooms, and kitchenettes. Some states have defined assisted living as analogous to apartments rather than as institutions resembling nursing homes. Others have chosen to license service providers in multiple settings, including conventional elderly housing, or congregate housing sites, as well as settings that may be licensed under residential care categories. Nevertheless, place of care should not be mistaken with type of care. Elders should not be forced to move to a nursing home either because of their disability levels or by virtue of public policies that deny them access to a residential setting. Frail older people should be allowed to remain in settings in which they can age in place and receive services in self-contained dwellings, in complexes that offer a full range of personal and nursing care, housekeeping, and congregate meals.

Spatial and physical elements and their attributes are critical components in people's relationships to settings. The physical elements are, after all, what is designed, built, and manipulated. The architectural framework can provide opportunities for independent action, control, privacy, and socialization. Therefore, places in which the elderly relocate in order to receive long-term care services should be designed to feel like private dwellings, where these qualities are commonly celebrated. Furthermore, the policy implications of the current situation call for encouraging state agencies to create a system for testing and disseminating experimental, creative combinations of housing and services. The system should be shaped to have less restrictive building codes and licensure restrictions to allow experimentation and development of new ideas for providing housing and care services in more humane and effective ways. It should be organized for oversight to monitor and document outcomes and should be followed by a research mechanism so that future generations of innovative housing and service combinations for frail elders can be improved.

Range of Services

Assertions and Imprints

Assisted living embraces a range of settings and residential services, which vary in sponsorship, size, environmental design, cost, residents, admission and retention policies, service, and staffing patterns. These substantial variations are, in part, a response to market forces and state regulations (see chapters 1 and 2). However, the disparity among the models creates some confusion and requires from elders and their decision influencers further investigation in each case to determine what each program means in practice (see chapter 3). Some care providers complain about the boundary blurring of services and fight for maintaining programmatic distinctions. Others regard the confusion about the definition of care services as an opportunity to bring new service options to the frail elderly, which is "the largest population in need of care and the people whose care, presently, is most formula driven, owing to the regulatory and reimbursement provisions in Medicare and in state Medicaid policies" (Kane, R. A., 1995:162).

Nevertheless, residents and their families choose assisted living for its two components, housing and services, which enhance each other and fill a gap in the continuum of care. The intensity of delivered services and style of delivery vary according to the program's orientation, to the individual consumer, and to the state in which the facility is located (see chapter 1). Still, standard services in assisted living commonly include the following: personal care to help residents with activities of daily living, two or three meals, housekeeping and laundry services, 24-hour on-site protective oversight, primary medical care (see chapter 10), activity programs for appropriate social stimulation, and transportation (see chapter 14). Not all residents need or desire the same type and level of care. Services are designed to suit resident needs and preferences; and as residents become more frail and require more care, they are assessed so that the level of care can be adjusted.

Assisted living is conceived as a way of serving people with a wide range of disabilities. As such, it serves those who become physically frail as well as those with cognitive impairments, many of whom are now in nursing homes. Service packages in communities designed for residents with dementia typically offer a higher level of protective oversight, special personal care geared toward persons with Alzheimer's disease, and activity programs directed to benefit these residents (see chapters 1, 7, 9, and 14). Care services for persons with dementia and hospice care in assisted-living settings further demonstrate the trend toward broadening the range of services in assisted living into the long-term care continuum as clients become more frail (see chapter 2).

Commentary

Most states now require an assessment of the resident's situation and mandate a plan of care that determines the required services. At the same time, most states link the required services to the agencies that provide them

(Mollica and Snow, 1996). Thus, the operating philosophy of assisted living calls for the development of unique and flexible service plans for specific residents to promote their strengths while minimizing the incapacitating effects of their weaknesses. Residents can choose the basic service program offered by the community or can pay for additional services to match their special needs. The various service options are typically delivered by the community staff or are contracted by residents with outside agencies. In addition, sponsors may subcontract services such as management, food, laundry, or personal care to vendors.

The model of care that is followed and the style in which the services are delivered continue to be crucial concerns, because the term *assisted living* embraces settings that provide very limited personal care as well as those that provide extensive services of this sort. The term encompasses settings that are characterized by high levels of comfort and privacy for residents and ones that offer their tenants only multiple-occupancy rooms and provide care only within constrained reimbursement standards (Kane and Wilson, 1993). Nevertheless, advocates of assisted living assert that, regardless of the model of care, the balance of power needs to shift from the professionals to the consumers. This power shift is an essential prerequisite for resident autonomy—a cornerstone in the care philosophy of assisted living. Accordingly, R. A. Kane (1995) argues that the setting has to be residential and "must be sufficiently private and self-contained to coincide with a reasonable definition of home; and the providers of service, whether they are home care agency personnel or staff of the residential program, must treat clients as tenants in their home rather than as residents of an institution" (167).

Several assisted-living communities are experimenting with a resident-oriented model of staffing, which divides staff into teams according to the groups of residents they serve, in contrast to the more common approach of dividing staff into functional crews. In the team-oriented approach, staff members do all housekeeping, food preparation, laundry, personal care, and programmed activities for a small group of residents. Working with smaller groups allows caregivers to center on individual residents in the spirit of resident-focused care. In addition to more effective communication between staff and residents and stronger group identity, the model promotes partnerships among residents, paid professional caregivers, and family members. Perhaps the only problem of this model is finding employees who are willing and able to perform the tasks in each of these areas to the level of quality desired.

Quality assurance of services requires a further vital component in the form of carefully constructed regulations that focus on consumer satisfaction. Some advocates of assisted living promote the idea of outcome-oriented regulations that address consumer satisfaction with services, setting, and autonomy—essential components of a resident's quality of life (Wilson, 1996). In many states, however, the controversy regarding regulations of services has centered on the provision of skilled nursing care. While many states promote the concept of aging in place by allowing provisions of skilled nursing services within assisted living, some nursing home operators oppose rules that allow services of this kind to be delivered outside the home or the nursing home setting. They are concerned about keeping the competition between nursing homes and other residential programs on a level playing field and complain that it is inequitable to regulate two settings differently if they have similar consumers. At issue, it seems, is not the higher good of residents but competition for clientele, a rivalry that often appears to be driven by less altruistic goals.

Resident Characteristics

Assertions and Imprints

At this time, a typical assisted-living resident in an average assisted-living community can be described as a single or widowed woman, 84 years of age, who was living alone before her entry into the facility. Residents' average yearly income tends to be in the middle to upper-middle range, or $20,000 to $50,000. The typical resident is in need of three types of self-maintenance assistance for everyday activities or acuity levels (see chapter 2). The following clinical profile of residents receiving reimbursement for assisted-living services is described in the Frail Elderly Act of the Medicaid Home and Community Care Options Act of 1990: they are 65 years old and older who need substantial assistance with two or three activities of daily living (ADLs) (see chapter 10) or elders with Alzheimer's or other cognitive impairments who cannot perform two of five ADLs (see chapters 7, 8, 9, and 14).

Residents of assisted living differ significantly due to the multiple models of care embraced by the broad definition. Wilson (1994), for example, classifies the models of assisted living as housing with services, assisted housing, and nursing home replacement. Residents of the first model are relatively independent and are able to self-direct, identify, request, and evaluate the services they need. In the second model, residents are characterized by more need for oversight and help to ensure that their needs are identified and services provided. Residents of this model ordinarily need assistance with personal care services, such as bathing, grooming, walking, eating, taking medications, and toileting. Residents of the nursing home replacement model are presumed to have significant service needs, which must be identified, organized, and evaluated by trained personnel. These residents are typically more frail than residents of the other models and are more limited in their ability to eat, walk, toilet, transfer, or self-direct their own care.

Many assisted-living arrangements serve people with cognitive impairments because almost half of all people over the age of 85 suffer from Alzheimer's disease or other kinds of dementia (see chapters 1, 2, 4, 7, 9, and 14). While some communities are specifically designed and operated to meet the specialized needs of people with Alzheimer's disease (see chapters 7, 8, 9, and 14), others do not separate this resident group from the rest of their population. As residents age in place, management of assisted-living communities face the need to plan for cognitive changes by training staff and adopting programs and policies to support their tenants. An Alzheimer's assisted-living program, with a special setting, program, and a trained staff, allows residents to remain in their own community as they progress through the stages of the disease.

Commentary

American society is characterized by diversity in income, education, geographic location, race, gender, and physical attributes. The elderly population in the United States, like the rest of the population, continues to diversify in socioeconomic, ethnic, linguistic, and political makeup. The anticipated increase in life expectancy and reduction in mortality rates will mean an increasing proportion of older people in racial and ethnic populations. Since there is no absolute melting pot of cultures and ethnic groups at any age, many questions arise when older people elect to move into a group setting. To meet the needs of a population with a growing assortment of languages, customs, and racial characteristics, housing arrangements such as assisted living will have to be sensitive to issues of cultural heritage (see chapter 6).

Beside racial and ethnic changes, future generations of elders can expect meaningful shifts in social and family structures and lifestyles, which, together with income and economic factors, will add to the diversity of future generations of older people. The typical family of the 1990s has fewer children, greater geographic mobility, a larger proportion of single-parent households, and more women in the workforce (Torres-Gil, 1992). The latter factor is expected to reduce the number of adult caregivers significantly, leading to increasing numbers of elders living alone. Elders who live alone have been found to seek out formal service systems for care. These changes will inevitably affect personal rituals and adaptation to life changes (see chapters 4 and 5) as well as access to services, equitable distribution of scarce resources, and financing of benefits. The main concern is, of course, the inability or refusal to recognize the rights, needs, dignity, or value of people of particular ages, races, and geographical or ethnic origins.

Most older Americans prefer to live in their own homes. When they are faced with the reality of being unable to remain in their own homes, they opt most often to live in an noninstitutional environment that retains many of the qualities of their private, independent living. Presented with options, elders respond favorably to assisted living regardless of price. Those who choose to move to assisted living rather than to other types of setting for long-term care demonstrate their appreciation for the values of independence, choice, and quality of life that this model promotes. Residents, their families, and other decision influencers seek services in settings that compensate for their declining competencies while fostering continued autonomy in choice of lifestyle. Assisted living is attractive to them because it strives to meet residents' needs rather than forcing them to adapt their lifestyle to fit an inflexible, institutional regime.

Business Relationships

Assertions and Imprints

While the focus of this book is not on the business relationships of assisted living, several authors address issues of this nature in their chapters. For example, as the match between supply and demand of assisted living fluctuates and as enrollment of Medicare beneficiaries in managed care plans grows, discussion of the potential linkages between assisted living and managed care proliferates (see chapters 2, 3, and 4).

The business relationship between provider and resident in assisted living differs from other business relationships in senior care. In many housing arrangements for the elderly, such as continuing care retirement communities or independent-living apartments, residents usually pay entrance fees or make large deposits in addition to the ongoing service fees. In contrast, assisted-living tenants commonly pay fees based upon a fixed monthly amount that covers room, board, utilities, and basic services. More services may be purchased for additional fees. In this business arrangement, neither the resident nor the provider have committed to lifetime care. The resident may choose to terminate the agreement and select housing and services elsewhere, just as in any other agreement between a tenant and a landlord.

Assisted living is a need-driven option; and yet, since older adults are provided with other choices, it is also a market-driven product. Consumer preference is the force driving the need and demand for assisted living. Thus, assisted living must respond to consumers' needs and, perhaps even more, to consumers' desires. In comparison to the nursing home, assisted living is seen as a more affordable and desirable option (see chapters 1, 2, 3, and 12), and the wish of elders to reside in assisted living creates the demand. Thus the market forces that propel consumer demand for assisted living are affordability, demographics, preference for a residential environment, and the inability of nursing homes to adapt to change (see chapters 1, 12, 13, and 15).

Labor costs in long-term care arrangements represent more than 60 percent of total operating expenses. For that reason, operators of assisted living use the resident-oriented team approach and encourage increased family involvement in the care of loved ones. Their goal is to meet residents' needs while keeping labor costs down. Although there may be more self-care support and family assistance in assisted living than in a nursing home, the cost of staff in assisted living continues to be high. The quality of staff is the single most important determinant of the success of service operation. Therefore, management of assisted living has to provide continuous and ongoing quality training and education to ensure quality of care (see chapters 9, 10, and 14).

Affordability is another significant issue in assisted living, since most programs have been developed for and marketed to relatively affluent elders, who pay for these services privately (see chapters 1, 2, and 3). At present, reimbursement to assisted living is limited. Unlike nursing home care, assisted living is not a covered health care service within the Medicaid payment structure. Consequently, assisted-living arrangements focus on self-pay elders, and as a result services are not easily accessible to low-income older adults. The concern is that moderate- to low-income older people cannot afford this long-term care model. However, several states have shifted Medicaid funding from nursing homes to assisted living, and Medicaid is becoming the primary source of financing for low-income assisted-living residents.

This trend will probably intensify state regulation of assisted living because public funds "inevitably lead to a regulatory response, especially when the funds are distributed to proprietary providers" (Kane, R. L., 1995:58). Thus, providers are challenged to develop, in cooperation with state regulatory agencies, a new model of regulations for service under which operations would be conducted. One hopes that the unfolding process will not repeat the blunder that derailed the regulatory process of nursing homes. At the same time, financing for construction and funding for services of assisted living have to be increased to target a range of income groups, which will allow frail elders to live in residential settings regardless of their income.

Commentary

Long-term care in nursing homes and other settings is extremely costly. Studies show that elders living alone are particularly at risk of becoming impoverished as a result of paying for long-term care. Clearly, there is a need for lower-cost alternatives. Assisted living holds promise as a cost-effective form of care that can effectively serve low-income people. Kane and Wilson (1993) argue that, of sixty-three assisted-living arrangements surveyed, "the majority of the rates, even at the high end, would cost substantially less than nursing home care for privately paying person in the same community" (48).

In the challenge to reduce health care costs, policy makers often identify managed care as a viable option. Managed care is not new to health care, but serving elderly people in assisted living through the governing factors of managed care is still a relatively new phenomenon. As a lower-cost way of providing services in a less restrictive setting, assisted living is perceived as an appropriate alternative that matches the objectives of managed care. At least thirty states were planning or developing managed care programs by the end of 1996. Planned services included acute and long-term care, and "most were considering combining Medicaid and Medicare services to create a fully integrated program" (Mollica, 1997:11). However, as networks of managed care develop relations with assisted living, problems of control may arise. At issue, for example, is the question of who will make the decisions about admission to or moving out of health care settings. In other words, who will control case management and care planning?

Managed care networks have been established to manage both the delivery of services and the financing of services. Thus, when reimbursement rates are capitated by states, it creates incentives for managed care organizations to contract with assisted-living providers for delivering services to residents. But controlling costs through managed care can turn into a calamity. While it is possible to "manage" costs of care by preventing admission to institutional health care settings or shorten younger patients' length of stays in hospitals, it is much more complex to control a frail elderly population with multiple chronic conditions, cognitive impairments, or terminal illnesses. The most common connection between assisted living and managed care, at this time, is through inclusion of programs as part of an integrated service delivery system. However, the manner in which care is paid for will determine what sort of care is given and, perhaps indirectly, what happens as a result. Despite potential problems, experts argue that "the emergence of assisted living in managed care has a significant potential and is likely to influence the direction of at least a segment of the assisted-living industry" (Mollica, 1997:21).

Long-term care services are greatly influenced by two types of regulatory forces: the obvious quality regulation and the less apparent but equally potent policies concerning public payment. "Payment affects both who and what are covered and, hence, what types of services are provided to whom" (Kane, R. L., 1995:58). By accepting public money through Medicare and Medicaid, both assisted-living providers and residents must submit to the dictates of others. From the consumer's perspective, there are more limitations, because not everything is covered. Frail elders who depend on public funds are limited by the options available to meet their needs and are constrained by the type of service for which they are eligible. Benefit packages may be limited, and consumers may be bound by the agencies that provide those services. Providers of care must often be certified to qualify for the provision of services, further limiting choice for consumers. Consequently, advocates worry that assisted living will develop into a two-class program, with extreme discrimination between luxurious settings for the wealthy and substandard accommodations for the poor. Existing state regulations and reimbursement mechanisms further encumber the development of assisted living and increase the administrative cost of existing programs, worrying developers and providers about particular regulations, such as fire protection standards, that might drive up the price of assisted living.

Clearly, assisted living must be recognized as a unique, humane, and cost-effective form of long-term care for it to achieve its potential. It will not and should not replace nursing homes entirely but should be allowed to flourish and to proliferate as a viable, lower cost, alternative to existing long-term care models, an alternative that may keep down both personal and national health care expenditures. The enthusiasm for assisted living reflects the public interest in such an alternative and the recognition that elder care policies can and must be reconstructed.

The Philosophy of Care

Assertions and Imprints

Perhaps the most fundamental aspect of assisted living is philosophy of care. More than the setting or the service components, this philosophy distinguishes assisted living from other forms of long-term care. The focus on individual preference and needs is perhaps the aspect that most characterizes this philosophy of care. At its best, assisted living holds promise to redefine the relationships between consumers and providers of long-term care. Rather than mandating that frail elders receive particular services in certain ways, the assisted-living philosophy of care advocates choice and independence. This shift in perception supports human values such as dignity and privacy, which are often disregarded in other aggregations of housing and services for frail or cognitively impaired elderly.

Part of the reason it is easy to violate these human principles, when individuals are dependent on help from others, is the confusion and misuse of concepts such as autonomy, reciprocity, and empowerment, as Wilson (1995) notes:

> Objectively defined, autonomy is the ability, willingness, and opportunity to make and act on decisions. Reciprocity implies a balance of giving and taking in relationships. Reciprocity demands that the individual's needs and preferences be balanced against the needs and preferences of others, including the caregiver. Empowerment is the redistribution or restoration of opportunities to promote reciprocity and autonomy for those in society labeled as disabled, disenfranchised, or dependent. Assisted living is uniquely positioned to support fundamental change to achieve empowerment of frail, often significantly impaired adults. (145)

Empowerment of residents can be achieved when individual elders take an active part in setting priorities, devising strategies to meet their needs, and accepting limits in services as part of their plan of care. The plan is negotiated by the individual, the service provider, and resident advocates, all

300

of whom are expected to reach a consensus. The process emphasizes the collaborative effort among the parties in analyzing needs and in searching for alternative solutions. "Such a process encourages integration, competency-based task assignment, service incrementalism, and familial involvement" (Wilson, 1995:146).

Nemeth and Roush (1994) write that the Assisted-Living Federation of America (ALFA) expects its members to comply with the following principles that outline the philosophy of care in assisted-living residences: providing quality care, with special attention to the individual's needs (see chapters 1, 4, 6, and 7); treating each resident with dignity and respect (see chapters 1, 8, and 12); encouraging independence for each resident (see chapters 1, 4, and 12); fostering resident choice of care and lifestyle (see chapters 4, 6, 11, and 13); protecting residents' right to privacy (see chapters 1, 4, 7, 12, 14, and 15); nurturing residents' spirits (see chapters 4, 6, 12, and 16); involving family and friends in care planning and implementation (see chapters 1, 4, and 14); providing a safe residential environment (see chapters 3, 12, 14, 15, and 16); and making the assisted-living residence a valuable community asset.

The intention of the philosophy of care in assisted living has been to support aging in place. However, while many operators believe and encourage this goal by helping residents to stay in assisted living, others make a clear distinction between the roles of assisted living and nursing homes. Provider opinions differ on the question of whether to take the risk and responsibility of extending aging in place in order to avoid placement in an institutional setting. In addition, some states regulate the policies for discharging or retaining residents, while in others the policies are more flexible and decisions are left to providers' discretion. Clearly, there is no one common philosophy of care. As a result, providers are expected to define their mission statement and to articulate their operating position distinctly.

Commentary

Autonomy is an ambiguous and multitextured concept not subject to narrow definition. It may pertain to privacy, free choice, individual liberty, and moral independence. Autonomy refers to the freedom to make decisions and to act on those decisions. Still, the two expressions—decisional autonomy and autonomy of execution—neglect the broader view that having autonomy gives meaning to life (Agich, 1993). Hofland (1990) suggests that there are at least three dimensions to personal autonomy that form a hierarchical continuum: the *physical* dimension, which relates to freedom of mobility, physical independence, and use of the least restrictive environment; the *psychological* dimension, which relates to control over one's environment and one's choice of options; and the *spiritual* dimension, which involves an expanded concept of self.

The paradox of autonomy and long-term care involves the contrast between the concept of autonomy that stresses independence and the dependence that characterizes long-term care. Indeed, defined narrowly, the very concept of autonomy in long-term care is an oxymoron. Long-term care is, by definition, designed for elders who suffer from disabilities or limitations that compromise their ability to function independently. Residents of long-term care settings are frequently dependent on others to assist in implementing their own decisions. Therefore, autonomy in a nursing home or an assisted-living residence cannot be equated with absolute independence. "The reality of long-term care apparently forces even the staunchest proponents of autonomy as independence to deal with the reality of an impaired decision-making capacity or incompetence that is an inevitable feature of long-term care" (Agich, 1993:10).

Thus, rather than asking whether a resident's choice is influenced by others and assuming that all such influences inhibit autonomy, the proper question is how institutional factors affect resident actions and whether these influences subvert resident control. Personal autonomy in a long-term care setting tends to be compromised for many reasons. The characteristics of other residents, staff, physical setting, programs, and public policies governing the facility may all limit autonomy. Nevertheless, the challenge for institutional long-term care is to develop substitutes for the activities that residents value but can no longer perform. In this context, assisted-living arrangements need to identify and establish conditions that encourage individuals to face distress and threats to the self that are the inevitable results of chronic conditions and functional declines that bring elders to long-term care in the first place. Respecting autonomy requires attending to what is significant and meaningful for these elders. It means that elders must be treated as individuals with personal histories steeped in a rich assortment of memories and experiences.

The cognitively impaired elderly present many challenges for those assisted-living arrangements that make efforts to support residents' autonomy. With approximately 75 percent of residents in long-term care facilities afflicted by some cognitive problems, the task is substantially complex (Beck and Vogelpohl, 1995). No condition of frailty has a more pervasive impact on the autonomy of elders than cognitive impairment. When mental capacity becomes restricted and resident judgment becomes questionable, caregivers may justifiably intervene to protect persons from decisions and behavior that are harmful. In assisted-living arrangements in which residents suffering from Alzheimer's disease reside together with other residents, another issue arises: How can the facility simultaneously protect the interests of all residents and staff? By granting more autonomy to cognitively impaired residents, the facility runs the risk of damaging the collective good of other residents. This is, perhaps, the most important reason for creating special care assisted living for people afflicted by dementia.

As an innovative model that centers its philosophy of care on resident autonomy, assisted living can and should provide positive messages and hope despite severe illnesses and grave impairments. Hope does not mean recovery or cure; instead, hope pertains "to the prospect of meaningful experience with others at those times when one most needs comfort and companionship" (Agich, 1993:113).

Further Reflections

Several broad trends have focused our attention on issues of assisted living as a new model of long-term care: the democratization of longevity, the increasing numbers of very old persons who are often physically or mentally impaired and require high levels of services and assistance, the ideological and fiscal crises of the welfare state, the rapid progress of biomedical technology, and the shift in attitudes toward consumers and therapeutic goals. In the late twentieth century, most Americans can expect to live a long, healthy, and vigorous life. Ironically, due to the accomplishments of the modern scientific enterprise in and its conquest of premature death from acute illnesses, most of us will suffer from chronic diseases before we die. Certain problems of aging, such as poverty, isolation, and treatable diseases, can and should be alleviated, but the gradual decline of physical vitality, the eventual path to death, is for many inescapable and only partly controllable. No amount of biomedical research or medical intervention can bring frailty and old age under the control of human will or desire (Cole, 1992).

Choosing to live with inherent limitations, even as we struggle against them, is the inevitable reality of frailty and vulnerability in old age. In a rapidly aging society, with those over the age of 85 constituting the most rapidly growing segment of the population, the necessity of considering what life means and what constitutes an acceptable quality of life is paramount. From that perspective, there remain the questions, What is the meaning of assisted living in view of the themes of aging, autonomy, and architecture? And why is it important?

Cole (1992), in *The Journey of Life*, notes: "In contemporary culture, *meaning* is generally used in one of two ways: as generalized theory of language or as intuitive expression of one's overall appraisal of living. The *scientific* questions about meaning are part of the human attempt to develop logical, reliable, interpretable, and systematically predictive theories. The *existential* questions about meaning are part of the human quest for vision within which one's experience makes sense" (xviii). Cole uses the term *existential* not in reference to any particular existentialist philosophy but in respect to the experience of human beings in this world, seeking "love and meaning in the face of death" (Barnard, 1988). The generative power of meaning as a concept evolves from the essential ambiguity between the scientific meaning and the existential (or experiential) meaning. Thus, throughout this book, authors are attuned to the scientific and existential meaning of aging, autonomy, and architecture in assisted living.

The scientific meaning is represented in this book by studies from the environment and aging perspective, which have proliferated in recent years. As a subfield within environment-behavior studies, environment and aging is plagued with problems similar to those that distinguish its source discipline. Inherent in environment-behavior studies is the assumption that studying the behavior of people and the social context in relation to buildings can elicit knowledge about these relationships that is generalizable to the level of conventional rules and theories for future application. Lang (1987), to cite an instance, differentiates between *positive* theory, which describes the world as it is, and *normative* theory, which presents the world as it ought to be. Normative theories are informed by positive theories and involve prescriptions for action through standards, design principles, and philosophies stemming from ideological positions on what the world should be like. However, the conceptual danger in this assumption in regard to design practice is in deducing an "ought" from an "is" without explaining why there is an obligation to design something for the future on the basis of what already exists (Johnson, 1994). At this time, there are very few descriptive positive theories consisting of statements and assertions that describe and explain the reality of assisted living and that are capable of extension to predictions of future reality. Hence, it is not feasible to provide sufficient generalizable knowledge about assisted living to generate normative statements about what assisted living ought to be.

The principal purpose of this book is to contribute descriptive theories to the public dialogue on assisted living. Rather than developing grand theory through abstractions and generalities, we choose to promote the exchange of ideas concerning innovative residential models of long-term care among a wide range of participants. This more modest course corresponds with the philosophy that generally rejects the view that theory mirrors reality. Theories, according to this direction, are only partial perspectives on their objects (Cole, 1993). Accordingly, it is unlikely that we will ever possess a precise prototype or blueprint for living that will include a comprehensive list of human needs that could be used in designing settings. Nevertheless, it remains true that both the way in which frail elders live and the settings they live in are products of the human mind and, as such, are subject to constant modification and improvement.

Furthermore, to gain a more dependable sense of how design will perform once it is built is a desirable objective. But to rely solely on scientific methods for this aspiration is to overlook both the limitations of science and the fact that prediction, in the classical sense of explicating cause-and-effect relationships, is not invariably the goal of science. Neither designers nor sponsors can know whether a setting for assisted living will facilitate particular behaviors or will fulfill certain perceived needs of frail elders, because no one can tell whether this is the case until after the design is built and occupied. On that account, we need to support the construction of several versions of assisted living to test new ideas and facilitate better care services. To set this course is not merely a challenge, as Rowles and Ohta (1983) note: "in larger sense it is a responsibility, for ultimately we are charged with nothing less than the potential for determining the milieu in which we all may grow old" (238).

Several chapters in this book allude to the existential meaning of aging, autonomy, and architecture of assisted living. Authors of these essays recognize that we are all vulnerable to chronic disease and that death is imminent. As Weisman (1997) puts it: "Old people have their own share of vulnerability and ambiguity to deal with, not always a function of age, but of uncertainty itself, a first cousin to anxiety and fear. I contend that death as a prospect is less distressing than dread of disability, helplessness, dependence, and dementia, about which prevention is notoriously uncertain and often inadequate" (288).

This vulnerability, once understood and accepted, can become an inspiration for providing compassionate care and for building realms of symbolic forms through which we can explore and express the meaning of human existence. The paradoxical nature of aging, with its tension between ambitions, dreams, and desires on the one hand and its declining physical being on the other, cannot be eliminated by the wonders of modern medicine, scientific rigor, or unsubstantiated verbiage. What we need is social criticism and public dialogue aimed at creating socially just, economically viable, and spiritually satisfying places in which we can care for frail elders. Opening the dialogue at a time that is opportune, this book is an instrument of commu-

304

nication and understanding as it relates to what we know about frail elders and their inhabitation. We are unabashed in recognizing the ambiguities of our aging and frailty; nonetheless, we are dauntless in illuminating the potential stratagem of assisted living as having virtue to us as human beings.

References

Agich, G. 1993. *Autonomy and Long-term Care*. New York: Oxford University Press.

Barnard, D. 1988. Love and death: Existential dimensions of physicians' difficulties with moral problems. *Journal of Medicine and Philosophy* 13:393–409.

Beck, C., and T. Vogelpohl. 1995. Cognitive impairment and autonomy. In L. Gamroth, J. Semradek, and E. Tornquist, eds., *Enhancing Autonomy: Concepts and Strategies*. New York: Springer.

Cole, T. 1992. *The Journey of Life: Cultural History of Aging in America*. Cambridge: Cambridge University Press.

———. 1993. Preface to T. Cole, W. Achenbaum, P. Jakobi, and R. Kastenbaum, eds., *Voices and Visions of Aging: Toward a Critical Gerontology*. New York: Springer.

Hofland, B. 1990. Introduction. *Generations* 14:5–8.

Johnson, P. 1994. *The Theory of Architecture: Concepts, Themes, and Practices*. New York: Van Nostrand Reinhold.

Kane, R. A. 1995. Expanding the home care concept: Blurring distinctions among home care, institutional care, and other long-term care services. *Milbank Quarterly* 73:161–86.

Kane, R., and K. Wilson. 1993. *Assisted Living in the United States: A New Paradigm for Residential Care for Frail Older Persons?* Washington, D.C.: American Association of Retired Persons.

Kane, R. L. 1995. The impact of long-term care financing on personal autonomy. In L. Gamroth, J. Semradek, and E. Tornquist, eds., *Enhancing Autonomy: Concepts and Strategies*. New York: Springer.

Lang, J. 1987. *Creating Architectural Theory: The Role of the Behavioral Sciences in Environmental Design*. New York: Van Nostrand Reinhold.

Mollica, R. 1997. *Managed Care and Assisted Living*. Washington, D.C.: American Association of Homes and Services for the Aging.

Mollica, R., and K. Snow. 1996. *State Assisted Living Policy, 1996*. Portland, Maine: National Academy for State Health Policy.

Nemeth, K., and D. Roush. 1994. Overview of the assisted living concept. In D. Roush and T. Grape, eds., *Integrated Senior Care: Assisted Living and Long-term Care Manual*. New York: Thompson.

Pynoos, J., and P. Liebig, eds. 1995. *Housing Frail Elders: International Policies, Perspectives, and Prospects*. Baltimore: Johns Hopkins University Press.

Regnier, V., and D. Hoglund. 1995. *Building Codes' Impact on the Environments of Older People*. Washington, D.C.: American Association of Retired Persons.

Rowles, G., and R. Ohta. 1983. Emergent themes and new directions: Reflection on aging and milieu research. In G. Rowles and R. Ohta, eds., *Aging and Milieu: Environmental Perspectives on Growing Old*. New York: Academic.

Torres-Gil, F. 1992. *The New Aging: Politics and Change in America*. Westport, Conn.: Auburn House.

Weisman, A. 1997. Ambiguity in aging. In S. Strack, ed., *Death and the Quest for Meaning: Essays in Honor of Herman Feifel*. Northvale, N.J.: Jason Aronson.

Wilson, K. 1994. Creating residential models of assisted living. *AAHSA Provider News* 9(6), June. Washington, D.C.: American Association of Homes and Services for the Aging.

————. 1995. Assisted living as a model of care delivery. In L. Gamroth, J. Semradek, and E. Tornquist, eds., *Enhancing Autonomy: Concepts and Strategies*. New York: Springer.

————. 1996. *Assisted Living: Reconceptualizing Regulation to Meet Consumers' Needs and Preferences*. Washington, D.C.: American Association of Retired Persons.

Index

AAHSA. *See* American Association of Homes and Services for the Aging

Activities, 84, 87, 90, 93, 243, 258; of daily living (ADLs), xix, 24, 145, 152, 156, 169, 171, 264, 296

Activity room, 257

Adaptability, 118–20

ADARDS, Tasmania, Australia, 104, 105

Adjustment, 83

Admission, 48, 145

ADS Senior Housing, 11

Aesthetic quality, 240

Affection, 18

Age, 68; identification theory, 49; segregation, 33, 55

Ageism, 34, 94

Aging, 90, 303; and environment, 96; autonomy, and architecture, xv; in place, xvii, 6, 68, 78, 144, 176–78, 185, 193, 291, 292, 295, 296, 301; philosophy of, 160; population, 22

Agitation, 248

ALFA. *See* Assisted Living Federation of America

Alzheimer's disease, 99, 102, 110, 112, 114, 119, 127, 129, 150–52, 296. *See* dementia(s)

Alzheimer's Disease Rating Scale, 152

American Association of Homes and Services for the Aging (AAHSA), 11, 143

American Seniors Housing Association (ASHA), 30

Anxiety, 304

Archetypal spaces, 116

Architects, 263, 282, 286

Architecture, xvii, 166, 167, 281, 282, 289, 293, 303

Asbury Place, Mount Lebanon, Pennsylvania, 252, 253, 256, 258–60

Assessment: model, xxi, 130; protocols, 130

Assisted living: affordability, xix, 26, 41, 43, 298; appearance, 192, 250; architecture, xxiii; attributes, xxiii, 145; availability, 32; classification, 23; concept, 11, 166, 278; as consumer-driven phenomenon, 35; costs and finance, 13, 273; definition, xix, 3, 37, 190, 292; demand for, 32, 43; demographics, 21–31; exterior appearance, 207–28; future, 11, 29, 50; growth, xix, 4, 22, 28; as long-term care alternative, xix, xviii, 3, 42; management and staff, 88; medicalization of, 50; models, 38, 130, 293; as needs-driven, 273, 298; Oregon's, 44; perception of, 207–28; for persons with dementia, xxi, xxii, 104, 110–29, 130, 138, 145, 146, (*see also* Dementia[s]); philosophy of care, 14, 45, 92, 145, 169, 170, 181, 185, 207, 239, 291, 295, 300; as place type, xxiii, 7, 185–206; policies, 187; primary care, xxii; residents, 47, 113, 164, 166–82, 203; setting, 18, 130, 155, 164, 195; staff turnover, 44; supply and demand, 21, 32

Assisted Living Federation of America (ALFA), xix, 30, 301

Attachment: emotional, 18; to place, 82, 89, 105

Australian: backyard, 104; life, 105

Autonomy, xx, xxiii, 46, 51, 74, 76, 78, 91, 101, 112, 125, 181, 185, 186, 190, 191, 193, 200, 251, 291, 293, 300, 301, 302, 303; and long-term care, xvi; and security, 192

Awareness and orientation, 135, 137, 138

Baby boomers, 40

Bachelard, G., 78

Balconies, 210

Behavior, xx; aggressive, 164; disruptive, 153

Behavioral: disorder, 153; needs, 111; pathology, 152; problems, 152

Board-and-care facilities, 41, 53, 54, 191

BOCA. *See* Building Officials and Code Administrators

Book of the Dead, The, 77

Breaking up the home, 167

Building: classification, 194, 195; features, 149; materials, 211, 219, 221, 222, 226; type, 186, 192, 193, 195, 196, 203, 207, 208

Building Officials and Code Administrators (BOCA), 14, 276
Business relationships, 291, 297

Care, 147, 208, 229, 278, 280; goals, 232; housing, 280; philosophy, 146; programs, 91; services, 291; and supervision practices, 47; system, 143
Caregiver, 39, 121, 123, 125, 154, 233, 241
Case-mix programs, 281
Categorization, 279, 280
Category-identifying methodology (CIM), 219
Catholic shrine, 102
Characteristics, 219; of culture, 92; of current residences, xix; of residents, 291
Child, Martha, 19
Choices, 76, 92, 143, 181, 186, 243, 265, 267, 279, 286, 289, 291, 300, 301
Chronic conditions, xxii
Chronic diseases, 303
Churchill, Winston, 70
Circulation paths, 243
Classification, 21, 195
Clusters, 239
Cognitive: decline, 233, 335; impairment, 47, 243, 293, 302
Color, 211; coding, 244, 248; contrast, 226
Comfort, 279
Comfortable place, 250, 252, 289
Common life experience, 98
Common spaces, 291
Communal spaces, 268, 270
Communal zone, 267; semi-communal zone, 267, 268
Communication systems, 16, 259
Community, 10, 65, 168, 233, 265, 301; -based care, 189; life, 101; solidarity, 89
Companionship, 174, 175
Compassion, 280, 304
Conceptual framework, 96
Conceptual model, xxi, 131
Confusion, 249; of product line, 34, 35
Congregate: facility, 266; housing, 130; settings, 91
Congruence, 107, 132
Construction codes, 292, 293
Consumer, xxii, 7, 278, 303; demand, xviii, 143; orientation, 203; perspective, xxii; preference, 5, 298; values, 291
Consultant, 265
Continuing care retirement communities (CCRCs), 130
Continuity of self, 97, 137

Continuum of care, 125, 146, 176, 178, 179, 292
Control, 47, 72, 76, 91, 92, 101, 139, 275, 286, 289, 299
Coopers & Lybrand LLP, 30
Copper Ridge, Sykesville, Maryland, 143–55, 252–60
Corrine Dolan Center, Chardon, Ohio, 231, 260
Cost-effective option, 26, 299
Courtyard, 242
Cueing: perceptible, 204; strategies, 243, 248; visual, 245
Cultural: context, 97; heritage, xx, xxi, 90–109, 92, 94, 97, 297; identity, 90; interpretation, 195; message, 95; norms, 94; religious and ethnic expressions, 95; responsiveness, 107
Culturally: based interventions, 96; meaningful experience, 98, 102–5; responsive environmental design, xx; responsive environments, 97; significant therapeutic experiences, 105
Culture, 92–94, 196; characteristic of, 93; and ethnic groups, 17

Daydreaming, 72
Daylight, 289
Death and dying, 63, 66, 76, 284, 290, 304; dignified, 77
Deathbed environment, 73, 77
Decorative features, 226
Dementia(s), xviii, 49, 99, 102, 116, 150, 163, 296; assisted living for, 13, 114, 125, 143–55, 229–61; care, xxii, 110–29, 143–55; diagnosis of, 152; facilities, xx, 27, 43, 73, 110–29, 139, 143–55, 199, 229–61; people with, 13, 17, 37, 43, 90, 110–29, 130, 131, 135, 136, 143, 146, 154, 192, 225, 229, 231, 232, 236, 237, 241, 243–45, 248, 249, 252, 260, 278, 294, 296, 302
Demographics, 27, 280, 298
Dependency, xvi, 6, 15, 177, 304
Depression, 151
Design, 120, 128, 191, 195, 229, 230, 236, 239, 241, 242, 244, 246, 257, 264, 267, 278; of assisted living, 262–77; concepts, 230, 284; criteria, 267; decisions, 247; elements, 121, 125; enablers, 105; features, xviii; of hospice, 278–90; implications, 249; intervention, 107; issues, 233; objectives, 267; perspectives, 203; for people with dementia, 229–61; process, 187, 230, 284, 286; of special care units, xxiv, 110–29, 247, 260
Designers, 76, 77, 95, 197, 198, 202, 282
Destination, 244

Developers, 198, 202
Diagnosis-related groups (DRGs), 5
Dignity, 63, 90, 112, 147, 185, 190, 191, 224, 236, 279, 281, 284, 286, 289, 300, 301
Diminutive property, 207, 210
Dining services, 149
Disability, 304
Discharge criteria and policies, 48, 168, 169, 177
Division of Geriatric Medicine, St. Louis University, 156–64
Dormers, 210
Dumbbell, or dog bone, design scheme, 17
Dutch doors, 15, 149, 245, 259
Dwelling, 65, 66, 198, 209

Eden alternative, 19, 51
Elderhaus, 102
Elderly, 214, 226; frail, 44, 45, 48, 156, 177, 187, 193, 207, 278, 292, 293; aged over 80 years, xv
Embracing property, 208, 209
Emotional attachment, 18
Empowerment, 300
Enclosure, 208, 209
Entrance, 249
Environment, 229, 282; and aging, 303; and behavior, xx, 64, 116, 128, 192, 197, 204, 303; demanding, 49; and health, 128; for older persons, 90, 97, 134
Environment-behavior (E-B) model, 137
Environmental: assessment: —models, 130–39, 162; —protocols, 136; attributes, xx, 8, 32, 186, 187, 192, 199; cueing, 244, 248; design, 96, 110, 111, 113, 120, 121, 241, 291; determinism, 128, 187; intervention, 97–99, 102, 105; precedent, 281; sampling, 212; standards, 229; stimulation, 135, 247, 248; type, 84
Essa Flory Center, Lancaster County, Pennsylvania, 278–90
Ethnicity, 97, 98
Ethnographic research, 207
Exit control, 113, 120, 121
Exterior image, 251

Factor analysis, 215, 219
Fair Housing Amendments Act (FHAA; 1988), 48
Familiarity, 18, 208, 243, 250–52
Family, 8, 18, 118–26, 146, 154, 190, 233, 237, 257, 265, 279, 289, 301; caregivers, 234; neglect, 34
Fear, 304
Federal: licensure, 203; regulations, 195, 203

Finishes, 250
Fire safety, 293
Flexibility, 230, 245, 246, 273
Flexible: rhythm, 233, 236, 237; service plans, 295
Folstein Mini-Mental State Exam, 161
Form, function, and space, 195, 196
Frail Elderly Act (1990), 296
Freedom: of choice, 145; of movement, 145; of will, 72
Friendships, 173
Functional: abilities, 137, 139; disabilities, xv
Furniture, 250, 252

Gardens, 18, 99; healing, 113, 115, 117, 120, 123; and outdoors, 289
Gardiner, Maine, 231, 260
Geriatric ghettos, 34
Gerontopia, 63, 78
Giza, Egypt, 95
Goethe, Johann Wolfgang, 65
Group: environment, 132; setting, 4
Guilt, 66

Health care, 111, 281, 282; costs, 299; industry, 52, 53
Health Care Financing Agency (HCFA), 13
Health maintenance organizations (HMOs), 52
Healthy and familiar, 100
Hearthstone Alzheimer Care, 125, 126
Helen Bader Center, Milwaukee, Wisconsin, 99
Helplessness, 304
Heritage, 94; Newton, Mass., 9; Village, Kankakee County, Ill., 262–77
Hierarchy, 236; of spaces, 246
Home, xx, xxii, 38, 41, 66, 72, 75, 81–84, 166–68, 177–80, 186, 189, 197, 198, 207, 226, 241, 251, 266, 281, 284, 286, 289; attributes, 82, 199; -based services, 41; health care, 39
Homelike, xxii, xxiii, 32, 53, 54, 180, 186, 197–99, 207, 214, 219, 221–26, 257, 289, 291; accessories, 78; ambiance, 81, 222, 241, 250; appearance, 212; attributes, 199; environment, 123, 179, 185, 276
Homeownership, 40, 41
Homeyness, xxiii, 179, 207–10, 212, 219, 222, 225, 226, 292
Hopelessness, 171
Hospice, xxiv, 68, 69, 278–90
Hospital, 52, 188, 189; -based care model, 5
Hotel, 84
House, 198, 229, 233, 257

Household, 266
Housing and service, xix, 6, 91
Human: experience, 278; presence, 209; scale, xxiii, 210, 212, 226; stress theory, 49

I Ching, xxv
Incontinence, 14; DRIP, 163
Independence, 10, 67, 113, 115, 120, 124, 125, 143, 145, 169, 175, 181, 185, 191, 231, 233, 245–47, 268, 286, 289, 291, 300–302; and dignity, 91; equation, 171
Independent living, 156
Individual, 133, 215; care, 91, 107; choice, xxiii; needs, 91
Individual-organization (I-O) model, 117, 118
Individuality, xviii, 8, 72, 91, 92, 147, 229
Informal property, 208, 211
Inhabitation, 305
Innovation, 278
Institution, 198, 199
Institutional: appearance, 55, 219, 224; care, 292; character, xvii; environments, xxiii, 191, 197, 199, 219, 226, 230, 241; long-term care, xvii, 302; routines, 231
Institutionalization, xix, xv, xvii, 6, 14, 190
Instrumental activities of daily living (IADLs), 24, 156, 171
Integrative model of place (IMP), 133, 135, 139
Interior design, 233
Isolation, 173

Japanese: home, 105; takanoma, 105
Jewish: home, 101; identity, 99; life, 101
John Douglas French Center, Los Alamitos, California, 231
Johns Hopkins University School of Medicine, 143

Kahn, Louis, 65, 66
Katz's activities of daily living, 161
Kitchen, 246, 258
Klaasen, Paul, 19
Kosher Oasis, 100, 101

Lake St. Charles (Missouri), 156–62
Landmarks, 211, 243, 244, 258, 243
Landscape-perception, 211
Landscaping, 222, 226
Lawton's instrumental activities of daily living, 161; model, 132, 133
Lefroy Hostel for Elderly Persons (Australia), 232
Lewin's model, 131

Licensing: regulations, 15, 21, 292, 293; requirements, 282; standards, 33
Life: -centering activities, 82; quality, 111, 126; richness, 120; routines, 124; safety standards, 282, 293
Life-quality (L-Q) model, xx, 119
Lifestyle, 90, 94; care, 298; groupings, 93; in long-term care settings, xvi; options, 265
Lighting, 243, 244, 247, 250, 252
Liminality, 168, 177
Loneliness, 173, 174, 177
Long-term care, 51, 54, 185, 186, 189, 203, 299–302; continuum, 156, 157; costs, xix, 5, 189; services, 185, 292; settings, xvii, 91
Low-income consumers, xviii, 53
"Luxury creep," 12

Managed care, 26, 51–53, 297, 299; organizations, 51
Managed risk, 47, 192
Management, 111, 117, 247, 298; interactions, 120; philosophy, 47
Market: forces, 264–65, 272, 273, 298; models, 191; perspective, 203; research, 265
Marketing, 146, 272, 274
Marriott Corporation, 11
Meadowview Lodge, Heritage Village (Illinois), 268–76
MEALS ON WHEELS, 161
Meaning, 76, 83, 116, 195, 197, 303; of aging, 304; of home, 166, 123, 291; of place, 196; and stimulation, 18
Meaningful environments, 94, 108
Medicaid, 27, 33, 39, 42, 43, 51–54, 189, 190, 281, 294, 296, 298
Medical: care, 150, 151, 153; conditions, 160–64; diagnoses, 161; director, role of, 164; environment, 67, 282; model, xvii, 45, 50, 52, 81, 91, 130, 185, 186, 188, 246; supervision, 282
Medicare, 39, 42, 51, 52, 160, 281, 294, 297, 299
Medications, 145, 163
Memory, 68, 81; boxes, 245; loss, 14; of place, 68
Milieu, 66, 68, 73, 74–76, 170; clinical, 63
Milwaukee Jewish Home, 100–101
Missouri, 157
Mnemonic property, 208
Models: of care, 295, 296; of primary care, 158
Multiphasic Environmental Assessment Procedure (MEAP), 132, 136

National Citizens' Coalition for Nursing Home Reform, 53

National Investment Conference (NIC), 21

Naturalness, xxiii, 212, 226

Nature, 211, 289

Need(s), 111; to move, 33; physiological, 111; of residents, staff, and operators, xxiii

Neighborhood, 267, 268; clusters of units, 18

Neuropsychiatric care, 150–53

New England home, 103

National Fire Protection Model Code (NFPA 101), 16

Noise level, 248

Noninstitutional: appearance, 251; environment, 143, 144, 229, 293; image, 250

Norbert-Schulz, Christian, 65

Normative activities of daily life, 147

Normative theory, 303

Nourishment, 111

Nurse: delegation, 44; nurse's station, 239, 246; practitioners (NPs), 159

Nursing home, xvi, xvii, 5, 6, 15, 18, 26, 34, 41–43, 45, 50, 52, 55, 68, 91, 130, 145, 146, 168, 185, 188, 189, 190, 194, 195, 230–33, 240, 246, 279, 282, 299; care, 41, 130, 146; facility, 232, 233, 240; lobby, 43; residents, 42, 131; substitute, 44

Occupancy, 273

Old age: and denial, 34; and uselessness, 172

Older adults, 156, 213, 297

Oneida: assisted living, 98; Indian culture, 99; long house, 98

Operable windows, 275

Oregon, 44

Organizational: context, 133; and physical environments, 107

Orientation, 139

OWP&P Architects, 262

Parking, 275

Participant sampling, 213

Path to safety, 158, 202

Patient-focused care, 78, 79

Patterns, 236, 237

Pennsylvania Dutch, 106

Perceptions, 207, 211, 214

Perceptual categories, 215, 216, 219, 222

Perkins Eastman Architects, 230, 252

Personal: care services, 130, 207; control, 137; environment, 132; and social history, 151

Personalization, 8, 82, 84, 107, 116, 208, 244, 268

Personhood, 117, 120

Physical: environment, xvii, 132, 166, 167, 179, 197, 200, 236, 239, 240, 265; features, 207, 212, 293; health, 175; plant, 37; properties, 208; restraints, 241; setting, 133, 179, 187, 199, 203, 229, 302

Physician's assistants (PAs), 159

Place, 63, 68, 70, 78, 79, 83, 132, 197, 210, 248, 283; experience, 68, 132, 135; knowing, 243; memories, 70; personal, 113, 114, 120, 122; type, 185–206,

Poe, Edgar Allan, 77

Positive theory, 303

Post-occupancy evaluation, xxiv, 274–76

Preference, xix, 32, 215–17, 219, 225, 298, 300

Presbyterian SeniorCare, Oakmont, Pennsylvania, 230

PricewaterhouseCoopers, 30

Primary care, 156–65; practice, 164; provider, 156–59, 164

Privacy, 10, 112, 122, 135, 137, 139, 185, 191, 233, 235–36, 249, 251, 265, 268, 289, 291, 293, 300

Private places, 122

Private zone, 266; semiprivate zone, 266, 268

Professional environmental assessment protocol (PEAP), 137–39

Program(s) 302; philosophy, 145, 186; and policies, 199, 200

Programming, 267, 268, 278

Project data, 283

Prosthetic model, 188

Provider(s), xxii, 7, 50, 146, 167–70, 177–81, 187, 202, 278, 290, 294, 297, 298, 300

Proximity, 28

Psychogeriatric Dependency Rating Scale, 152

Public: payment, 299; policies, 293, 302

Purpose, 117, 118, 120

Quality: assurance, 295; of care, 32, 45, 46, 191, 239, 279, 298, 299, 301; domestic, 250; of life, xxii, 45–48, 93, 108, 110, 127, 130, 139, 203, 231, 240, 284, 295, 303; of a person's life, 229; and quantity of stimulation, 137

Real-worldness, 118–20

Reciprocity, 88, 300

Reese, Lower, Patrick & Scott, Ltd. (RLPS), 282, 283

Regulation(s), xxiv, 6, 14, 36, 145, 189, 191, 203, 277, 282, 292, 298, 300

Regulatory: guidelines, 46; philosophy, 53; standards, 50; statements, 18

Rehabilitation services, 160

Reimbursement, 203, 299, 300

Religion, 98, 99

Religious: corner, 100; ritual, 101

Reminiscence, 68

Resident(s), xviii, 32, 88, 123, 125, 126, 163, 167–74, 176–81, 190, 199, 233, 234, 239–42, 246, 247, 266, 267, 275, 279, 296, 297, 302; -centered model, 91, 295; characteristics, 296; room, 27, 244, 245; turnover rate, 44

Residential, xvii, 64, 229, 230, 250–52; ambience, 257; appearance, 4, 8, 192, 250, 291; attributes, 17, 197, 200; care facilities, 48, 157, 200–202; care settings, 26, 131; character, xix, 4, 192, 251; environment, xviii, xx, 14, 81, 113, 115, 120–24, 177, 237, 239, 241, 298; model, 32, 81, 185, 186, 192, 291, 304; places, 124; qualities, 116, 233, 249, 251; setting, xxi, 93, 148, 196, 197, 278, 291, 293

Responsibility, 46, 118, 120

Restraints, 247

Retirement, 281; communities, 86, 89, 216

Richness of life, 118, 119

Risk, 46, 247

Ritual(s), 83, 90, 168, 198; personal, xx, 81–89

Rosewood Estate (Minnesota), 3, 4, 11

Routine, 83, 189, 198, 229

Rules, 86

Rummaging, 241, 242

Safety, 45, 51, 111, 135, 139, 243, 246, 258, 267, 301; and security, 137, 143

Satisfaction, 240

Scale, 8, 215, 233, 238, 291, 295

Security, 175, 192, 231, 233, 243, 245, 246, 259; and autonomy, xv; outdoors space, 149, 257

Sedgewood Commons, Falmouth, Maine, 102, 104

Segregation, 49

Self-: actualization, 66, 111; determination, 72; expression, 107; history, 70; identity, 89, 90; rule, 72; worth, 90

Sense: of autonomy and control, 107; of institutional, 225; of place, 68

Sensory: comprehensibility, 113, 115, 120, 125; cues, 258; stimulation, 248, 289

Service, 32; costs, 33, 37; range, 291, 293

Shared: life experience, 102; residences, 85

Shelter, 111, 209; and care setting, 32

Signage, 244, 245

Single-family home, 209, 210, 251
Size, 238, 255; of resident units, 27
Skilled care, 266; facility, 286
Smoking room, 99
Social, 139; contact, 137; context, 133; environment, 132; exchange theory, 49; interaction, 135, 242; life, 173, 233, 234; model of care, xvii, xix, 32, 45, 46, 48, 50, 52; roles, 236; spaces, 113, 114, 120, 122; structure, 90; ties, 174
Sociocultural context, 96
Space, 196; structure, and order, 197
Spatial: organization, 90; relationships, 84, 86
Staff, 148, 199, 229, 237, 239, 240, 242, 246–48, 258, 295, 302; education, 154; exit/entrance, 249; room, 240, 241; shift changes, 248; suitability, 118–20; training, 16, 145, 154
State government, 54
Stimulation, 9, 233, 247
Storage, 241
Strategic plan, 273
Stress, 240
Suburban, 280, 281
Sundowning, 248
Sunrise Assisted Living, 11, 18, 19, 42
Supplemental Security Income (SSI), 41, 54

Supportive protection, xxiii, 208, 212
Swedish experiments, 13
Symbolism, 97, 196, 208

Takanoma, 105, 106
Technology, 6, 16, 247
Temporality, 87
Terminal condition, 279, 282
Territory and privacy, 116. See also privacy
Therapeutic, 68, 230; bathers, 259; building type, 191; environment, xvii, 187, 209; goals, xxi, 90, 96, 97, 100, 101, 134–36, 139, 186, 191, 291, 303; intervention, 148; needs, 64; philosophy, 189; programs of care, 278; resource, 92; setting for care, 190, 278
Therapeutic Environment Screening Scale (TESS), 137
Third-party payers, 42
Thomas, W. I., 202
Time, 83, 243
Tinnetti Gait and Balance Test, 162
Town center, 267
Training, 154, 298
Tranquilizers, 163
Transition, 167, 168
Type, 194

U.S. Bureau of the Census, 22

Units, 32, 238
Unobtrusive surveillance, 247
Urinary incontinence, 163
Usefulness equation, 171
Uselessness, 170–73

Van Gogh, Vincent, 77
Variability, 36, 207, 211
Varnhem, Sweden, 13
Visitors, 242, 267
Vulnerability, 304

Walking: circuits, 243; paths, 113, 114, 120, 121
Wandering, 49, 121, 161, 164, 233, 241, 242; areas, 243; path, 242
Wayfinding, 116, 233, 243, 276
Weiss Institute, Philadelphia Geriatric Institute, 136
Woodside Place, Oakmont, Pennsylvania, 106, 230–60, 278

Yankee Healthcare, 231
Yesavage Geriatric Depression Scale, 161

Library of Congress Cataloging-in-Publication Data
Aging, autonomy, and architecture : advances in assisted living /
    edited by Benyamin Schwarz and Ruth Brent.
        p.   cm.
      Includes index.
      ISBN 0-8018-6033-4 (pbk. : alk. paper)
        1. Congregate housing—United States.   2. Life care communities—
United States.   3. Frail elderly—Dwellings—United States.
4. Architecture and the aged—United States.   I. Schwarz, Benyamin.
II. Brent, Ruth.
HD7287.92.U54A375   1999
363.5'946'0973—dc21   98-49451
                                                                CIP